AF825905

M. Schein   L. Wise

Controversies in Surgery

Springer-Verlag Berlin Heidelberg GmbH

Moshe Schein   Leslie Wise

Controversies in Surgery

Volume 4

With 43 Figures and 23 Tables

Springer

MOSHE SCHEIN, MD, FACS, FCS (SA)
Professor of Surgery, Weill Medical College of Cornell University;
Attending Surgeon, New York Methodist Hospital,
Brooklyn, New York, USA

LESLIE WISE, MD, FACS, FRCS (Eng)
Professor of Surgery, Weill Medical College of Cornell University;
Chairman, Department of Surgery, New York Methodist Hospital,
Brooklyn, New York, USA

ISBN 978-3-540-41103-1

Library of Congress Cataloging-in-Publication Data
Controversies in surgery, volume 4/[edited by] Moshe Schein, Leslie Wise. p.; cm.
Includes bibliographical references and index.
ISBN 978-3-540-41103-1 ISBN 978-3-642-56777-3 (eBook)
DOI 10.1007/978-3-642-56777-3
1. Surgery. I. Schein, Moshe. II. Wise, Leslie.
[DNLM: 1. Surgical Procedures, Operative. WO 500 C7639 2001]
RD31.C753 2001 617 - dc21 00-068783

This work is subject to copyright. All rights are reserved, whether the whole or part of the material is concerned, specifically the rights of translation, reprinting, reuse of illustrations, recitation, broadcasting, reproduction on microfilm or in any other way, and storage in data banks. Duplication of this publication or parts thereof is permitted only under the provisions of the German Copyright Law of September 9, 1965, in its current version, and permission for use must always be obtained from Springer-Verlag. Violations are liable for prosecution under the German Copyright Law.

http://www.springer.de

© Springer-Verlag Berlin Heidelberg 2001
Originally published by Springer-Verlag Berlin Heidelberg New York in 2001

The use of general descriptive names, registered names, trademarks, etc. in this publication does not imply, even in the absence of a specific statement, that such names are exempt from the relevant protective laws and regulations and therefore free for general use.

Product liability: The publisher cannot guarantee the accuracy of any information about dosage and application of operative techniques and medications contained in this book. In every individual case the user must check such information by consulting the relevant literature.

Printed on acid-free paper SPIN 10782719 24/3130/Di 5 4 3 2 1 0

Dedication

This book is dedicated to our wives, Amal and Heidi,
and our children, Dan, Julian, Nicky, Omri, Tania and Yariv.

Preface

"When a thing ceases to be a subject of controversy, it ceases to be a subject of interest."

WILLIAM HAZLITT (1778–1830)

This is the fourth volume in a series which we started in 1997. In 1976, Varco and Delaney edited a "surgical bestseller" entitled *Controversy in Surgery*. This was followed by a second volume in 1985. The immense success of these books among both surgical trainees and experienced surgeons, and their wide international appeal, supported the editors' notion that a view of controversy is integral to teaching. However, despite major advances in surgical science and practice, no other similar publication has since been put together with the objective of addressing major controversies in surgery. The aim of this series is to address such deficiency by covering the most crucial current controversies in general, vascular and trauma surgery. Since almost everything is controversial in surgery, we will be able to tackle different issues almost each year.

The editors have selected a nationally/internationally recognized authority for each topic. Most books available today are either "North American," "British-Commonwealth" or "British-European," contributing to the constant transatlantic rivalry. Our series specifically aims to bridge this "culture gap" and includes North American, British, European, and other authors while maintaining a cohesive structure. This will hopefully also broaden the appeal of such a book across both sides of the Atlantic and beyond.

Each author has been asked to define and briefly discuss the current major controversies in his/her respective field within the confines of a single short chapter: "You have limited space; tell us what the essential controversies are; share your insight with us!" Each contribution has then been reviewed by another expert in the specific field who provides a brief "balancing" commentary. Finally, at the end of each chapter, the editors add a comment.

This series is aimed not only at surgical trainees preparing for the American Surgical Boards, but also for those preparing for the Royal Colleges' examinations in the UK, and other higher examinations elsewhere. It will be most valuable reading before oral examinations, providing the candidates with important insight and perspective and broadening their scope of knowledge with a "user friendly" and concise text. We believe that it will also appeal to the practicing surgeon who has only a limited amount of reading time. Residents in training and the "thinking" medical student will also find this book useful and fun to read because it conveys a large amount of knowledge in a highly concentrated fashion. In addition, the book will serve as an ideal source to prepare for teaching rounds or seminars on "controversies".

New York, February 2001 MOSHE SCHEIN, LESLIE WISE

Contents

List of Contributors

ADAMS, CHARLES A., JR., MD
Surgical Resident, Department of Surgery, UMD-New Jersey Medical School, Newark, NJ, USA

ARROYO, VICENTE, MD
Liver Unit, Institute of Digestive Diseases, Hospital Clinic, Barcelona, Spain

BALCH, CHARLES M., MD, FACS
Departments of Surgery and Oncology, Johns Hopkins University Medical Center, Baltimore, MD, USA

BARIE, PHILIP S., MD, FCCM, FACS
Professor of Surgery and Chief, Division of Critical Care and Trauma, Weill Medical College of Cornell University, Surgical Intensive Care Unit, New York-Presbyterian Hospital, New York, USA

BARTSCH, D., MD
Department of Surgery, Philipps-University of Marburg, Marburg, Germany

BASSI, CLAUDIO, MD
Surgical and Gastroenterological Department, Endocrine and Pancreatic Unit, University of Verona and Borgo Roma University Hospital "G. B. Rossi", Verona, Italy

BATALLER, RAMÓN, MD
Liver Unit, Institute of Digestive Diseases, Hospital Clinic, Barcelona, Spain

BEN EL KADI, HASSEN, MD
Fellow, Laparoscopic Vascular Surgery, Department of Surgery, Laval University, Québec City, Canada

BENJAMIN, IRVING S.
Professor of Surgery, Guy's, King's and St. Thomas' School of Medicine, King's College, London, UK

BOYERS, JUDGE SEYMOUR
Counselor At Law, New York, USA

BREMNER, CEDRIC G., MD, FACS
Professor of Surgery, Department of Surgery, University of South California, Los Angeles, CA, USA

BROLIN, ROBERT E., MD, FACS
Professor of Surgery, UMDNJ-Robert Wood Johnson Medical School,
New Brunswick, NJ, USA

BURPEE, STEPHEN E., MD
Chief Surgical Resident, Lenox Hill Hospital, New York, NY, USA

CARRILLO, EDDY H., MD, FACS
Associate Professor, Department of Surgery, University of Louisville, Director,
Trauma Service, University of Louisville Hospital, Louisville, KY, USA

CIOFFI, WILLIAM G., MD, FACS
Professor of Surgery, Division of Trauma and Critical Care, Brown University
School of Medicine, Providence, RI, USA

CLAVIEN, PIERRE-ALAIN, MD, PHD, FACS
Professor of Surgery, Division of General Surgery, Duke University Medical Center,
Durham, NC, USA

CONDON, ROBERT E., MD, MS, FACS
Professor of Surgery (Emeritus), Medical College of Wisconsin, Clyde Hull,
Washington, USA

DEITCH, EDWIN A., MD, FACS
Professor and Chairman, Department of Surgery, UMD-New Jersey Medical School,
Newark, NJ, USA

DENNIS, JAMES W., MD, FACS
Associate Professor of Surgery, Chief, Division of Vascular Surgery,
University of Florida Health Science Center, Jacksonville, FL, USA

DION, YVES-MARIE, MD, MSC, FACS, FRCS
Associate Professor of Surgery, Laval University, Clinical Researcher,
Québec Biomaterials Institute, Québec City, Canada

EFRON, JONATHAN E., MD
Clinical Fellow, Department of Colorectal Surgery, Cleveland Clinic,
Fort Lauderdale, FL, USA

ELDAR, SAMUEL, MD
Associate Professor of Surgery, The Technion Institute of Technology,
Chief of Surgery, Bnai Zion Medical Center, Haifa, Israel

FAHOUM, BASHAR, MD, FACS
Director of SICU, Department of Surgery, New York Methodist Hospital, Brooklyn,
New York, USA

FALCONI, MASSIMO, MD
Surgical and Gastroenterological Department, Endocrine and Pancreatic Unit,
University of Verona and Borgo Roma University Hospital "G. B. Rossi",
Verona, Italy

Farndon, John R., FRCS
Professor of Surgery, University of Bristol, Co-Editor British Journal of Surgery, Bristol, UK

Fingerhut, Abe, MD, FACS
Chief of Surgery, Centre Hospitalier Intercommunal, Paris, France; Clinical Professor of Surgery, University of Louisiana State Medical Center, New Orleans, LA, USA

Fong, Yuman, MD, FACS
Professor of Surgery, Department of Hepatobiliary Surgery, Memorial Sloan Kettering Cancer Center, New York, NY, USA

Franco, Dominique, MD
Chief, Department of Surgery, Hôpital Antoine Béclère, Clamart, France

Fromm, David, MD, FACS
Penberthy Professor and Chairman, Department of Surgery, Wayne State University, University Health Center, Detroit, MI, USA

Frykberg, Eric R., MD, FACS
Professor of Surgery, Chief, Division General Surgery, University of Florida Health Science Center, Jacksonville, FL, USA

Gagner, Michel, MD, FACS
Chief, Division of Laparoscopic Surgery, Professor of Surgery, Mount Sinai University, Medical School, New York, NY, USA

Gair, Anthony H.
Counselor At Law, New York, NY, USA

Garden, O. James, FRCS
Regius Professor of Clinical Surgery, Department of Clinical and Surgical Sciences (Surgery), Royal Infirmary, Edinburgh, UK

Gecelter, Gary R., MD, FACS
Chief, Division of General Surgery, Department of Surgery, Long Island Jewish Medical Center, New Hyde Park, NY, USA

Gentilello, Larry M., MD, FACS
Associate Professor of Surgery, Associate Director Trauma Intensive Care Unit, Harborview Medical Center, University of Washington, Seattle, WA, USA

Godellas, Constantine V., ND
Academic Program Coordinator, Department of Surgery, Rush-Presbyterian St. Luke's Medical Center, 1653 W. Congress Parkway, Chicago, IL 60612

Gorecki, Piotr J., MD
Attending Surgeon and Director of Advanced Laparoscopy, Department of Surgery, Nassau County Medical Center, Assistant Professor, State University of New York at Stony Brook, East Meadow, NY, USA

Gracia, Carlos, MD, FACS
Director, California Laparoscopic Institute, San Ramon, CA, USA

GUPTA, SANJAY
Clinical Lecturer in Surgery, Guy's, King's and St. Thomas' School of Medicine, King's College, London, UK

HAGLUND, ULF, MD, PHD, FACS
Professor and Chairman of Surgery, University Hospital, Uppsala, Sweden

HARRINGTON, DAVID T., MD, FACS
Associate Professor of Surgery, Division of Trauma and Critical Care
Brown University School of Medicine, Providence, RI, USA

HASSOUN, ZIAD, MD
Liver Unit, Centre Hospitalier de l'Université de Montréal (CHUM),
Hôpital Saint-Luc, Montreal, Québec, Canada

HAU, TONI, MD, PHD, FACS
Chief and Professor, Nordwest-Krankenhaus, Sande, Germany

HINDER, RONALD A., MD, FACS
Professor and Chairman, Department of Surgery. Mayo Clinic, Jacksonville, FL, USA

HIRSHBERG, ASHER, MD
Associate Professor of Surgery, Michael DeBakey Department of Surgery, Baylor College of Medicine, One Baylor Plaza, Houston, TX, USA

HORGAN, SANTIAGO, MD, FACS
Assistant Professor of Surgery, Division of General Surgery, University of Illinois College of Medicine at Chicago, Chicago, IL, USA

KALIMI, ROBERT, MD
Surgical Resident, Long Island Jewish Medical Center, New Hyde Park, NY, USA

KAMINSKI, DONALD L., MD, FACS
Professor of Surgery, Department of Surgery, St. Louis University School of Medicine, St. Louis, MO, USA

KARGER, THOMAS, Dr.
S. Karger Publishers, Basel, Switzerland

KATKHOUDA, NAMIR, MD, FACS
Professor of Surgery, University of Southern California School of Medicine,
Chief, Division of Emergency Non-Trauma and Minimally Invasive Surgery,
Los Angeles, CA, USA

DE KEMP, ARNOUD
Director, Division Sales/Marketing & Corporate Development
Springer-Verlag, Tiergartenstraße 17, 69121 Heidelberg

KLAUSNER, JOSEPH M., MD, FACS
Director, Department of Surgery B, Tel Aviv Sourasky Medical Center,
Professor of Surgery, Sackler Medical School, Tel Aviv, Israel

KLYACHKIN, MICHAEL, MD
Vascular Fellow, Department of Surgery, SUNY, Stony Brook, New York, USA

Koea, Jonathan, MD
Fellow, Department of Hepatobiliary Surgery, Memorial Sloan Kettering Cancer Center, New York, NY, USA

Krukowski, Zygmunt H., PHD, FRCS
Consultant Surgeon, Aberdeen Royal Infirmary, Professor of Surgery, University of Aberdeen, Aberdeen, Scotland

Laitman, Cynthia J., PHD
Managing Editor, Annals of Surgery, Department of Surgery, University of Wisconsin, Madison, WI, USA

Landau, David, MD, FACS
Assistant Professor of Surgery, Department of Surgery, Division of Vascular Surgery, University of Illinois College of Medicine at Chicago, Chicago, IL, USA

Leitman, Michael, MD, FACS
Chief, Surgical Critical Care, Department of Surgery, Lenox Hill Hospital, New York, NY, USA; Visiting Clinical Associate Professor of Surgery, State University of New York - Health Science Center at Brooklyn, NY, USA

Lev-Chelouche, Dina, MD
Department of Surgery B, Tel Aviv Sourasky Medical Center, Tel Aviv, Israel

Lipschitz, Jeremy, MB, BCh, FCS(SA), FRCS(C)
Assistant Professor, University of Manitoba, Section Head General Surgery Health Sciences Center and St. Boniface General Hospital, Winnipeg, Canada

Lynch, Thomas G., MD
Department of Surgery, University of Nebraska Medical Center and Omaha VAMC, Omaha, Nebraska

Massad, Malek, MD, FACS
Assistant Professor of Surgery, Division of Thoracic Surgery, University of Illinois College of Medicine at Chicago, Chicago, IL, USA

Matter, Ibrahim, MD
Consultant Surgeon, Department of Surgery, Bnai Zion Medical Center, Haifa, Israel

Mavor, Eli, MD
Division of Emergency Non-Trauma and Minimally Invasive Surgery, Department of Surgery, University of Southern California School of Medicine, Los Angeles, CA, USA

McGuire, Hunter H., Jr., MD, FACS
Professor of Surgery (Emeritus), Medical College of Virginia, Chief of Surgical Services, VA Hospital, Richmond, VA, USA

Meakins, Jonathan L., MD, FACS, FRCSC, DSc
Surgeon-in Chief, McGill University Health Center, Professor and Chair of Surgery, McGill University, Montreal, Quebec, Canada

MESSINA, LOUIS M., MD, FACS
Professor and Chief, Division of Vascular Surgery, Department of Surgery, University of California, San Francisco, CA, USA

NATHENS, AVERY B., MD, PHD
Assistant Professor of Surgery, Harborview Medical Center, Seattle, WA, USA

NYHUS, LLOYD M., MD, FACS
Professor of Surgery Emeritus, Department of Surgery, Division of General Surgery, University of Illinois College of Medicine at Chicago, Chicago, IL, USA

ORGAN, CLAUDE H., JR., MD, FACS
Professor and Chairman, Department of Surgery, University of California, Davis, Editor-Archives of Surgery, Oakland, California, USA

PAPADIA, FRANCESCO, MD
Department of Surgery, University of Genoa School of Medicine, Genoa, Italy

PATTERSON, EMMA J., MD
Department of Surgery, Mount Sinai University, Medical School, New York, NY, USA

PEDERZOLI, PAOLO, MD
Surgical and Gastroenterological Department, Endocrine and Pancreatic Unit, University of Verona and Borgo Roma University Hospital "G. B. Rossi", Verona, Italy

PELLETIER, SHAWN J., MD
Surgical Resident, University of Virginia Health Systems, Charlottesville, VA, USA

POMIER-LAYRARGUES, GILLES, MD
Liver Unit, Centre Hospitalier de l'Université de Montréal (CHUM), Hôpital Saint-Luc, Montreal, Québec, Canada

PORIES, WALTER J., MD, FACS
Professor of Surgery and Biochemistry, East Carolina University School of Medicine, Greenville, NC, USA

PRINZ, RICHARD A., MD, FACS
The Helen Shedd Keith Professor and Chairman, Department of Surgery, Rush-Presbyterian St. Luke's Medical Center, 1653 W. Congress Parkway, Chicago, IL 60612

PRUETT, TIMOTHY L., MD, FACS
Director of Transplant Program, Professor of Surgery, University of Virginia Health Systems, Department of Surgery, Charlottesville, VA, USA

RASMUSSEN, IB, MD, PHD
Department of Surgery, University Hospital, Uppsala, Sweden

RDIGER, HANNES A., MD
Research Associate, Division of General Surgery, Duke University Medical Center, Durham, NC, USA

Richardson, J. David, MD, FACS
Professor and Vice Chairman, Department of Surgery, University of Louisville, Louisville, KY, USA

Ricotta, John J., MD, FACS
Professor and Chairman, Department of Surgery, SUNY, Stony Brook, NY, USA

Rikkers, Layton F., MD, FACS
Professor and Chairman, Department of Surgery, University of Wisconsin Medical School, Clinical Science Center, Madison, WI, USA; Editor in Chief of the Annals of Surgery

Rodriguez, Joaquin A., MD
Fellow, Department of Surgery, Mayo Clinic, Jacksonville, FL, USA

Rothmund, Matthias, MD, FACS
Chief and Professor, Department of Surgery, Philipps-University of Marburg, Marburg, Germany

Saadia, Roger, MD, FRCS (ed)
Professor of Surgery, University of Manitoba, Health Sciences Center and St. Boniface General Hospital, Winnipeg, Canada

Schneider, Darren B., MD
Fellow in Vascular Surgery, University of California, San Francisco, San Francisco, California, USA

Schreiber, Martin A., MD
Michael DeBakey Department of Surgery, Baylor College of Medicine, One Baylor Plaza, Houston, TX, USA

Scopinaro, Nicola, MD
Professor of Surgery, University of Genoa School of Medicine, Genoa, Italy

Seigler, Hilliard F., MD, FACS
Professor of Surgery and Immunology, Department of Surgery, Duke University Medical Center, Durham, NC, USA

Sherlock, Dame Sheila
Department of Surgery, Royal Free Hospital, London, UK

Smith, Christopher T., MD
Fellow in Colon and Rectal Surgery, Department of Surgery, St. Louis University School of Medicine, St. Louis, MO, USA

Spain, David A., MD, FACS
Associate Professor, Department of Surgery, University of Louisville, Director, Surgical Critical Care, University of Louisville Hospital, Louisville, KY, USA

Stein, Hubert J., MD, Priv. Doz.
General and Thoracic Surgeon, Oberarzt, Chirurgische Klinik und Poliklinik, Klinikum rechts der Isar, Technische Universität München, Munich, Germany

STONEY, RONALD J., MD, FACS
Professor of Surgery, Division of Vascular Surgery, University of California, San Francisco, CA, USA

THEISEN, JÖRG, MD
Resident, General Surgery, Chirurgische Klinik und Poliklinik, Klinikum Rechts der Isar, Technische Universität München, München, Germany

THOMPSON, JON S., MD, FACS
Professor of Surgery, Department of Surgery, University of Nebraska Medical Center, and Omaha VAMC, Omaha, NE, USA

TYLER, DOUGLAS, MD, FACS
Associate Professor of Surgery, Department of Surgery, Duke University Medical Center, Durham, NC, USA

WEXNER, STEVEN D., MD, FACS
Chief of Staff, Chairman and Residency Program Director,
Department of Colorectal Surgery, Chairman, Division of Research and Education, Cleveland Clinic Florida, Fort Lauderdale, FL, USA

CHAPTER 1

Surgical Publishing in the Twenty-First Century

Journals

Claude H. Organ Jr.

> "If it has been in print and especially if it has been peer reviewed, it shouldn't be in print again."
> Donald Kennedy, PhD [1]

Introduction

The death of biomedical journals is perhaps premature. Electronic publication is currently being used increasingly in parallel to the traditional paper format [2]. The importance of the story of Rip Van Winkle was not that he slept for 20 years, but that he slept through a revolution. As surgeons, and particularly as editors, we must not sleep through this revolution and be more than marginally involved with these changes. Editors and journals must become more sensitive of and responsive to this rapidly evolving journalistic culture. In recent years our lexicon has become saturated with concepts such as the Inglefinger rule, the fair use doctrine and safe harbor guidelines. The electronic news media (ENM) have made us more acutely aware of the importance of issues surrounding intellectual property.

Are We at the End of the Paper Literacy Era?

ENM has not as yet become the gold standard of publication. This editor is uncertain as to the extent science citation indices will be impacted by ENM when compared to traditional print publications. However, in the future, electronic publications will exercise a much more influential role. Although ENM is in its embryonic stage, the publication industry is not yet prepared to have it take over the role of traditional journals. Several advantages of electronic surgical publishing are:

- The volume of information (memory) is infinite.
- The transfer of information conserves time.
- The reader may preselect topics of primary interest.
- Ease and diversity of use.

- Interactivity between the journal and reader will allow rapid comment and response.

The problems that editors and journals increasingly face with the competitive edge of ENM are paper costs, physical space, accessibility and relevance. The advantages of ENM apply to changing concepts of library design in today's market as we give rise to the virtual library. This revolution is consumer driven and stimulated by the advent of inexpensive computers and their capacity to store larger amounts of information.

The Internet and World Wide Web have already expanded our access to and utilization of information including third world countries. House officers, surgeons and patients are aggressively utilizing these technological advancements. It is a frequent occurrence now to have a surgeon, resident, medical student or patient respond, when asked where they obtained their information, to state, "I found it on the Internet." The EM publication process now involves textbooks, papers, magazines, newspapers etc. Ultimately the electronic media will depend upon the acceptance by peers [3].

Many of our colleagues contend that there is too much information to consume already with minimal reading time. The availability of a pre-print before formal publication is a real concern. *The New England Journal of Medicine* (NEJM) and the *British Medical Journal* are opposed to electronic pre-prints. Should the public trust only those findings published in peer review journals? This will be no easy task. Pre-publication peer review will become an even greater problem with ENM where readers will review a manuscript before publication. Several institutions have addressed this concern (MIT publication "Fostering Academic Integrity").

Editors and authors will be burdened with concern for misappropriation of intellectual property. Post-publication reviews pose similar problems. *Once ideas become public, then theft, scholarship and plagiarism too often follow close behind.* Of the many issues confronting ENM, the most difficult will be peer review and intellectual property. The Inglefinger rule, authored by the previous editor of the NEJM, states that the NEJM would not publish a manuscript whose results were made public before appearing in their journal. Editorial concerns about redundant ("salami") publications will multiply with ENM. Communicating ideas electronically to a worldwide audience will make it difficult to establish ownership. The author either establishes a claim that converts his/her work into intellectual property or disposes of that claim through some contractual agreement. The author owns, through copyright, his/her expression of ideas. The mechanism for establishing ownership of a new product, process, or technology is very different: the process of publication supports the claim of priority for anything contained in the work that is patentable [1]. The entry of information into the ENM gains great publication exposure but intellectual property will need a better focus. Issues of intellectual property ownership will continue in the ENM during the twenty-first century [4].

Reproduction of information even for educational use and even where nothing is being charged for the materials is limited. The Fair Use Doctrine permits the copying and distribution of limited amounts of material for educational purposes. Most universities and publications have warned individuals to stay cautiously within the "Safe Harbor" guidelines particularly with reference to educational purposes.

Evidence to date does not support the conclusion that we are at the end of the era of paper literacy. Peer review is achieved through participation but not consensus. In the twenty-first century the quality of journals will continue to be governed by editorial judgment, peer review and relevance. Additional independent journals will continue to be launched; time and journal content will dictate their survival. A long-term commitment, high editorial standards, and a clear mission statement will give a journal substance. Such a statement is found in the *Archives of Surgery*: "To promote the art and science of surgery by publishing relevant peer-reviewed clinical and basic science information to assist the surgeon in optimizing patient care. The *Archives of Surgery* will also serve as a forum for the discussion of issues that involve ethics, teaching, surgical history, and socioeconomic concerns."

Regardless of access, whether ENM or traditional, editorial boards will need to be more active, diversified, and responsible. Only then will surgical journals in the twenty-first century have improved impact factor ratings and higher citation indices.

References

1. Kennedy D (1997) Academic duty. Harvard University Press, Cambridge, p 195
2. Young AE (1996) The future of surgical journals in the electronic publishing age. Br J Surg 83:280–290
3. LaPorte RE, Merier E, Ahazaws S, Sauer F, Gambia C, Shenton C et al. (1995) The death of biomedical journals. BMJ 310:1387–1390
4. McLeod SD, Grier JP (1996) Knowledge or noise. Arch Ophthalmol 114:1269–1270

Books

Jonathan L. Meakins

Since the invention of movable type and the development of the Gutenberg press, books have been the major, perhaps even the principal form of recording, documenting, and communicating ideas. The last 10 years of the twentieth century have introduced a whole variety of other forms of communication – particularly as related to science and surgery, specifically computers and the Internet. For purposes of this discussion, I exclude radio and television as media, clearly of communication, but more attuned to sound bytes than to in-depth analysis, reasoning and clear debate. While debate on controversial issues can unquestionably take place in these ether media, there are circumstances more akin to scoring points and winning in the short term rather than resolving issues. While quick wit certainly enlivens the printed page, it scores more points in television and radio where the basic issues tend to be lost in the joys of entertainment.

The recreational book industry is thriving. One needs only to note the increased number of quality newspapers, which are including book review sections as an integral part of their weekend editions. The number of books appears to be proliferating. Bookstores in airports, on the streets, and in high rent districts are continuing to proliferate and there is intense competition for the sale of these books and for contracting high-profile, popular authors. There is, in addition, a continuing demand for nonfiction books for the layman covering all manner of subjects from the most profound science to economics to the recreational components of life including gardening, hiking, traveling, etc.

The increasing numbers of readers have raised the profile of book awards including the Booker Prize in Britain, the Goncourt Prizes in France, the Governor General Prizes in Canada, the Pulitzer Prizes in the United States, as well as others around the world. The interest is such that it is not only the authors receiving the prizes who benefit, but all on the short list. Indeed the judging panels publish the short lists of authors considered, thereby enhancing sales and the reputations of all those authors. A good deal of this is hype and designed to augment sales to the occasional devaluation of the final winner - there being so much discussion in the press about the various merits of the short list that it is occasionally impossible for the eventual winner to feel highly valued.

Where does medical and surgical publishing of textbooks fit into this overall enhancement or increase in the world of publishing? The likelihood that recreational books will remain with us is high. Reading for recreation is not at a desk - it is in a lounge chair, on the beach, at the cottage, etc. These books rarely go through multiple editions, they are occasionally reprinted and if they become classics, fancy editions will certainly be published subsequently. But the text remains what was originally published. What Will wrote in the sixteenth century remains the same in the twenty-first century.

What surgical text remains static? The reality is that none worth its salt. Therefore, the questions that must be posed with respect to the future of surgical texts include: Who needs textbooks? Is the text a reference such that it defines the state of art in some point in time? What does the reader require from a surgical book? Should books be on paper, on CDs, on the net? What is the difference between a single author and a multiple authored text? Whose idea was the book?

If we address who needs the book and whose idea the book was, the answers are one of three: the publisher, the author (editors), or the reader. The publisher needs the book to stay in business. The authors need the book usually for their academic careers, and I suspect that all too often the readers have the book on a bookshelf where it remains a decorative part of their office or library.

If the text becomes a classic reference, it will stay valuable for a protracted period of time. The difficulty in medicine and in surgery is that, as we are all told in medical school, half of what we know will be obsolete in the next 5–10 years. Unfortunately, the fact that we do not know which half will be obsolete questions the importance of the dogma that is inherent in a textbook. This therefore brings out the advantages of the ability to rapidly update or edit a book, which is much easier to do when it is published as a loose leaf, on a CD, or on the Internet.

The time to publish a text is exemplified by the timelines required for this particular book. We were notified in July of the opportunity to participate with a hard deadline of 1 December in order that the publication would be ready for the American College meeting in the following October. In reality, when a large textbook of medicine or surgery is being prepared, the publishers will not consider starting the copy-editing process until between 90% to 99% of the chapters are in hand. This can, of course, lead to enormous delays. The editing for content, quality of writing, and duplication is in general exclusively the editor's responsibility. Most publishers pay lip service to these issues. It may require as long as 1 year to 18 months from all chapters arriving to when the printed book is finally published. Therefore, chapters which arrive exactly on time and those which arrive at some time later for large, multi-authored medical books lead to an inherent time lag of information and datedness for those chapters which arrive first. There may be as long as a 4-year time gap between the concept and the identification of authors to the time at which the book is finally in print and for sale. This inevitably leads to inaccuracies as the nature of movable knowledge is that it evolves and that therefore a text is inevitably out of date by the time it is printed. This time lag becomes particularly evident in rapidly changing areas such as chemotherapy, gene therapy, the recent explosion in minimal access surgery, immunology, critical care, etc. This returns us to the concept: should texts be published on paper or through some other medium?

The textbook publishing industry is undergoing a major consolidation at the present time where we see large publishers merging, the number of publishers of journals and textbooks being dramatically reduced for all of the market-driven reasons that we see consolidation in other industries. Added to these reasons for consolidation are the competition that comes from computers and the ability to communicate via the Internet or publish via CDs.

The reading public has no real idea of what goes into the production of a multi-authored text. In the 1980s, I was approached by several publishers to do "books." At that time, not having done one before, it seemed like fun, and the idea of having done a "book" was somewhat glamorous. The bait was my ego plus the promise of potential revenue. Designing the book is creative and, if the field is understood, interesting. It turns out that getting "the" good authors is often difficult. However, having the chapters in by the deadline is the real trial. As noted, the publisher will not help with editing content and will not copy edit until all chapters are in hand. In addition, they are generally not interested in standardizing the quality of writing and the quality of information. Therefore, as an editor, you are responsible for reading, editing, and controlling the quality of all chapters. The reality turns out that the writing in multi-authored texts is uneven: some chapters will be much too long, key areas will not be covered, reference lists will often be old, the material may be a rehash of previously published work not entirely brought up to date. In all of these settings, authors are frequently married to their own words and *will not* allow a word to be changed. This leads to great trials for the editor who, because of time constraints, may be unable to standardize the quality of writing, the nature of the information, and so on.

The financial side of publishing is also blurred, at least in its initial stages, by our wish to be the editor or author of a book. In multi-authored texts, generally speaking, the authors of chapters receive very little support, if any, and that will be deducted from the royalties of the editor. So, it is possible to lose money if you support your authors. After a couple of these experiences, publishers eventually stopped asking for books as our conversations evolved along the following lines: if the publishers make money from the book and the editor is the marketable commodity, should not the editor be as fairly reimbursed as the publisher? My answer was always: "of course." Nevertheless, the publishers felt that the answer was: "not really." They took their cut first and there would therefore be little support for the text. At this point, we inevitably agreed to disagree and they fortunately went off looking for another editor.

The key controversies which will evolve relate to how the Internet integrates with the evolution of new knowledge and how the ability to combine the use of digital video imaging and text, particularly in the surgical domain, will evolve such that books must compete with the dynamic images which will mean so much to surgeons. As visual people, surgeons learn in large part by watching and recall as a function of the imagery to which we are exposed. I have no illusion that, in time, textbooks will disappear. However, the nature of non-journal surgical publishing is going to change. My own sense is that 5 years from now, classic "major subject" texts will remain but in both paper and electronic form; atlases will remain, but most other medical publishing of "books" will be electronic with downloading capability and outstanding indexing.

Publishing in the Internet Age

Thomas Karger

In 1890, Samuel Karger founded S. Karger Publishers in Berlin with the intent of making a collection of compendia to be used as reference works by students and practicing physicians. In short, he intended to share medical knowledge. Before long, his reference books were widely distributed across Europe and beyond the continent. More than one century later, Karger Publishers, now based in Basel, continues to uphold the doctrine of its founder – although in a very different world. In the Internet Age, the dissemination of medical knowledge has taken a vastly different shape: today medical findings are accessible to anyone with a modem and a computer screen. However, the intent and results of our work remain the same.

For over 110 years, Karger's business has been connecting resource to reader. We are a link in a long chain that has been far-reaching from its inception and has since become a closely knit network spanning the globe.

The Changing Role of the Publisher

The function of the publisher has traditionally been to collect, evaluate, edit, produce, and distribute information for its authors and readers. The advent of advanced information technology and the Internet has impacted every step of this process. Source data collection can now be conducted electronically, thus expediting the pace of information processing. Even the vitally important peer review phase has been accelerated by electronic means. Internet-based software enables editors and reviewers to share manuscript files and make recommendations for editing changes and manuscript acceptance. Feedback and re-evaluation can be conducted with greater efficiency due to the high velocity of information exchange.

Production has also taken a new shape. Electronic journal production is concurrent with our traditional hard copy production. At Karger, articles for publication are prepared in a universally applicable data format. Once page lay-out is complete, the production path of electronic and print media diverges. The printed page production is nearly finished, with only the physical printing and distribution process ahead, whereas the electronic production path has just begun.

The electronic version of a journal is formatted for publishing on Karger's web site and on partner sites around the world. E-journal data is archived in a formatting language that permits conversion into the various forms required by the production department and external electronic partners. Software applications shape this raw data into new electronic products for use on our web site. Abstract information, links to cited references, table of contents alerting, customized web channels, Internet news services for medical professionals, and other electronic dissemination methods reflect the new ways people use medical information. Together with electronic partners, we build solutions for the market, namely broader gateways to full-text articles facilitating wide-spread access for all, bibliographic links to cited source materials from other publishers, and enhanced search tools for more optimal search results.

Finding the Data Afloat

The Internet Age has perhaps had the greatest effect on how potential readers access our publications. Readers and researchers can uncover valuable medical information not only by reading a physical copy of a journal found in a medical library or on a clinician's desk, but also by searching a widely cast network of electronic databases. As pools of electronic resources expand, the reader is engulfed in a sea of knowledge: effectively navigating these waters is the key to success in conducting research on the Internet. The search criterion is the rudder with which one directs a search for pertinent information. These criteria, coupled with an intelligent search engine, determine the depth, breadth, and direction of a query. Databases with well-equipped search tools empower the reader to discover hidden treasures and concise details on any given topic. Databases lacking precise search tools can toss the reader almost randomly from one crest to another.

Article of Record

As the electronic journal strives to overtake the print journal as the primary citation source, the electronic version of an article as the mainstay of the research process is taking on escalating importance and may very well entirely wipe out the concept of "journal" as we know it today. Increasingly, the unit of information sought by researchers is becoming more concise; in other words, the research journal as an information unit is losing its significance to the single article. The electronic (e)-article is easier to locate and can hold additional information such as three-dimensional or moving images. Once this e-article has value-added research significance, it may well surpass print and become the article of record. E-articles may be printed on demand based on research needs, leaving the traditional subscription to a collection of articles within a journal - printed or electronic - by the wayside. No one can accurately predict if and when such a complete changeover will occur. However, it is important to note that, as long as the print journal is published, it will maintain its place as a reliable and essential resource, even if it no longer holds the potency it once had - not unlike radio after the introduction of television.

Our role in this industry is defined but changing. New rules may change the means, but not the goals. The all-important factor is to maintain the openness and flexibility necessary to adapt quickly to important innovations, while avoiding the pitfalls of following every new trend. Not all of the predictions resulting from the advent of the Internet, in this industry or others, will actually occur. Sensible evaluation of developments is required for healthy progression into the next stage of business, whatever that may be.

We have spent the past century as a publisher working to connect people who want to share their knowledge with those who want to learn. As new partners add links to our communication network, it becomes fuller, more complete, and more effective. As the electronic media gain momentum, we will see a more highly defined, uniquely specialized role for printed books and journals - one that responds to the specific needs of the changing market. Our common goal remains bringing authors and readers together, as well as making information more accessible to all who seek it. As society benefits from the advancements we help bring to the medical profession, our closely knit network of information turns into a tapestry rich with knowledge, organized in an intelligent, practical system for communication equal to itself in intricacy and interrelation. Having been fortunate enough to be in the publishing industry for 50 years, I now stand back to view the complete picture and take pleasure in the information landscape I behold.

Invited Comment - Germany

Arnoud de Kemp

The basic role of the scientific publisher in the Internet age is not changing. It is the scope of publishing that is changing. Primary content may become multimedia enriched, but the same or an even stricter selection and reviewing (evaluation) process is required. All other functions of a publisher are related to this core function. The editorial and production process as well as physical distribution have changed or will change due to new technologies, the convergence of media and the Internet.

(Arnoud de Kemp is a Deputy Member of the Board responsible for Marketing, Sales and Logistics, including electronic media. For more information: dekemp@springer.de)

Technologies that have entered the publishing houses are digital workflow, manuscript tracking systems, editorial management, digital rights management, conversion and indexing software. Repositories are being built where manuscripts are stored in a medium-neutral format and structured according to document type definitions (dtd). These are all enabling or facilitating technologies that increase efficiency and speed, but do not change the function of publishing, which is to make relevant facts and experiences known.

The most important challenge is to increase the accessibility and retrievability of information. At first sight (but only at first sight), this has little to do with publishing. Books and journals, as they were produced and distributed over the centuries, more or less disappeared in libraries. The only way to find them was by using a catalogue or a list of currently held periodicals. Little was done to describe the content. If more than three authors, the other authors disappeared under "et al.". The standard catalogue description of a book was and is very limited and does not provide any information about different articles. Periodical literature was not disclosed at all. Here, the so-called abstracting and indexing services started to produce secondary publications with short descriptions of articles, subject classifications and keywords, that became more important with the increase of journal publications. Last but not least, handbooks provided an overview of all relevant literature in a defined period.

Almost all abstracting and indexing publications were available online, long before WWW was invented and the Internet was rolled out. This has greatly improved the information about new as well as old articles and their authors. It was still problematic to get the full copy as one had to go to a library to borrow it or write to the author. The restricted availability created the need for document delivery services and special lending libraries. The most prominent is the British Library Document Supply Centre in Boston Spa, York, United Kingdom. The fact that electronic versions of print publications, especially journals, can be offered on the Internet is changing the scope of publishing dramatically. Of course, anybody can use the same Internet as a platform for offering information and there are heated discussions about whether publishers will survive or not. Publishers however, with their knowledge and new craftsmanship in editing and processing, have a unique chance to offer the same information in a new way: structured, indexed, layered and henceforth much more accessible and retrievable by search engines, indexes and an unlimited number of users.

Searching and identifying relevant information on the Internet is not that easy. It is a common fact nowadays that all search engines together reach less than 35% of the information offered in approximately 1 billion pages. Approximately two more billion pages are "hidden" behind fire walls and can only be retrieved with permission (passwords). In order to offer a quality seal, STM publishers have developed the DOI (Digital Object Identifier), which helps to find, identify, secure, link and trade original articles. As a rule, the publisher guarantees the originality of the material.

At Springer-Verlag, we are already applying the DOI to those articles that are ready for publication but not yet assigned to an issue with page numbers. In so doing, we can already publish these articles in its electronic form (Online First). The DOI can be used in citations, references and links and will be printed with the article. The electronic version of the printed article then replaces the Online First version. The DOI is independent of time and location and, as such, a permanent identifier.

Articles will not replace the journal any more than journals will be replaced by the Internet. The need for printed documentation in library collections will continue to be there, although there may be fewer libraries and smaller collections. The quality of the article content is guaranteed by editorial policy, editors and their peer reviewers. A journal represents quality selection of primary findings and experiences among specialists. Publishers of all kinds organize and finance this activity. In addition to traditional marketing, sales and distribution, servers offer electronic content. This content may or will become enriched. We offer abstracts with images (enhanced abstracts) and offer authors an opportunity also to publish supplements to their articles. These can be color slides, video and sound sequences, statistical material, simulations, manuals, etc.

The most interesting development in publishing is called "CrossRef". It is an initiative of the International Association of Scientific, Technical and Medical Publishers (STM) to create links systematically between the bibliographic references of their articles. Today (February 2001) over 40 publishers are participating and more than 1 million articles are registered for linking.

The Springer online information service is called LINK. LINK offers online versions of more than 500 journals and, increasingly, book series and reference works from different publishers. Content is offered in ten subject libraries. For medical content it is possible to search in LINK and in Medline simultaneously. The information can be searched at different levels. Monthly, more than 18 million documents are downloaded under the protection of passwords and IP registration.

We had to invest heavily in the development of new document types, workflow procedures, server technology, indexing and search software – and in human resources. For the last ten years we have been experimenting with new publication forms and formats, and we have participated in research and developing programs. One of the first digital libraries was the Red Sage Project with medical journal content in San Francisco. Our mission is to continue to offer the highest quality in information. The Internet supports this.

Invited Comment – USA

Cynthia J. Laitman · Layton F. Rikkers

Increasing Access to Information

For centuries the possession of knowledge was considered appropriate only for an elite segment of the population. With the invention of the printing press in the fifteenth century, it was feared that this new technology would bastardize knowledge by making it more accessible to the masses. While, happily, we have evolved, stratification of knowledge persists in medicine. The sheer volume of new information makes it impossible for everyone to know everything. However, with the advent of electronic media, everyone who needs to know and who has access to a computer can know, regardless of politics or financial constraints or geography. Universal access democratizes the possession of knowledge. This can only bode well for surgeons and their patients, wherever they may be.

Source Credibility and Peer Review

That said, the need for source credibility becomes even more important as the Internet expands in use and influence. Anyone with computer access and the will to do so can establish an Internet site. As George Lundberg has put it, "the Internet can be the ultimate vanity press. You can be writer, editor, and publisher all at the same time and fake all the information" [1]. Whose information do we trust? Peer review has been and continues to be the means by which science is judged. We have established a system for print publication that, if not perfect, is at least functional. Claude Organ correctly points out that electronic publication of medical information poses new concerns about adequate peer review. It also imposes added responsibility on all of us to be active and discriminating receivers of information.

Timeliness

Closely aligned with adequate peer review is the issue of timeliness. As George Lundberg, editor-in-chief of Medscape, stressed, the speed with which an electronic format can disseminate new information cannot possibly be matched by traditional print production. He says that Medscape's submission-to-publication time can be measured in weeks rather than the 6–12 months or more typical of print journals [2]. However, weighted against pure speed of publication are considerations of medical practice, patient safety, and public policy issues [3]. The time it takes before publication to evaluate and authenticate new medical information ultimately serves the interests of health care consumers more truly than the speed with which the data are made public. The trick, of course, is balancing "the competition between timely release of medical findings and validity" [4].

Proliferation of Print Journals

During the past 30 years, the estimated number of scholarly journals has quintupled [5]. Partly driven by medical specialization and partly by the ever-increasing volume of knowledge, this trend has been reflected by the increasing number of surgical specialty journals. The point has been made that anyone with sufficient perseverance can eventually find a journal to publish almost anything. In addition to opening the door to poor quality material, the proliferation of specialty journals makes it more difficult for a diversified audience to access information.

Since publication is, after all, a business, with profit as the bottom line, will electronic media affect the financial dynamics of print publication and ultimately the proliferation of surgical journals? We believe that, by its presence, electronic media will accentuate a dynamic tension between necessary and desirable print publication and what is simply not profitable to print.

Conclusion

The three essays presented in this volume, dealing with various aspects of medical publication, essentially beg the same two questions:

- Is electronic publishing going to supplant print publication in academic medicine?
- Is electronic publishing going to compromise the transmission of medical information?

The answer to the first question is "no." As Dr. Meakins points out, there will always be a market for print media, because it continues to serve its purposes. However, as Dr. Organ describes, electronic media can augment print medical publications in incalculably useful ways not before possible. The answer to the second question is "probably not" as we develop new means of quality control. Concerns of "bastardizing" information by broadening access to senders of information as well as to receivers is no more valid in the twenty-first century than it was in the fifteenth century. As Dr. Karger put it, the intent and results of our work remain the same, regardless of the means of delivery.

References

1. Lundberg G (1999) Lecture at the University of Wisconsin, Madison, March 29
2. Lundberg G (1999) Medscape editorials, April 14
3. Relman AS (1999) The NIH "biomed proposal," A potential threat to the evaluation and orderly dissemination of new clinical studies. NEJM 340:1828–1829, June 10
4. Glueck, Michal (1999) Commentary: peer review vs. timeliness: a delicate balancing act. Medscape General Medicine, {HYPERLINK http://www.medscape.com/Medscape}www.medscape.com/Medscape, June 11
5. Abel R (1999) The national enquiry into scholarly communication: twenty years after. Publishing Research Quarterly. Spring, pp 3–19

Invited Comment – UK

John R. Farndon

> "There's something special about people who are interested in the printed word. They are a species all their own – learned, kind, knowledgeable and human."
> Nathan Pine
> Bookseller

There's something special about receiving your monthly issue of a journal. Having just finished reading number 26 of volume 341 of the *New England Journal of*

Medicine and Surgery (1812 title!) – what comfort and reliability there is in the front cover, what pleasure in being able to jump from a paper showing advantages for coronary artery stenting to one showing that primary care physicians are irrelevant and inappropriate (I paraphrase!). What delight to see figures which encapsulate iron metabolism and lipoprotein receptor mechanisms in half-page color boxes and thrown in for good measure, a restful photograph of Alaska (I thought Alaska was a state – the illustration suggests it is only a mountain and a few pine trees). How refreshing to see three corrections declared.

Surely these pleasures and delights could have been achieved in any of the surgical journals we read but perhaps there would have been no need for corrections.

"To err is human but to really foul things up requires a computer."
Farmers' Almanac for 1978
Capsules of Wisdom

Can you really say you enjoy sitting in front of that flickering screen?: log-on name?; password?; messages unread – 3,142 (nobody ever wrote me a letter); oh no, he's sent a document in Word 6; – the choppy seas of electronic searching.

Hold on a minute!

"For they are a very forward generation, children in whom there is no faith."
Deut. 32:20.

There is a threat in change, something new that we do not understand, perhaps do not like or cannot use or manipulate to our advantage. Although we have had television for about 50 years the wireless still provides an excellent entertainment and information service. With time, new patterns of dominance may emerge but I doubt if books will disappear.

"Books are the carriers of civilization."
Barbara Tuckman, born 1912
American historian

Enlightened publishers will use electronic means to hasten the process of publication. The dogma of earlier textbooks will be reinforced by categorized quality of references. Authors who embrace electronic sources of information will produce work in a timely fashion (some hope!). At the end of the day, remember that most of our knowledge was established by book reading and learning.

"The true university of these days is a collection of books."
Thomas Carlyle, 1881–1975

Remember also that treatment options demanded by patients will not always be driven or informed by book, journal or electronic information. The mechanisms by which laparoscopic cholecystectomy was widely used before publication of randomized trials are complex but be assured it was not due to factors considered in these chapters or commentary.

Most journals with their publishers are embracing electronic means of publishing in parallel with paper copy. What are the challenges/threats/advantages?

Quality-assured domains must be established where the peer review process continues. There is no reason why referees and editors cannot continue in their roles before posting articles onto the Net. There will be relaxation of the Ingle-finger rule, e.g., "posting an audio-recording of an oral presentation at a medical meeting on the Internet, with selected slides from the presentation, will not be considered prior publication." N Engl J Med 1999; 341:1956.

A more serious challenge is how to get rid of the rubbish, salami and identical sausages. Does your journal with an acceptance rate of 20% really want to take this article which got the thumbs down from three referees by our journal? How about posting rejected articles onto the Net with the referees' comments?!

The measurement of quality is a challenge currently and many feel that citation index and impact factor may not be the best measures. Work found to be fraudulent will be frequently cited. Membership-linked subscriptions may artificially boost perceptions of a journal. Compulsory presentation of manuscripts emanating from meetings may bias publication. Measurement of quality and reliability will be a major challenge.

Many of our journals are parochial. Looking west down the Severn Estuary from my office in Bristol, there beyond Ireland, I can just see the United States of America. Electronic publication reduces these barriers. We don't want to see them disappear. We would not want to see one surgical journal – *The Global Surgical Journal*! Who would be the editor?!

How to conclude? Take care! Change can be challenging, disturbing and stressful. We are aware of the new animal 'Publication electronicus.' Let us study it carefully and see how best we can allow it to fit into our ecosystem without it devouring all other living beings. I am sure we do not want it to become extinct until we have at least seen whether we can eat it. In all events, avoid "future shock"!

> "Future shock (the dizzying disorientation brought on by the premature arrival of the future) – the shattering stress and disorientation that we induce in individuals by subjecting them to too much change in too short a time."
> Alvin Toffler, 1928–
> American writer
> In *Horizon Summer*, 1965

Invited Comment – France

Abe Fingerhut

At the time when the amazon.com Time person of the year Jeff Bezos is making millions selling everything from strings to beans, when e-commerce has opened a new era, e-medical publication seems to be in its babbling stages. As television and billboards have been zoomed into expensive, prehistoric costly advertisement media, so books *seem* to be doomed. Some interesting figures show that the average daily visits for some web sites (period ending December 1999) are: amazon.com 1,262,000; cd.now.com 307,000; and Barnes and Nobles.com 282,000. In the parlance of the web, medical books and journals might soon be "clicks and bindings" [1].

Who Needs the "Classical" Book?

Although I agree with Dr. Meakins that the recreational book industry is thriving and that bookstores are proliferating, the medical writing profession might be in for a different fate. One main reason (and not the least) for this, which was perfectly highlighted by Dr. Meakins in the second part of his chapter, is that our knowledge is forever increasing, and nowadays it increases with e-speed. In order to keep up with the "last" trial, the "last" meta-analysis, the "latest" reference list for one's upcoming article, nothing is better than to be able to hook up directly with the e-National Library or another e-site and "e-scoop" what is needed.

So who needs the "classical" book? Although less profitable in the short term, the publisher will be happy with the e-book as well as the hard copy. He will have to. The authors, if their e-article is cited and referenced, and can be used for their academic careers, will not take issue with the change. The reader, on the other hand, although he or she might be happy to get the work done more cursorily through the online zapping, still might want to keep a hard copy on their office bookshelf or in their library.

E-publications

Electronic publication should offer new opportunities for improving both the quality of research and that of research reports. This might be through "open," real time peer review of protocols and their publication as well as improved correspondence between the reviewer and the writer.

As suggested by A.E. Young in his editorial [2], e-publication might enhance the publication of several forms of manuscript that have progressively disappeared from most journals, that is, manuscripts with tons of raw data, which usually gave such pimples to editors that many were never even sent to reviewers. These, as well as case reports, and negative finding reports, otherwise blackballed from the roster of the contents of many journals, might then have a chance to reappear. On the negative side as far as I am concerned, he also suggested that editors might be tempted to simply grade and publish *all* submitted work, but with a grading system. This, in my opinion, is dangerous, for just to see something in print is somehow the proof that it exists and what is written can be used. Even a low grade will not prevent the material from being used to support an idea or reinforce personal beliefs (without the grading being mentioned, of course). This is a step backwards away from the evidence-based scientific world in which we wish to remain. One might even see in these cases a "popularity score" arise, based on the number of "hits." However, the "popularity" does not necessarily correspond to its scientific value. Instead of throw-a-ways, this would be glance-a-way information. No thank you, we do not want that.

Interactivity

"Interactivity," on the other hand, is something readers have always sought for. Once the paper is "e-published," comments and questions can be added and "attached" immediately by the reader to the author(s), and if he, she or they are available, a true conversation can take place. I would disagree, however, that this should replace the actual peer review system.

However, interactivity can also be applied to the conception and the actual writing of the paper. Peer reviewers can be contacted and, once their comments have been formulated and addressed to the editor, he, or she, in turn, can address the issues to the writer. Corrections and modifications can be made in real time, either to the editor, or directly to the reviewer, and the text is (nearly) immediately ready for impression. If and ever we come to this, then the impact factor will have to be transformed into the "hit factor."

Electronic Editing

Electronic editing will help the potential writer. Online editing is better and more expedite because spelling and most grammar are no longer a major problem, and mailing and correspondence with authors, editors and/or corrections and editing have become instantaneous. There is instant gratification to see the work in "print"; this is "author-friendly." In addition, indexing references at the end of the article is simple, and changing from one reference system to another (because the article was refused in one journal and accepted in another) becomes a game rather than a hardship. References can be updated in a glance of the eye. In the future, one can easily imagine that the "instructions to authors" will be in electronic format and all the author has to do is to fill in the spaces, specifically designed to the journal or book format.

Non-English-Speaking Authors

Another foreseeable advantage of e-publishing might be the help provided for non-English-speaking authors. English is undoubtedly the language most widely and universally used to diffuse scientific knowledge and in particular, medicine. One problem that has constantly been on the minds of many authors whose mother tongue is not English is how to balance his or her list of publications in English with that in his or her mother tongue. Most if not all high-ranking journals, the ones with the high impact factors, are in English. On the other hand, non-English-speaking authors need to publish in their own language, for obvious reasons. One solution was taken by the long-standing German journal, founded in 1860 by Bernhard von Langenbeck from Berlin, the *Langenbecks Archiv für Chirurgie*, which decided to go to English a few years ago, and is now called *Langen-*

beck's Archives of Surgery. Another solution is represented by bilingual journals, only a few of which have survived through the years. One example is the *Annals of Vascular Surgery*, founded in 1986. This solution, however, is costly, and worked only because the promoter of this adventure, Edouard Keiffer, was so well known and was able to undertake and accomplish the enormous work load the journal entailed. Another reason was that the journal received sufficient sponsorship and was able to remain on its feet, financially speaking. Electronic publication might be an elegant solution to this problem for many national journals (and authors) that want to continue to publish in their mother tongue as the cost of space for the translation would no longer be a major problem. This might also help to avoid the problem of double publications that arises from time to time.

Although the computer, hardware essential for the transmission of e-publication, has become cheaper, it, and the telephone lines necessary for world-wide diffusion, are behind the mail services, however slow and erratic they may be. Mail services, however, are more expensive, so that developing countries could favor diffusion of information through the telephone rather than paper.

Another major problem is the fact that reading on a screen is awful for the eyes and brain. Reading on paper is easier for our optical machines and the soft matter attached to them.

Pirating

Pirating, the once feared plague of vinyl records, has become the foe again. As suggested by Dr. Organ, literature theft and plagiarism might be enhanced by e-publishing. No one will quibble with the notion that hundreds if not thousands of knowledgeable souls are ready (if not doing it already) to import any and all information on the web to personal (or lucrative) goals. Although most journals only offer the contents "online," several "specialists" are able to enter the e-files of journals and diffuse not only the list of contents but also the entire article with references. Staying with the "Safe Harbor" guidelines or abiding to the "Fair Use Doctrine" might hold for some, but not for all. But, any of us who have traveled to some of the so-called developing countries know that the paper or hardcover textbooks in medicine have been "pirated" for many years. All of us have seen the Harrison or the Schwartz classical textbooks, on "bible paper," for just 25% of the best price available in any book store in the United States: why fool ourselves about the electronic age?

References

1. Greenfeld KT (1999) Clicks and bricks. Time, Dec 27
2. Young AE (1996) The future of surgical journals in the electronic publishing age. Br J Surg 83:280–290

Editorial Comment

We are proud to open this volume of *Controversies in Surgery* with contributions from the editors of three leading surgical journals: Claude Organ (*Archives of Surgery*), John Farndon (*British Journal of Surgery*), and Cynthia Laitman and Layton Rikkers (*Annals of Surgery*). Thomas Karger – from S. Karger AG Publishing House in Basel – eloquently offered the publisher's perspective and Drs. Meakins and Fingerhut – both truly "international" academic surgeons – gave us the viewpoint of surgeons who read and write.

The contributors dealt adequately with the "hot topic" of the role of the printed material in the increasingly "electronized world." Be that as it may, we still see our residents carrying handbooks, reading heavy texts in their rooms and printing onto paper the material they find from Internet searches. Perhaps the small portable Rocket eBook (already available at B&N.com) will replace paper books sooner or later – we hope later. But think about it: in bed or on the beach – with an e-book? What an unromantic idea!

Editors Versus Publishers

Dr. Meakins provides us with an honest and personal glimpse into the often unhappy and frustrating experiences of surgeons who dare to undertake the task of editing a major multi-author book. Having gathered our own "wisdom" on this topic we would like to add to Dr. Meakins' story, to serve perhaps as an advice to readers who wish to undertake book projects in the future. From the first step, the aspiring book editor is wedged between the publishers and the contributing authors.

The medical publishers of today are a "difficult crowd"; having to perform in a world of ever-increasing competition, and decreased revenues, they want you the editor – to do all the work for almost nothing in return, except having your name on the cover of the book. Unless you are a leading "giant" in your field, the publisher will let you feel that he is doing you a favor. Never ever start a book without a signed contract, as in today's world of constant mergers your publisher of today may not exist next week. A signed contract however is not an insurance card; we experienced a publisher who decided not to publish our book a year after such a contract was indeed signed. As Dr. Meakins alluded to – forget about money; you may spend many hours over many years never seeing a cent unless your book is a huge bestseller – which in the limited realm of surgical publishing is most unlikely. So you do it for the "fun and fame" – nothing more!

Editors Versus Contributors

Procuring contributors for your book involves a whole science – which has been poorly described hitherto – so read carefully. The ideal contributing author for your multi-authored book is a "famous giant" in his field and an accomplished writer (he has to be one, otherwise he would not be "famous"). Typically, however, the giants are constantly over-committed – a fact which has the following potential consequences.

- *The "refusnik".* The giant may refuse your invitation up front. When editing a book, which requires 60 authors, you'll get five immediate refusals. Initially, your feelings may be hurt – "what, my book is not important enough for him?" – but later on you'll understand that a polite decline is an honest act which saves you time and frustrations.
- *The over-committed giant* accepts your invitation and immediately delegates the task of writing to his junior colleague. This is fine as long as the giant meaningfully controls the final product. Occasionally, however, it is not so and all you get is a text written by the junior without any touch of novelty and wisdom you expect from the giant. Thus, some giants would commit their name to a sub-optimal chapter they hardly had the time to review.
- *A few giants may engage in self-plagiarism.* This is not uncommon and sadly understandable. Having been invited to write numerous chapters and reviews on his topic of main interest, the giant is forced to use his "mouse" to click and paste onto the new chapters whole segments from his previous work. As long as the new chapter is good this is not a disaster – as self-plagiarism of purely educational material (as books are) is not considered an ethical misconduct.
- *The "fugitive" giant.* Even giants may first accept the invitation to contribute and then totally ignore all your efforts to procure the chapter from them. Your "reminder" letters, e-mails and even phone calls are never returned and you'll never see their chapter. You start wondering how they ever became giants. The incidence of such mini-tragedy is fortunately rare – around 5% per book, but when it occurs it is time-consuming and may significantly delay your book submission to print. Being a fugitive contributor is a major crime! How to deal with it is another controversy.
- *Giants are often late.* Characteristically, they start writing the chapter for you only when the deadline arrives.

Most giants, however, will provide you with excellent, well-written and well-polished chapters – on schedule. Reviewing their final product you'll understand why they became giants and are considered so.

An alternative to the giants are "upcoming talents." Those are younger but talented academicians who strive to build their names. You can identify them in MEDLINE search, during society meetings, in journals and in major textbooks – where their names are usually overshadowed by their "giant-mentor" co-authors. Not unexpectedly, however, youngsters tend to emulate their giant-mentors including the exhibition of the above-stated pitfalls.

Practical Tips for the Inexperienced Editor

- Strive for a balanced combination of giants and upcoming talents; give a chance to relatively unknown surgeons – they may surprise you with the quality of their product. In order to satisfy your publisher, at least half of the contributors have to be giants.

- Maintain a list of "excellent contributors" and use them repeatedly. This is, however, impossible when your books focus on an ever-changing set of topics. Similarly, have a black list of those who are habitually late and/or poor writers. Try not to use them again. Of course, never invite a fugitive contributor again. On the other hand, you may invite a "refusnik" again to contribute – your new invitation may be of a greater interest to him or perhaps he now has more time.
- Always get yourself a few "spare" chapters for every book and you will not have to worry about "no shows" anymore.
- Always overestimate the time required to produce a book. You will never have all the chapters on your desk earlier than 6 months after the declared deadline.

Dr. Meakins concludes with a pessimistic financial note: "If the publishers make money from the book and the editor is the marketable commodity, should not the editor be as fairly reimbursed as the publisher?" This is a good question which unfortunately will remain "rhetorical" for as long as there will be "suckers" (as us probably) who agree to do more and more for almost nothing – except "fun and fame" – publishers won't have any reason to change. Why should they?

Redundant Publications

Another crucial and controversial issue relevant to "surgical publication" which was not mentioned by the contributors is that of "redundant publications." A redundant publication is a publication that duplicates another, or few – previous, simultaneous, or ensuing – publications by the same author or group or, alternatively, could have been combined into one paper. The medical community considers it bad practice because it distorts scientific findings and wastes the time, effort and resources of journals, editors, reviewers, readers, libraries and electronic data bases. Recently we set out to assess the incidence, spectrum and salient characteristics of redundant publications in three leading surgical journals (*Surgery*, *British Journal of Surgery*, and *Archives of Surgery*). We developed a grading system to define several types of redundant publications: A "dual"; B "potentially dual"; C "salami-slicing." A total of 660 articles were screened leading to 158 (24%) "suspected" papers – representing some form of a redundant publication. Twenty-three (14.5%) of the "suspected" papers were defined as dual publications, 53 (33.5%) as potentially dual publications, and 82 (52%) as products of salami-slicing. Clearly, our study shows that at least one out of five "original" articles published in leading surgical journals represents some form of redundancy. Current online search technology provides an effective tool for identifying and tracing such publications, but is not used routinely as part of the peer review process. Redundancies occur in several well-defined patterns; the phenomenon is widespread and cuts across the entire spectrum of surgeons in the United States and abroad. Redundant publications must be recognized not as a mere nuisance but as a real threat to the quality and intellectual impact of surgical publishing. It therefore behooves editors, reviewers, writers and readers to cooperate in creating effective filter mechanisms to screen for redundancy and to eliminate this phenomenon.

Many books are available on "*how to write and publish*" in science – none, however, is aimed specifically at surgeons. During 2000, the *British Journal of Surgery* has published a series of articles on "how to publish for surgeons." Surgeons who wish to write and publish should consult these pages which are freely available on the Internet [http://www.blackwell-synergy.com/issuelist.asp?journal=bjs].

CHAPTER 2

Malignant Melanoma

Surgical Management: The Role of Intraoperative Lymphatic Mapping and Sentinel Lymph Node Biopsy

DOUGLAS TYLER · HILLIARD SEIGLER

Intraoperative lymphatic mapping and sentinel lymph node biopsy is a technique that was initially described in 1992 by Donald Morton [1]. This technique is based upon the concept that each area of skin drains to a specific lymph node, the so-called sentinel lymph node, within a regional nodal basin before it drains to additional lymph nodes within that basin. Each area of skin drains to different sentinel lymph nodes and many areas of skin may have sentinel lymph nodes in more than one nodal basin. In theory, by accessing the status of the sentinel lymph node one should be able to determine whether metastatic disease has occurred to that regional basin. As it was initially described, Dr. Morton and colleagues utilized an intradermal injection of a blue dye called 1% lymphazurin blue, which was preferentially taken up by the lymphatics to try and identify the sentinel lymph node. By making a small incision over the regional lymph node basin, they could visually identify a blue afferent lymphatic channel and one or two lymph nodes that accumulated the blue dye within them. Using the lymphazurin blue dye alone, a blue lymph node could be identified approximately 85%–90% of the time. In the initial study, when the blue lymph node was identified it was removed and followed by a complete lymph node dissection. An examination of the blue lymph nodes in comparison to the other lymph nodes present in the nodal basin supported the concept that the blue lymph node was indeed the sentinel lymph node. When the sentinel lymph node was negative, it was extremely rare to have any additional lymph nodes positive, and if the sentinel lymph node was positive, it was the only positive lymph node about 85%–90% of the time.

Several centers have gone on to validate the sentinel lymph node concept for melanoma and help to refine the technique [2–10]. Preoperative lymphoscintigraphy helps to ensure that the appropriate nodal basins are being mapped and helps to identify any in-transit lesions. Utilization of a hand-held gamma probe intraoperatively in conjunction with either reinjection of the radiolabelled colloid or using the residual radioactivity from the radiolabelled colloid injected as part of the original lymphoscintigraphy has become another method of sentinel lymph node identification. When the radiolabelled colloid is used together with the blue dye injection, the sentinel lymph node identification rate increases to 99%. Using the combination of radiolabelled colloid and blue dye, intraoperative lymphatic mapping and sentinel lymph node biopsy can be done through very small incisions, using local anesthesia, on an outpatient basis. As this minimally invasive technique has become validated and more widely available, several issues have been raised as to exactly what does intraoperative lymphatic mapping do for patients and which patients should this technique be offered to.

What Does Intraoperative Lymphatic Mapping and Sentinel Lymph Node Biopsy Do for Patients with Melanoma?

The technique of intraoperative lymphatic mapping and sentinel lymph node biopsy has become a powerful tool to more accurately stage patients with melanoma [11]. By identifying one or two lymph nodes that are at the highest risk of harboring metastatic disease, a pathologist can carry out types of analyses that are not practical or cost-effective to perform on the 10–30 lymph nodes that might be present in a routine elective lymph node dissection. Routine histology with H&E stain allows the detection of one tumor cell in a population of 10,000 normal cells. By performing serial sectioning and immunohistochemistry on one or two sentinel lymph nodes, one tumor cell in a population of 100,000 normal cells can be detected. The application of molecular biology techniques to the sentinel lymph node, looking for evidence of tumor protein production using reverse transcriptase-polymerase chain reaction technique (RT-PCR) for melanoma markers such as tyrosinase, MAGE, MART, and/or gp100, can allow the detection of one tumor cell in a population of 1 million normal cells.

Although the significance of a positive PCR result has been debated, two recent studies have demonstrated that patients whose sentinel lymph node is histologically negative but PCR-positive have a statistically worse prognosis than those with histologically negative, PCR-negative nodes, but the prognosis is statistically better than patients whose sentinel lymph node is histologically positive and PCR-positive [12, 13]. In these studies, the PCR status of the lymph node was the most significant predictor of survival even over tumor thickness and ulceration. Therefore, utilization of intraoperative lymphatic mapping and sentinel lymph node biopsy in patients with melanoma can provide extremely accurate staging information and important prognostic information for both the patient and physician. This technique in and of itself does not improve survival but it does help identify patients with evidence of nodal metastasis that may become candidates for therapeutic lymph node dissections and considered for adjuvant therapies because of their high risk for developing recurrent disease.

Who Should Be Offered Intraoperative Lymphatic Mapping and Sentinel Lymph Node Biopsy?

Melanomas Less than 1 mm

Although the prognosis for patients with thin melanoma is excellent, approximately 10% of these patients will die of their disease [14]. Several studies have tried to determine the characteristics of thin lesions that are more likely to metastasize [14–17]. Features of regression, ulceration, and/or discordant Clark level of IV or V are generally associated with a worse prognosis in this subgroup of patients. Intraoperative lymphatic mapping may be another way to further evaluate patients with thin melanomas whose primary tumors have poor prognostic features. Although there are currently no data to suggest that this group of patients would receive a survival benefit from a therapeutic lymph node dissection based upon a positive sentinel lymph node, they would be candidates for adjuvant therapies either in the form of interferon or immunotherapy trials. Some of these patients may also qualify for the Multicenter Selective Lymphadenectomy Trial, which would enroll patients with melanomas greater than 1 mm or patients with thin melanomas if they have a discordant Clark level of IV or V. This trial randomizes patients to wide local excision alone vs. wide local excision in conjunction with sentinel lymph node biopsy [18]. If the sentinel lymph node biopsy is positive, patients go on to receive a therapeutic lymph node dissection (see Fig. 1). Our institutional policy is to offer intraoperative lymphatic mapping and sentinel lymph node biopsy to patients with thin melanomas if their primary lesion is associated with regression, ulceration, and/or a discordant Clark level and they are interested in some form of adjuvant therapy should their sentinel lymph node be positive.

Melanomas Between 1 and 4 mm

Much controversy has surrounded the appropriate management of patients with intermediate thickness melanomas with regard to lymph nodes. It is thought by some that patients in this group have a higher probability of having regional nodal disease (15%–60%) than metastatic disease (8%–15%), and as such may in theo-

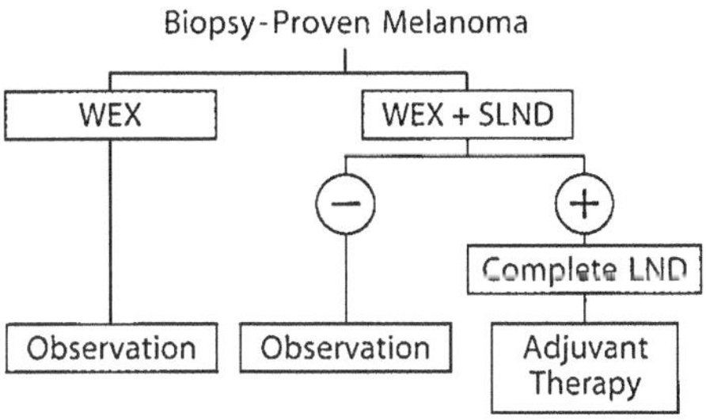

Fig. 1. Algorithm for Multicenter Sentinel Lymphadenectomy Trial
WEX: wide excision

ry benefit from removal of regional lymph nodes [19]. At the time intraoperative lymphatic mapping and sentinel lymph node biopsy was first described, there were only a few retrospective studies that demonstrated a survival advantage to prophylactically or electively removing the regional lymph nodes [20, 21]. In addition to a few large retrospective studies that showed no benefit to elective removal of the regional lymph nodes in this patient population, there are three prospective, randomized clinical trials that failed to show any benefit [22–25].

To address many of the concerns raised by the initial randomized prospective clinical trials, the Intergroup Surgical Trial was initiated and accrued 781 patients between 1983 and 1991 [26]. This study stratified patients by tumor thickness, ulceration and site. At the most recent analysis it has greater than 5-year follow-up in all patients and a mean follow-up of 10 years [27]. Although there was no overall survival advantage to elective lymph node dissection when the entire group of patients was examined, there did appear to be some groups of patients who benefited from lymph node dissection as identified by subgroup analysis. The analysis of prospectively stratified groups demonstrated significant reductions in mortality for patients with nonulcerated lesions (29%), extremity lesions (27%), and lesions with Breslow thickness between 1 and 2 mm (35%). In addition, although not stratified prospectively, age appeared to be an important factor in that patients younger than 60 years showed improved survival from elective lymph node dissection.

Although the Intergroup trial has demonstrated some survival advantages to certain subgroups of patients with intermediate thickness melanoma, the majority of patients with intermediate thickness melanoma (70%–80%) do not have micrometastatic disease and thus would not benefit from lymph node dissection. Since lymph node dissection is not without its morbidity, many surgeons have been hesitant to perform elective lymph node dissection on patients to potentially benefit a few. A recent study from the John Wayne Cancer Institute of over 500 matched patients comparing elective lymph node dissection to selective lymph node dissection (intraoperative lymphatic mapping and sentinel lymph node biopsy with lymph node dissection performed if the sentinel lymph node was positive) found no differences in the incidence of tumor-positive dissections, tumor recurrence or survival, suggesting that the two procedures are therapeutically equivalent [28].

Current Studies

There are currently two clinical trials examining the role of intraoperative lymphatic mapping and sentinel lymph node biopsy in patients with intermediate thickness melanoma: the Multicenter Selective Lymphadenectomy Trial as described above and the Sunbelt Melanoma Trial [19]. The Sunbelt Melanoma Trial (see Fig. 2) enrolls patients with melanoma between 1 and 4 mm and attempts to incorporate molecular pathologic staging (PCR) in an attempt to determine whether early intervention with lymphadenectomy and/or interferon alpha-2b will improve survival. All patients undergo intraoperative lymphatic mapping and sentinel lymph node biopsy. The sentinel lymph node has a small piece removed for

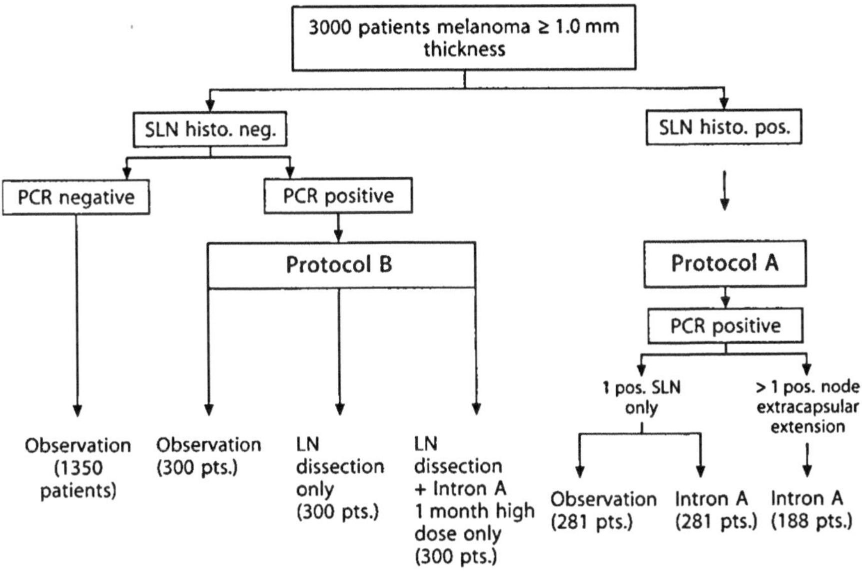

Fig. 2. Algorithm for Sunbelt Melanoma Trial

PCR analysis and the rest of the lymph node is examined with serial sectioning and immunohistochemistry. Patients with a histologically positive sentinel lymph node undergo completion nodal dissection. If the sentinel lymph node is the only positive lymph node, then the patient is randomized to observation or adjuvant high-dose interferon for 1 month. If the sentinel lymph node is histologically negative, then PCR analysis is performed and if positive patients are randomized to observation, completion lymphadenectomy, or completion lymphadenectomy plus 1 month of high-dose interferon.

Our current practice is to encourage patients with intermediate thickness melanomas to participate in the Sunbelt Melanoma Trial, a trial that is active at over 50 centers nationwide. For patients who do not qualify or do not desire to participate in this trial, we take a more selective approach to evaluating regional lymph nodes. Generally we reserve intraoperative lymphatic mapping for patients who would desire participation in an adjuvant therapy trial if their lymph nodes were positive or if their primary melanoma has characteristics that would suggest that they might have a survival benefit from lymph node dissection. This would include patients less than 60 years old who have nonulcerated lesions.

Melanoma Lesions Greater than 4 mm

Most studies suggest that this patient population has a very high chance of harboring distant metastatic disease and as a result no survival benefit has ever been demonstrated for patients undergoing elective regional lymph node dissection. Our approach to this patient population has been to perform a staging work-up consisting of chest, abdomen and pelvic CT scan. If no metastatic disease is identified, then we have offered intraoperative lymphatic mapping and sentinel lymph node biopsy to these patients if they were interested in participating in an adjuvant therapy trial should their sentinel lymph node be positive. The additional benefit of performing a sentinel lymph node biopsy in this patient population is that those individuals who have a negative sentinel lymph node have an excellent prognosis - much better than would be expected for the group of patients with thick melanomas as a whole [29]. The ability to give patients this type of prognostic information is another reason for offering these patients this technique.

Conclusions

In conclusion, intraoperative lymphatic mapping and sentinel lymph node biopsy are powerful tools for accurately staging patients with malignant melanoma. More accurate staging as provided by this technique will not only provide better prognostic information but also allow better stratification of patients in future clinical trials. Current clinical trials utilizing this technique are designed to determine whether earlier therapeutic intervention based upon molecular pathology of the sentinel lymph node will improve survival.

References

1. Morton DL, Wen DR, Wong JH, et al. (1992) Technical details of intraoperative lymphatic mapping for early stage melanoma. Arch Surg 127:392–399
2. Ross MI, Reintgen D, Balch CM (1993) Selective lymphadenectomy: emerging role for lymphatic mapping and sentinel lymph node biopsy in the management of early stage melanoma. Semin Surg Oncol 9:219–223
3. Reintgen D, Cruse CW, Wells K, et al. (1994) The orderly progression of melanoma nodal metastasis. Ann Surg 220:759–767
4. Gershenwald JE, Colome MI, Lee JE, et al. (1998) Patterns of recurrence following a negative sentinel lymph node biopsy in 243 patients with stage I and stage II melanoma. J Clin Oncol 16:2253–2260
5. Albertini JJ, Cruse CW, Rapaport D, et al. (1996) Intraoperative radiolymphoscintigraphy improves sentinel lymph node identification rate for patients with melanoma. Ann Surg 223:217–224
6. Kapteijin BAE, Nieweg OE, Liem I, et al. (1997) Localizing the sentinel lymph node in cutaneous melanoma: gamma probe detection versus blue dye. Ann Surg Oncol 4:156–160
7. Krag DN, Meijer SJ, Weaver DL, et al. (1995) Minimal-access surgery for staging of malignant melanoma. Arch Surg 130:654–658
8. Leong SPL, Steinmetz I, Habib FA, et al. (1997) Optimal selective sentinel lymph node dissection in primary melanoma. Arch Surg 132:666–673
9. Mudun A, Murray DR, Herda SC, et al. (1996) Early stage melanoma: lymphoscintigraphy, reproducibility of sentinel node detection, and effectiveness of the intraoperative gamma probe. Radiology 199:171–175
10. Thompson JF, McCarthy WH, Bosch CM, et al. (1995) Sentinel lymph node status as an indicator of the presence of metastatic melanoma in regional lymph nodes. Melanoma Res 5:255–260
11. Wang X, Heller R, VanVoorhis N, et al. (1994) Detection of submicroscopic lymph node metastasis with polymerase chain reaction in patients with malignant melanoma. Ann Surg 220:768–774
12. Shivers SC, Wang X, Li W, et al. (1998) Molecular staging of malignant melanoma: correlation with clinical outcome. JAMA 280:1410–1415
13. Bostick PJ, Morton DJ, Turner RR, et al. (1999) Prognostic significance of occult metastases detected by sentinel lymphadenectomy and reverse transcriptase-polymerase chain reaction in early stage melanoma patients. J Clin Oncol 17:3238–3244

14. Slingluff CL, Vollmer RT, Reintgen DS, et al. (1998) Lethal "thin" malignant melanoma. Ann Surg 208:150–161
15. Park KG, Blessing K, McLaren KM, et al. (1993) A study of thin malignant melanomas with poor prognosis. Br J Plast Surg 46:607–610
16. Blessing K, McLaren KM, McLean A, et al. (1990) Thin malignant melanomas with metastasis: a histological study and survival analysis. Histopathology 17:389–395
17. Massi D, Franchi A, Borgognoni L, et al. (1999) Thin cutaneous malignant melanomas: identification of risk factors indicative of progression. Cancer 85:1067–1076
18. Morton DL, Chan AD (1999) Current status of intraoperative lymphatic mapping and sentinel lymphadenectomy for melanoma: is it standard of care? J Am Coll Surg 189:214–223
19. McMasters KM, Sondak VK, Lotze MT, et al. (1999) Recent advances in melanoma staging and therapy. Ann Surg Oncol 6:467–475
20. Balch CM, Soong S-J, Murad TM, et al. (1979) A multifactorial analysis of melanoma II: prognostic factors in patients with stage I melanoma. Surgery 86:343–351
21. McCarthy WH, Shaw HM, Milton GW (1985) Efficacy of elective lymph node dissection in 2347 patients with clinical stage I malignant melanoma. Surg Gynecol Obstet 161:575–580
22. Slingluff CL, Stidham KR, Ricci WM, et al. (1994) Surgical management of regional lymph nodes in patients with melanoma. Experience with 4682 patients. Ann Surg 219:120–130
23. Veronesi U, Adamus J, Bandiera DC, et al. (1982) Delayed regional lymph node dissection in stage I melanoma of the skin of the lower extremities. Cancer 49:2420–2430
24. Sim FH, Taylor WF, Ivins JC, et al. (1978) A prospective randomized study of efficacy of routine elective lymphadenectomy in management of malignant melanoma. Cancer 41:948–956
25. Cascinelli N, Morabito A, Santinami M, et al. (1998) Immediate or delayed dissection of regional lymph nodes in patients with melanoma of the trunk: a randomized trial. WHO melanoma programme. Lancet 351:793–796
26. Balch CM, Soong S-J, Bartolucci AA, et al. (1996) Efficacy of an elective lymph node dissection of 1 to 4 mm thick melanomas for patients 60 years of age and younger. Ann Surg 224:255–266
27. Balch CM, Ross M, Soong S-J, et al. (1999) Long term results of a prospective randomized trial involving elective regional lymph node dissection in patients with intermediate thickness melanomas. Abstract 3. Proceedings of the Society of Surgical Oncology. Orlando, March 5
28. Essner R, Conforti A, Kelley MC, et al. (1999) Efficacy of lymphatic mapping, sentinel lymphadenectomy, and selective complete lymph node dissection as a therapeutic procedure for early-stage melanoma. Ann Surg Oncol 6:442–449
29. Heaton KM, Sussman JJ, Gershenwald JE, et al. (1998) Surgical margins and prognostic factors in patients with thick primary melanoma. Ann Surg Oncol 5:322–328

Nonsurgical Modalities

Dina Lev-Chelouche · Joseph M. Klausner

The worldwide incidence of melanoma has reached epidemic proportions, increasing at a rate greater than for any other human cancer. Treatment is based mainly on surgical measures; however, early detection and prevention are the mainstays of a good outcome. Moreover, nonsurgical modalities may also have an important role to play in the adjuvant, palliative and even the therapeutic set-up.

Can Melanoma Be Prevented?

In an attempt to prevent the development of melanoma, its causative factors need to be understood. Two of the main hypothesized risk factors are genetic susceptibility and sun exposure.

It was only in 1983 that the first formal genetic analysis suggested an autosomal dominant mode of inheritance for both melanoma and the then newly described melanoma precursor, dysplastic nevi [1]. Subsequent genetic studies have assumed this model to be correct, although when viewed in aggregate, the data are inconsistent. At present, clinical predictive genetic testing for mutations in melanoma genes is available commercially, but its use is limited by the uncertainty as to how test results might affect the management of melanoma-prone family members.

Currently, management recommendations include monthly skin self-examination, clinical skin examination once or twice a year, and a low threshold for simple excision of pigmented lesions. In the future, identification of the exact molecular basis of genetic determinants governing the pathogenesis of normal nevi, dysplastic nevi and melanoma might enable their prevention via genetic engineering techniques.

There is a strong correlation between sun exposure, mainly intermittent intense exposure to ultraviolet (UV) radiation, and the development of melanoma [2, 3]; as one moves closer to the equator, the incidence of melanoma in white-skinned populations increases dramatically. This observation emphasizes the importance of protecting and educating populations as to the harmful effects of UV radiation. The use of sunscreens is widely advocated as a preventive measure against sun-induced melanoma. Several arguments have been raised in opposition to this inference [4–6]. Published melanoma case-control studies have not consistently demonstrated a protective effect of sunscreens. Moreover, some studies have even shown a harmful effect with an increased risk of melanoma suggested as being either secondary to sunscreen interference with cutaneous vitamin D synthesis or by the longer time spent in the sun while using such sunscreens. Uncertainty will remain until the usefulness of sunscreens is convincingly demonstrated in well-controlled studies. As the dust settles around this issue, it would be prudent to remind patients to lower their exposure to sunlight whether or not they use sunscreen products.

There is no doubt that public awareness and early diagnosis of lesions has led to improved survival rates, as more and more lesions are diagnosed at an earlier stage. The percentage of thin melanomas (<0.76 mm) making up the total number of melanomas diagnosed has increased from 9.4% in the 1970s to 31.5% in 1989 [7].

Adjuvant Treatment for Malignant Melanomas: Does It Exist?

Stage is the most important prognostic factor in melanoma patients. For patients with "thin" melanoma (AJCC stage I), surgical excision of the primary lesion with adequate margins is the only treatment recommended and carries very high survival rates. However, for patients with thicker primary lesions or patients who present with, or subsequently develop, regional lymph node metastases, there is a significant risk of developing recurrent, distant metastatic disease, even after adequate surgical intervention. The decreased survival rate in patients with thick primary lesions or regional metastases is attributable to the presence of occult systemic metastases at the time of surgical intervention, and adjuvant therapy is based on the premise that treatment will be more effective when tumor burden is small.

The following groups of melanoma patients are deemed to be at high risk for developing recurrent disease and should be considered candidates for adjuvant therapy:

- Patients with thick primary melanomas
- Patients with AJCC stage disease with clinical (macroscopic) or pathological (microscopic) nodal metastasis
- Patients with in-transit metastases (AJCC stage III) or satellite nodules or local recurrence (AJCC stage II)
- Patients with stage IV melanoma who have been rendered disease-free by surgical resection of metastases (either soft tissue nodal or visceral)

If highly effective and/or minimally toxic treatment strategies were available, patients with intermediate thickness primary melanomas (between 1 and 4 mm thick) might also be considered candidates for adjuvant therapy. Furthermore, patients who are at high risk for developing recurrent disease may be identified in the future by an assay for detecting melanoma cells in peripheral blood and lymph nodes, which is based on the amplification of mRNA for tyrosinase or other melanoma-specific markers by the reverse transcriptase-polymerase chain reaction (RT-PCR) [8].

The question as to whether there is any effective adjuvant therapy for patients with resected high-risk melanomas has been investigated many times over the past few decades [9–12]. The earliest studies were conducted with a series of nonspecific immunostimulants. BCG, the bovine mycobacterium used as a tuberculosis vaccine, can induce regression in up to 80% of cutaneous melanoma metastases when injected intralesionally. Even more striking is the fact that up to 20% of uninjected lesions regress. Tremendous interest in the adjuvant use of BCG arose following the suggestion of its benefits in nonrandomized trials. However, despite initial enthusiasm, no benefit was demonstrated in at least nine subsequent prospective randomized trials. Adjuvant use of *C. parvum*, another nonspecific microbial immunostimulant, also looked promising on the basis of retrospective studies. Again, prospective, randomized trials failed to substantiate this agent's efficacy. Levamisole, another nonspecific immunostimulant, showed no benefit in three out of four randomized trials. One Canadian study demonstrated a trend in favor of levamisole, and this agent is still used by some centers for adjuvant therapy for melanoma. Other agents tested in the adjuvant setting, but found to be of no benefit in randomized trials, include: vaccinia melanoma oncolysates, DTIC therapy alone or with other agents, transfer factor, thymostimulin, 156 prinosine, megestrol acetate, and retinoids. These studies clearly demonstrated the need for new and improved adjuvant approaches, as well as the critical importance of prospective, randomized trials to ultimately prove or disprove the clinical efficacy of such therapies.

The first statistically significant results of a prospective, randomized, adjuvant trial in high-risk melanoma patients were reported with interferon alpha-2 and will be discussed further, as will radiotherapy, chemotherapy, isolated limb perfusion, and immunotherapy, in the adjuvant and nonadjuvant set-up.

Radiation Therapy for Malignant Melanoma

In 1936, Paterson, a leading authority on radiation therapy at that time, considered malignant melanoma to be a radio-resistant tumor and therefore radiation was regarded "futile" in this disease. Although later reports demonstrated beneficial effects of radiation in this disease, the resolution of the controversy came from in vitro studies which revealed that melanoma cells are relatively less sensitive to radiation only at lower doses [13]. Indeed, several clinical studies used larger doses per fraction ($\geqslant 4$ Gy) and obtained high response rates in a variety of primary and metastatic sites and high in-field control rates in patients receiving elective or adjunctive regional radiation [14–16].

The primary management of malignant melanoma remains surgical. However, there is strong evidence to indicate that radiation therapy is a valuable alternative on rare occasions, such as large facial lentigo maligna melanomas, which may involve wide surgical resection and extensive reconstruction, medically inoperable patients, or those who refuse surgery. Radiation has been used as a supplement to limit the extent of excision and thereby reduce cosmetic deformity. A number of studies have defined subsets of melanoma patients at high risk for local recurrence post-surgery, such as thick melanomas or desmoplastic melanomas, who might benefit from adjunctive therapy for the primary tumor bed.

Available data indicate the need for improving regional control rates in patients with multiple or large nodes and those with extranodal disease. The data also suggest that improvement in regional control rates could potentially translate into improved survival in the small subset of patients who are at high risk of failure. Published studies of the role of adjuvant radiation therapy in the management of regional metastases of malignant melanoma are few but show a definitely lower local recurrence rate of around 10% following adjuvant radiotherapy as opposed to 25% for those who did not receive radiation therapy [17].

Radiotherapy is widely used and accepted for local palliation. In view of poor systemic agents for distant failures, radiation is an important tool in the management of symptomatic metastases. It is routinely used in lung, bone, brain, lymph node, and subcutaneous nodule failures. Response rates of 50% for skin lesions and 30% for brain lesions have been reported.

New data indicate that hyperthermia enhances the response of metastatic lesions to radiation. On-going research with a variety of experimental strategies offers the possibility of further increasing the utility of radiation therapy in the management of this disease.

The Role of Chemotherapy in Melanoma

Adjuvant chemotherapy trials were initiated in the 1970s after dacarbazine (DTIC) was shown to have a 20% response rate in the metastatic setting. The early trials included small numbers of patients and evaluated chemotherapy alone and in combination with immunotherapy with conflicting results, some showing improved disease-free survival while others were unable to show a significant benefit from chemotherapy or chemoimmunotherapy when compared to surgery alone.

To clarify the question, larger trials were conducted within cooperative groups. The largest multicenter, randomized trial was performed by the World Health Organization (WHO) and included 761 evaluable patients with Clark's level III–V truncal primaries and pathologically negative lymph nodes or with primary lesions from any other site with positive lymph nodes [18]. Patients were randomized into four groups including DTIC alone, BCG alone, DTIC + BCG, or observation. After a median follow-up of 41 months, no difference in disease-free or overall survival rates was detected between the groups. Other smaller trials using varying dosages and combinations of chemotherapy have been unable to show any benefit when compared to observation alone following resection of all evident disease.

There has been interest in adjuvant vindesine, a vinca alkaloid, following a non-randomized study which showed significant benefits with respect to time to first relapse and survival time after lymph node dissection, and overall survival in the treatment arm group in comparison to the control group [19]. This needs to be confirmed in a randomized control trial.

Adjuvant high-dose chemotherapy with autologous bone marrow rescue in 39 patients with AJCC stage III disease did not show any benefit in terms of survival relative to systemic chemotherapy [20].

Systemic chemotherapy for advanced melanoma has yielded poor response rates. Various treatment regimens have been proposed to date, all with unfavorable results. Chemotherapeutic single-agent regimens give objective response rates of up to 20% with DTIC as the most effective single agent. Combination chemotherapy regimens result in objective response rates as high as 55%. However, most of these regimens have resulted in short-term response and poor survival. The addition of immunotherapy to combination chemotherapy increases toxicity but not survival [21].

Regional Therapy for Malignant Melanoma

Isolated limb perfusion (ILP) has been establishing its role in the management of malignant melanoma for the past 40 years. ILP enables the administration of very high doses of chemotherapeutic drugs, 10–20 times higher than those administered systemically without exposing the patient's systemic circulation to these drugs. There are two clinical situations in which ILP is considered. The first is as an adjuvant treatment following complete removal of primary melanoma in high-risk patients and the second as therapeutic ILP in the presence of recurrent or regionally metastatic melanoma.

The concept of adjuvant ILP in melanoma is a very appealing one; high-risk tumors (1.5 mm and deeper) have probably shed tumor cells into the surrounding skin and lymphatic channels. The "standard care" – wide excision (WE) of the lesion with about 2-cm margins – does not address this risk. Perfusion of the entire limb with high doses of a chemotherapeutic drug can result in eradication of these tumor cells. However, hard evidence that this concept is true is lacking. Most studies report retrospective, single institutional experience [22–24]. The controls are historical and there is significant variability in dosage, technique and the use of hyperthermia.

The question of adjuvant ILP in melanoma and its impact on survival has been addressed by three randomized trials [25–27]. The first two done more than a decade ago presented relatively small series from single institutions. In a study conducted by Ghussen et al. [25], the advantage of ILP was so significant that the investigators stopped randomization, considering that it was not ethical to continue the trial. This study was criticized on two issues; its small size, less than 20 patients per stage of melanoma in each arm, and, secondly, the higher than expected survival in the perfusion group, 98% 5-year survival including 66% patients with stages II and III melanoma. In the second prospective study by Hafstrom et al., where 69 patients were randomized, there was an improved local recurrence rate and disease-free survival in the perfusion group, but overall survival did not improve significantly [26].

The third study is a recently published large, multi-centric study sponsored by the European Organization for Research and Treatment of Cancer (EORTC), the WHO and the North American Perfusion Group (NAPG) [27]. It comprised 832 melanoma patients (>1.5 mm thickness) from 16 centers. Patients were randomized to undergo WE alone or WE and ILP with melphalan and mild hyperthermia. Lymph node dissection was optional, but the same policy was applied to patients with or without ILP. The treatment groups were matched for age, gender, anatomical location, Breslow thickness, presence of ulceration and previous biopsy. Data analysis performed at a median of 6.4 years demonstrated a transient effect of ILP in terms of regional recurrence; the rate for in-transit metastases was reduced in the perfused group from 6.6% to 3.3% with an improved disease-free interval of 75% at 6 years relative to 62% in the untreated group. However, these effects were nullified by the higher rate of distant metastases in the ILP group (12.9% vs. 9.7%). Most importantly, the overall survival was practically identical in both groups and subgroup analysis also did not reveal any survival benefit. This study indicates that adjuvant ILP is not justified.

The issue of adjuvant ILP following a complete excision of local recurrence or in-transit metastases is different and has not been fully addressed. Ghussen et al. reported increased survival in a small group of stage III patients treated by complete excision of all measurable disease and ILP, compared to those treated by surgical excision alone [28]. However, Hafstrom et al. could not confirm such an advantage in their series [26]. Undoubtedly, a large-scale controlled study addressing this issue is required.

The biological rationale behind the performance of therapeutic ILP in patients with regional melanoma metastases relies on the fact that about 40%–50% of melanomas occur in the extremities and 10%–20% of tumor recurrences or in-transit metastases are confined to the affected limb. Although the prognosis of these patients is poor, the disease remains regional and in some cases allows long survival. The best evidence for this is contained in two studies in which major amputations were performed in patients with multiple in-transit metastases resulting in 42% and 21% 5- and 10-year survival, respectively [29].

The results of therapeutic ILP with melphalan for recurrent or in-transit melanoma metastases vary considerably [30–35]. Typically, time period to maximal response is approximately 7–8 weeks. Response rates range from 48%–100% and complete remission (CR) rates from 10%–82%. The largest series in therapeutic

ILP with high-dose melphalan, which also reflects the acceptable response rate, is the multicenter Dutch study [34]. The overall response was 79% with 54% CR.

The variation in response rates probably reflects patient selection, perfusion technique and drug concentrations. Klasse et al. [34] performed a detailed analysis of prognostic factors associated with CR in a group of 120 patients. CR was achieved in 54%. They concluded that the absence of lymph node metastases, leg (compared to foot or arm) location, and a double perfusion were associated with a higher CR rate.

Patients experiencing partial remission (PR) following ILP may still benefit from the procedure since the disease is usually arrested for a period and the time to progression may be of several months duration. The duration amongst complete responders ranges from 8 to 20 months. In the large Dutch study [34], it was a median of 9 months. Double perfusion did not result in a longer recurrence-free interval. It is generally accepted that long-term survival (>10 years) and cure is a reasonable goal in some 25%–30% of patients experiencing CR following ILP with melphalan. A number of chemotherapeutic drugs other than melphalan were used via ILP. *Cis*-platinum was evaluated due to its increased tumor concentration when delivered under hyperthermic conditions. Response rates were comparable to melphalan [30] but the duration was shorter [37].

DTIC is the most active single agent in melanoma. It was therefore tested in ILP although a passage in the liver is necessary for its conversion to the active metabolite. Didolkar et al. demonstrated a 76% response rate in a group of 32 patients [38]. However, others demonstrated only a 33% response rate [39].

The initial report of 100% response (90% CR) using the combination of TNF, melphalan and IFN-γ by Lienard and Lejeune [40] caused great interest in this combination therapy, and several centers embarked on trials to study the effect and specific contribution of TNF. Besides the high CR rate, close to double that of melphalan alone, the pattern of response was different; tumors became soft and even necrotic within hours to a few days.

IFN-γ was added to the original protocol following the observation that it upregulates TNF receptors on the membrane of both the tumor and endothelial cells [41]. However, a phase III study comparing the response to ILP with melphalan and TNF, with or without IFN-γ, showed no significant difference between the two regimens [27]. Based on this study, most centers stopped using IFN-γ.

Since its introduction, ILP with TNF and melphalan is being performed in centers in Europe, the USA and Israel [42–45]. In a multi-center European study (groups from Lausanne, Groningen, Amsterdam and Rotterdam), 53 patients – of whom 34 were stage IIIA (in-transit metastasis), 15 stage IIIAB (same plus lymph node metastasis) and 4 stage IV – were treated by TNF and melphalan. The response rate was 100% with 91% CR. The authors compared their results to a group of 103 matched historical controls treated at the same institutions by ILP with melphalan alone; the response rate was 77.6% with 52% CR. Duration of response was similar in both groups [45].

Our own experience within a phase II study in 43 melanoma patients, 28 of whom (65%) had bulky disease (tumor measuring >3 cm in diameter or >10 lesions), shows an overall response of 86% with 60% CR. The CR rate was significantly lower in patients with high disease volume [43].

In order to establish whether ILP with TNF and melphalan is advantageous over melphalan alone, a multi-center prospective randomized trial including 11 cancer centers from Europe and Israel was initiated in 1997. Its aim is to focus not only on response rates but specifically on duration of response, local recurrence and survival.

A phase III trial at the National Cancer Institute (NCI) in Bethesda, Maryland, compared perfusions with TNF-melphalan-IFN-γ combination to ILP with melphalan alone. The experimental arm had 80% CR compared to 61% in the melphalan-alone arm. The duration of response was identical. Subgroup analysis disclosed that the advantage of TNF was more significant in patients with high tumor burden [46]. In a second NCI trial, two groups of patients who were not eligible for the above-mentioned phase III study received ILP with TNF and melphalan. One group consisted of 17 patients who had previously failed ILP with melphalan. Reperfusion with TNF was associated with an overall 94% response rate and 65% CR [47].

In conclusion, the role of ILP in melanoma has recently been refined. Adjuvant melphalan perfusion is not justified for routine use in primary melanoma. Its role following the excision of metastatic disease should be evaluated. Therapeutic ILP is the most effective therapy for local recurrence or in-transit metastasis. The addition of TNF caused a marked increase in the response rates; however, the long-term effect of TNF is yet to be determined.

Melanoma – A Target for Immunotherapy?

Since melanoma was first described in 1787, its biological behavior has suggested that the immune system may play a significant role in its development. Over the ensuing years, there has been increasing evidence that melanoma is one of the more immunogenic of human solid tumors [48–51]. It is well known by clinicians that cutaneous melanoma can demonstrate partial or even complete regression of the primary lesion, thus giving rise to the classic diagnostic features of variation in color and irregular borders. These characteristics have been attributed to a spontaneous host anti-tumor phenomenon. Laboratory investigators have shown that blood from melanoma patients contains antibodies against tumor antigens and that patients with localized melanoma or those who have undergone spontaneous regression of their primary melanoma have a significantly higher incidence of anti-melanoma antibodies than those with advanced metastatic disease. Cytotoxic T lymphocytes that kill tumor cells in vitro in an immunologically specific manner have been isolated from melanoma patients. These tumor-reactive cytotoxic T lymphocytes can produce tumor regression after expansion in vitro and re-injection into the same patient. From other clinical studies, it is known that 3%–15% of cutaneous melanomas are first diagnosed as lymphatic or visceral metastases with no physical evidence of a primary tumor. The ability to cure a subgroup of these patients by surgical resection suggests that immunological mechanisms are capable of destroying residual micrometastatic disease.

All these observations lend credence to the notion that melanoma tumors express antigens that can serve as targets for immunotherapy and there has been significant effort towards treating melanoma employing various immunological modalities. To date, there has been only limited success with such treatment, as will be described further.

Interferon-α

Cytokines are defined as proteins produced by cells in response to antigenic stimuli that mediate cellular effector function. Interferons are cytokines and possess the potential for activity in melanoma based on their direct cytostatic and cytotoxic activity against tumor cells, their capacity to activate host defense mechanisms, such as NiK cell and macrophage-mediate cytotoxicity, and their ability to alter tumor cells by upregulating HLA and tumor antigen expression. Natural and recombinant interferons have been used in the treatment of melanoma since the early 1980s. Despite numerous studies of interferons alone and in combination with chemotherapy, their role in the management of melanoma is still not entirely clear. Limited studies with IFN-α and IFN-β suggest that they have minimal activity in patients with metastatic disease or in the adjuvant setting [52, 53].

Over the past 12 years, studies of the treatment of metastatic melanoma with IFN-α have been conducted with the cytokine used as a single agent or combined with chemotherapy [54, 55]. A reasonable summation of these different studies is that IFN-α alone induces a response rate of approximately 10%–20% with approximately 25% of the responses being complete remissions. Duration of response is approximately 6 months or less.

This antitumor activity of IFN-α-2 in metastatic melanoma led to the simultaneous initiation of several trials of IFN-α-2 for the prevention of melanoma relapse. The breakthrough article published by Kirkwood et al. in 1996 represented a significant advance in the treatment of melanoma [56]. This multicenter, randomized trial, which tested adjuvant, high-dose interferon in high-risk melanoma patients, showed that it can improve both disease-free and overall survival rates. Although the improvement in survival was modest, this was the first randomized adjuvant therapy trial after two decades of testing to clearly and significantly affect the natural history of melanoma. Multivariate analysis corroborated the positive effect of interferon-α on overall survival. The results of the ECOG trial resulted in the American FDA acknowledging and approving IFN-α as "an adjuvant treatment to surgery in patients with malignant melanoma who are free of disease but at high risk for systemic recurrence." However, the fact remains that high-dose interferon is toxic. In the Kirkwood trial, 67% of patients had severe toxicity, there were two drug-related deaths, and 26% of patients discontinued treatment. Furthermore, the treatment was very costly (approximately $30,000 for a year of therapy).

Other investigators have explored adjuvant IFN-α therapy for high-risk melanoma. However, even large-scale studies, such as the WHO, NCCTG, EORTC and even a second follow-up study by Kirkwood, have not shown the same encouraging results and no statistically significant differences in survival rates were found [57, 58].

All these factors suggest that patients who benefit from IFN-α may be restricted to a subset that includes those who: (1) do not have extracapsular nodal invasion,

(2) are able to tolerate high-dose IFN-α, and (3) preferably begin therapy within 30 days of surgery. The question as to optimal duration, dosage, and route of therapy, and as to whether it can be applied to intransit, cutaneous or occular melanoma, remains unanswered. Pending further evaluation, many clinical oncologists will still have to solve the dilemma as to the selection of patients for this promising but toxic and costly therapy.

Interleukin-2

The discovery that interleukin (IL)-2 induces the activation and proliferation of cytotoxic, promiscuous, killer lymphocytes, hereafter referred to as lymphokine-activated killer (LAK) cells, has initiated an entirely new era in the field of immunotherapy. Initially, LAK cells were shown to possess the capacity to kill autologous and allogeneic tumor cells but not normal cells. After in vitro demonstration of LAK cell activity, the administration of LAK cells plus IL-2 to tumor-bearing animals demonstrated that several different tumor types could be controlled by this therapy. Shortly thereafter, Rosenberg and co-workers demonstrated that patients receiving IL-2, stimulated and in vitro-expanded LAK cells, plus high-dose IL-2, experienced a substantial proportion of remissions [59, 60].

Although the initial report on high-dose IL-2 with LAK cells reported response rates of 50% for melanoma, subsequent reports were less encouraging. The IL-2 LAK cell working group reported an overall response rate in melanoma of approximately 15% and an update from the NCI reported a complete and partial response rate of 23% for LAK cells plus IL-2 and 13% for IL-2 alone [59]. In a subsequent update, there were 21% responses among patients treated with IL-2 plus LAK cells, of which somewhat less that half were complete remissions, and 24% responses (all partial) among patients treated with high-dose IL-2 alone [61]. Other groups have reported a 22% response rate, mainly partial remissions in patients treated with the standard high-dose IL-2 regimen.

The major limitations on the use of IL-2 relate to its toxicity. It is clear that high-dose IL-2 is more active than low-dose IL-2, but the severe toxicity limits its use. Approximately 5% of patients have experienced a fatal outcome, usually related to myocardial infarction or arrhythmia. High-dose IL-2 induces a capillary leak syndrome with major shifts of fluid out of the vascular compartment, resulting in septic shock-like syndrome and multiorgan failure.

Because of its toxicity, patient selection for high-dose IL-2 therapy is very strict, excluding patients with impaired performance status or organ function, and those with large tumor burdens. Therefore, we can assume that the proportion of all metastatic melanoma patients who could benefit is quite small, certainly less than 20%.

Thus all regimens of IL-2 treatment, including high dose alone, high dose with LAK or IL-2 cells, low dose alone, and low dose plus chemotherapy, should continue to be investigated. However, since IL-2 has been approved for use in renal cell carcinoma, physicians are free to use it in the management of malignant melanoma. It can be recommended for patients in good physical condition, with normal performance status, and no significant major organ disease such as cardiovascular disease. The use of IL-2 therapy may be considered for patients with metastatic disease as a back-up or second- or third-line therapy. An occasional patient may have very gratifying complete or major partial remission of long duration.

Melanoma Vaccines: A Promising Tool?

Active specific immunotherapy in the form of vaccines in now an accepted, albeit still experimental, method of treating melanoma. The development of melanoma vaccines is currently the focus of numerous investigations, particularly in patients who are at high risk for recurrence and death, such as those with metastases to regional lymph nodes or with clinically evident disseminated melanoma.

Early clinical trials with melanoma vaccines were generally disappointing, which may be explained in part by the fact that patients selected for vaccine therapy usually had advanced, bulky disease, and the adjuvants used were of limited effectiveness. The results of more recent studies, conducted in patients with surgically resected disease, are more promising.

The first attempts at vaccine therapy for melanoma involved irradiated allogeneic cultured melanoma cells with or without BCG. One experience is with the polyvalent melanoma vaccine developed by Morton et al. prepared from three allogeneic melanoma cell lines selected for their high expression of protein and ganglioside antigens which are immunogenic in melanoma patients [62]. The cells are administered admixed with BCG as an adjuvant. Vaccine treatment stimulated antibody and DTH responses to melanoma in over 60% of patients, although the specificity of these responses was not clear. Clinical responses were observed in 22% of 40 patients with AJCC stage IV disease and median survival time increased threefold in comparison to historical controls. Median survival of 61 vaccine-treated patients with surgically resected stage IIIA melanoma was 43.9 months vs. 28.7 months for 126 historical control patients. Overall 5-year survival increased from 10% to 28% in patients with stage IIIA and from 7.5% to 23% in patients with stage IV melanomas in comparison to historical controls.

These and other investigations of allogeneic whole cell vaccines have not shown significant benefit in randomized trials [63]. Possible drawbacks of the allogeneic vaccine approach include uncertain relevance of antigens in the vaccine to individual patient's melanomas and uncertainty as to whether a relevant immune response was induced. Thus, an anti-melanoma immune response may be generated to targets that are not present on the patient's specific tumor or simply to other components of the vaccine that are not melanoma associated.

The use of autologous tumor vaccines could ensure that antigens of specific immunological importance are included in the vaccine. One significant problem with this approach is the necessity of obtaining a relatively large amount of tumor to produce the vaccine. This requirement not only restricts the eligible patient population but also mandates it to include those patients who have a higher disease burden

In addition, as opposed to readily available vaccines derived from allogeneic cultured melanomas, quantities of autologous vaccines are necessarily limited by the amount of tissue obtained. Nevertheless, several small randomized trials of autologous tumor vaccines have been conducted in resected melanoma patients [64, 65]. No objective benefit from such treatment was observed.

The concept of the viral oncolysate was formulated to provide an alternative means of vaccine preparation that may improve sensitization to tumor cell antigens. This particular type of active specific immunotherapy, by infecting allogeneic tumor cells with vaccinia or other cytolytic viruses, results in a lysate with viral antigens that can initiate an antiviral immune response that will aid in the recognition of tumor-associated antigens. A prospective randomized trial of vaccinia melanoma oncolysates in patients with AJCC stage III melanoma demonstrated a trend towards increased survival that did not reach statistical significance in a subset of male patients less than 57 years of age with one to five positive lymph nodes. The control group in this study received live vaccine virus alone [66, 67].

In an effort to develop vaccines of defined specificity, several investigators have attempted to identify the most prevalent tumor-associated antigens on melanoma cells using panels of monoclonal antibodies. These studies have shown that carbohydrates, specifically glycolipids, may represent the best targets for vaccines that elicit an antibody response. Livingstone has conducted a series of trials using purified gangliosides administered either alone or combined with different adjuvants [68, 69]. A double-blind randomized study has been conducted in AJCC stage III melanoma patients pre-treated with cyclophosphamide and given either a GM2 vaccine + BCG or BCG alone [69]. There was no significant difference in either disease-free or overall survival between the two groups, but an encouraging trend in favor of the vaccine-treated patients was present. Outcome was significantly better in those patients who developed an antibody response to the vaccine. It has now been found that conjugating the GM2 to KLH and giving the construct with QS-21 as an adjuvant significantly augments antibody response, suggesting that this may provide a more effective vaccine.

Another approach is to use small peptides that are recognized by anti-melanoma T cells as a vaccine. Through a series of elegant transfection experiments, Coulie et al. have identified and isolated the genes that encode several such peptides, the MAGE series of melanoma-associated antigenic peptides [70]. Although silent in normal tissues, these peptides are expressed in many malignant melanomas. These antigens are recognized by cloned cytotoxic T cells, indicating that they are T-cell antigens and suggesting that they are immunogenic in man. Clinical trials are now performed to determine whether MAGE and other melanoma-associated peptides such as MART-1, BAGE, and those derived from tyrosinase or GP100 can stimulate effective antitumor immune responses in man. A limitation of this approach is that since the recognition of these peptides is HLA restricted, only a small fraction of melanoma patients are candidates for therapy with such vaccines. Lastly, it is unlikely that immune response directed towards a single epitope or to a single antigen will be sufficiently potent to result in tumor cell kill.

Various approaches to vaccine preparation and delivery have been used to overcome practical constraints such as limited immunogenicity, breaking tolerance, and production of adequate quantities of vaccine. The advent of DNA immunization has the potential to solve many of these problems. It is now known that the introduction of bacterial plasmid DNA intramuscularly or intradermally can stimulate both specific T cell and antibody responses [71]. The inherent antigenicity of bacterial DNA, in part owing to recently identified immunostimulatory sequences and the effective contextual presentation of the encoded antigen with proper co-stimulatory molecules, suggests that DNA immunization is a promising approach to cancer immunotherapy.

The results of current clinical trials of melanoma vaccines are encouraging, but not conclusive. To establish the true effectiveness of vaccines in the treatment of malignant melanoma, several large, prospectively randomized phase III trials are currently being constructed.

Summary

Melanoma poses an increasingly important health problem. Although surgery can be curative in the early stages of the disease, a large number of patients with deep primary lesions or nodal involvement are destined to develop distant metastases. The outlook for patients with melanoma metastases beyond regional lymph nodes remains bleak. Median survival in most series ranges from 6 to 10 months with 5-year survival rates of under 4%, a figure which has remained unchanged for the past 22 years.

These facts provide a strong rationale for prevention and there is no doubt that public awareness and early diagnosis can lead to improved survival. Although many nonprospective trials have suggested the efficacy of a variety of adjuvant therapies when compared with historical controls, these results have almost always been disproved in more controlled, prospective trials. Only recently, with the approval of high-dose IFN-α and the development of promising vaccines, does effective adjuvant therapy appear to be becoming a reality. Based upon the limitations and toxicity of currently available therapies, there is a need for the continued development of more active adjuvant and therapeutic treatment regimens for melanoma.

References

1. Greene MH (1999) The genetics of hereditary melanoma and nevi: 1998 update. Cancer 86 [Suppl 2]:2464–2477
2. Rusonis ES, Rusonis PA, Miller C, Oken HA (1999) Skin cancer detection and prevention: a community program promoting sun-safe behaviour. Md Med J 48(7):169–172
3. Weinstock MA (1998) Issues in the epidemiology of melanoma. Hematol Oncol Clin North Am 12(4):681–698
4. La Vecchia C (1999) Sunscreens and the risk of cutaneous malignant melanoma. Eur J Cancer Prev 8(4):267–269
5. Bigby M (1999) The sunscreen and melanoma controversy. Arch Dermatol 135(12):1526–1527
6. Weinstock MA (1999) Do sunscreens increase or decrease melanoma risk: an epidemiologic evaluation. J Invest Dermatol Symp Proc 4(1):97–100
7. Gallagher RP, Becky M, McLean DI, et al. (1990) Trends in basal cell carcinoma, squamous cell carcinoma and melanoma of the skin from 1973 through 1987. J Am Acad Dermatol 23:413–420
8. Mellad OB, Colomer D, Casel T, et al. (1996) Detection of circulating neoplastic cells by reverse transcriptase polymerase chain reaction in malignant melanoma: association with clinical stage and prognosis. J Clin Oncol 14:2091–2097

9. Barth A, Morton DL (1995) The role of adjuvant therapy in melanoma management. Cancer 75(2):726–734
10. Johnson TM, Yahanda AM, Chang AE, Fader DJ, Sondak VK (1998) Advances in melanoma therapy. J Am Acad Dermatol 38:731–741
11. Demierre MF, Koh H (1997) Adjuvant therapy for cutaneous malignant melanoma. J Am Acad Dermatol 36:747–764
12. Dickler MN, Coit DE, Meyers ML (1997) Adjuvant therapy of malignant melanoma. Surg Oncol Clin North Am 6(4):793–812
13. Barranco SC, Komsdahl MM, Humphrey RM (1971) The radiation response of human malignant melanoma cells grown in vitro. Cancer Res 31:830–833
14. Habermalz HJ, Fischer JJ (1976) Radiation therapy of malignant melanoma: experience with high individual treatment doses. Cancer 38:2258–2262
15. Johanson CR, Harwood AR, Cummings BJ, et al. (1983) Radiotherapy in nodular melanoma. Cancer 51:226–232
16. Overgaard J (1980) Radiation therapy of malignant melanoma. Int J Radiat Oncol Biol Phys 6:41–44
17. Gear FB, Ang K (1996) Radiation therapy for malignant melanoma. Surg Clin North Am 76(6):1383–1398
18. Veronesi Y, Adamus J, Aubert C, et al. (1982) A randomized trial of adjuvant chemotherapy and immunotherapy in cutaneous melanoma. N Engl J Med 307:913–916
19. Retsas S, Quigley M, Pectasids D, et al. (1994) Clinical and histological involvement of regional lymph nodes in malignant melanoma: adjuvant vinclesine improves survival. Cancer 73:2119–2130
20. Meisenberg BR, Ress M, Wedenburgh JJ, et al. (1993) Randomized trial of high dose chemotherapy with autologous bone marrow support as adjuvant therapy for high risk, multi-node-positive malignant melanoma. J NIH Cancer Inst 85:1080–1085
21. Agarwala SS, Ferri W, Gooding W, Kirkwood JM (1999) A phase III randomized trial of dacarbazine and carboplatin with and without tamoxifen in the treatment of patients with metastatic melanoma. Cancer 85:1979–1984
22. Rege VB, Leone LA, Soderberg CH, et al. (1983) Hyperthermic adjuvant perfusion chemotherapy for stage I malignant melanoma of the extremity with literature review. Cancer 52:2033–2039
23. Fletcher JR, White CR, Fletch WS (1986) Improved survival rates of patients with acral lentiginous melanoma treated with hyperthermic isolation perfusion, wide excision and regional lymphadenopathy. Am J Surg 151:593–598
24. Franklin H, Koops HS, Oldhoff J, et al. (1988) To perfuse or not to perfuse? A retrospective comparative study to evaluate the effect of adjuvant isolated regional perfusion in patients with stage I extremity melanoma with a thickness of 1.5 mm or greater. J Clin Oncol 6(4):701–708
25. Ghussen F, Kruger I, Groth W, et al. (1988) The role of hyperthermic cytostatic perfusion in the treatment of extremity melanoma. Cancer 61:654–659
26. Hafstrom L, Rudenstam CM, Blomquist E, et al. (1991) Regional hyperthermic perfusion with melphalan after surgery for recurrent melanoma of the extremities. J Clin Oncol 9:2091–2094
27. Lienard D, Eggermont AM, Kroon BBR, et al. (1998) Isolated limb perfusion in primary and recurrent melanoma: indications and results. Semin Surg Oncol 14:202–209
28. Ghussen F, Kruger I, Smalley RV, et al. (1989) Hyperthermic perfusion with chemotherapy for melanoma of the extremities. World J Surg 13:598–602
29. Jaques DP, Coit DG, Brenman MF (1989) Major amputation for advanced malignant melanoma. Surg Gynecol Obstet 169:1–6
30. Hafstrom L, Jonsson PE (1980) Hyperthermic perfusion of recurrent malignant melanoma of the extremities. Acta Chir Scand 146:313–318
31. Bulman AS, Jamieson CW (1980) Isolated limb perfusion with melphalan in the treatment of melanoma. Br J Surg 67:660–662
32. Kroon BB, Geel AN van, Benckhuijsen C, et al. (1987) Normothermic isolation perfusion with melphalan for advanced melanoma of the limbs. Anticancer Res 7(3 Pt B):441–442
33. Skene AI, Bulman AS, Williams TR, et al. (1990) Hyperthermic isolated perfusion with melphalan in the treatment of advanced malignant melanoma of the lower limb. Br J Surg 77:765–767
34. Klaase JM, Kroon BB, Geel AN van, et al. (1994) Prognostic factors for tumor response and limb recurrence-free interval in patients with advanced melanoma of the limbs treated with regional isolated perfusion using melphalan. Surgery 115:39–45

35. Bryant PJ, Balderson GA, Mead P, et al. (1995) Hyperthermic isolated limb perfusion for malignant melanoma: response and survival. World J Surg 19:363–368
36. Klein ES, Ben-Ari GY (1987) Isolation perfusion with cisplatin for malignant melanoma of the limbs. Cancer 59:1068–1071
37. Hoekstra HJ, Koops HS, Vries LG de, et al. (1993) Toxicity of hyperthermic isolated limb perfusion with cisplatin for recurrent melanoma of the lower extremity after previous perfusion. Cancer 72:1224–1229
38. Didolkar MS, Viens ML, Suter CM, et al. (1990) Phase II study of isolation perfusion with DITC in stage IIIa–IIIab melanoma of the extremity. Proc Am Soc Clin Oncol 9:276
39. Cavaliere R, Cavaliere F, Deeraco M, et al. (1994) Hyperthermic antiblastic perfusion in the treatment of stage IIIA–IIIB melanoma patients. Comparison of two experiences. Melanoma Res 4:5–11
40. Lienard D, Ewalenko P, Delmotti JJ, et al. (1992) High dose recombinant tumor necrosis factor alpha in combination with interferon gamma and melphalan in isolation perfusion of the limbs for melanoma and sarcoma. J Clin Oncol 10:52–60
41. Aggarwell BB, Eessalu TE, Hass PE (1985) Characterization of receptors for tumor necrosis factor and their regulation by gamma-interferon. Nature 318:665–667
42. Fraker DL, Alexander HR, Andrich MP, et al. (1996) Treatment of patients with melanoma of the extremity using hyperthermic isolated limb perfusion with melphalan, tumor necrosis factor, and interferon-gamma: results of a tumor necrosis factor dose-escalation study. J Clin Oncol 14:479–489
43. Gutman M, Lev-Chelouche D, Abu-Abeid S, Inbar M, Klausner JM (1998) Isolated limb perfusion with tumor necrosis factor and melphalan for locally advanced malignant melanoma. 9th Congress of the European Society of Surgical Oncology, Lausanne, 3–6 June
44. Hohenberger P, Kettelhack C (1998) Clinical management and current research in isolated limb perfusion for sarcoma and melanoma. Oncology 55:89–102
45. Lejeune FJ (1995) High dose recombinant tumour necrosis factor (rTNFα) administered by isolation perfusion for advanced tumours of the limbs: a model for biochemotherapy of cancer. Eur J Cancer B1 A:1009–1016
46. Fraker DL, Alexander HR, Bartlett DL, et al. (1996) A prospective randomized trial of therapeutic isolated limb perfusion (ILP) comparing melphalan (M) versus melphalan, tumor necrosis factor (TNF) and interferon-gamma (IFN): an initial report (abstract). Soc Surg Oncol 49:6
47. Barlett DL, Ma G, Alexander HR, et al. (1997) Isolated limb reperfusion with tumor necrosis factor and melphalan in patients with extremity melanoma after failure of isolated limb perfusion with chemotherapeutics. Cancer 80:2084–2090
48. Morton DL, Malmgren RA, Holmes EC, et al. (1968) Demonstration of antibodies against human malignant melanoma by immunofluorescence. Surgery 64:233–240
49. Morton DL, Eilber FR, Malmgren RA, et al. (1970) Immunological factors which influence responses to immunotherapy in malignant melanoma. Surgery 68:158–164
50. Mukheryi B, Chakraborty NG, Sivanadham M (1990) T-cell clones that react against autologous human tumors. Immunol Rev 116:33–62
51. Topalian SL, Solomon D, Rosenberg SA (1989) Tumor specific cytolysis by lymphocytes infiltrating human melanomas. J Immunol 142:3614–3725
52. Thompson JA, Cox WW, Lindgren CG, et al. (1987) Subcutaneous recombinant gamma interferon in cancer patients: toxicity, pharmacokinetics and immunomodulatory effects. Cancer Immunol Immunother 15:47–53
53. Meyskens FL Jr, Kopecky KJ, Taylor CW, et al. (1995) Randomized trial of adjuvant human interferon gamma versus observation in high-risk cutaneous melanoma: a South-West Oncology Group Study. J Natl Cancer Inst 1710–1713
54. Cregan ET, Schaid DJ, Ahmann DL, et al. (1988) Recombinant interferons in the management of advanced malignant melanoma. Updated review of five prospective clinical trials and long-term responders. Am J Clin Oncol 11:652–658
55. Falkson CI, Falkson G, Falkson HC (1991) Improved results with the addition of interferon alpha-2b to dacarbazine in the treatment of patients with metastatic malignant melanoma. J Clin Oncol 9(8):1403–1408
56. Kirkwood JM, Strawderman MIT, Ernstoff MS, et al. (1996) Interferon alpha-2b adjuvant therapy of high-risk resected cutaneous melanoma. The Eastern Cooperative Oncology Group Trial EST 1684. J Clin Oncol 14:7–17
57. Cascinelli N, Bufalino R, Morabito A, Mackie R (1994) Results of adjuvant interferon study in WHO melanoma programme. Lancet 1:913–914

58. Creagan ET, Dalton RJ, Ahmann DL, et al. (1995) Randomized surgical adjuvant clinical trial of recombinant interferon alpha-2a in selected patients with malignant melanoma. J Clin Oncol 13:2776–2783
59. Rosenberg SA, Lotze MT, Muul LM, et al. (1987) A progress report in the treatment of 157 patients with advanced cancer using lymphokine-activated killer cells and interleukin-2 or high dose interleukin-2 alone. N Engl J Med 316:889–896
60. Rosenberg SA, Yang JC, Topalian SL, et al. (1994) Treatment of 283 consecutive patients with metastatic melanoma or renal cell cancer using high-dose bolus interleukin-2. JAMA 271:907–913
61. Rosenberg SA, Lotze MT, Yang J, et al. (1989) Experience with the use of high-dose interleukin-2 in the treatment of 652 cancer patients. Ann Surg 210:474–484
62. Morton D, Hoon D, Nizze J, et al. (1992) Polyvalent vaccine improves survival of patients with metastatic melanoma. Ann Surg 216:463–482
63. Terry WE, Hodes RJ, Rosenberg SA, et al. (1982) Treatment of stage I and II malignant melanoma with adjuvant immunotherapy or chemotherapy; preliminary analysis of a prospective randomized trial. In: Terry WD, Rosenberg SA (eds) Immunotherapy of human cancer. Elsevier-North Holland, New York, pp 252–257
64. McIllmurray MB, Embleton MJ, Reeves WB, et al. (1977) Controlled trial of active immunotherapy in the management of stage IIB malignant melanoma. Br Med J 1:540–542
65. Aranha GV, McKhann CF, Grage TB, et al. (1979) Adjuvant immunotherapy of malignant melanoma. Cancer 43:1297–1303
66. Wallack MK, Sivanandham M, Whooley B, et al. (1996) Favorable clinical responses in subsets of patients from a randomized, multi-institutional melanoma vaccine trial. Ann Surg Oncol 3:110–117
67. Wallack MK, Sivanandham M, Ditaranto K, et al. (1997) Increased survival of patients treated with a vaccinia melanoma oncology site vaccine. Second interim analysis of data from a phase III, multi institutional trial. Ann Surg 226:198 206
68. Livingston PO (1992) Construction of cancer vaccines with carbohydrate and protein (peptide) tumor antigens. Curr Opin Immunol 4:624–629
69. Livingston PO, Wong GYC, Adulri S, et al. (1994) Improved survival in stage III melanoma patients with GM2 antibodies: a randomized trial of adjuvant vaccination with GM2 ganglioside. J Clin Oncol 12:1036–1044
70. Coulie P, Weynets P, Muller C, et al. (1993) Genes encoding for antigen recognition on human tumors by autologous cytolytic T lymphocytes. Ann NY Acad Sci 690:113–119
71. Raz E, Tighe H, Sato Y, et al. (1996) Preferential induction of a Th1 immune response and inhibition of specific Igt antibody formation by plasmid DNA immunization. Proc Natl Acad Sci USA 93:5141–5144

Invited Comment

CHARLES M. BALCH

Sentinel Lymphadenectomy

The section by Drs. Tyler and Siegler from Duke Medical Center nicely summarizes four decades of controversy about the management of clinically negative lymph nodes in patients with cutaneous melanoma. In my view, much of the debate at this point has subsided for three reasons: *first*, the long-term results of the Intergroup Surgical Trial have now been published demonstrating even more definitively than before that intermediate thickness, nonulcerated melanoma patients have a statistically improved cure rate with elective node dissection; *second*, the technological advance of sentinel lymphadenectomy has supplanted, for the most part, the need for elective node dissection in most patients, and *third*, research about prognostic factors predicting the risk of nodal metastases and survival outcome has reached a point of agreement that has fostered a major revision of the melanoma staging classification.

The long-term results of the Intergroup Melanoma Surgical Trial have demonstrated, for the first time, that prospectively defined groups of melanoma patients have a significant reduction of mortality if they have an elective node dissection compared to those whose initial management was clinical observation of the nodal basin and a later therapeutic lymphadenectomy for clinically apparent nodal metastases, an event that took place on an average of 16 months after the diagnosis [1]. Presumably, this 16-month delay in treating established metastases allowed further growth and dissemination at distant sites for the minority of patients who developed clinically evident nodal metastases. Among the prospectively stratified subgroups of patients, 10-year survival rates favored those patients with elective lymph node dissection (ELND), with a 30% mortality reduction for the 543 patients with nonulcerated melanomas (84% vs. 77%, $P=0.03$), a 30% mortality reduction for the 446 patients with tumor thickness of 1.0 to 2.0 mm (86% vs. 80%, $P=0.03$), and a 27% reduction in mortality for 385 patients with extremity melanomas (84% vs. 78%, $P=0.05$). Of these subgroups, *the presence or absence of ulceration should be the key factor for making treatment recommendations with regards to ELND for patients with intermediate thickness melanomas.*

Over the past few years, there has been a worldwide validation of the staging accuracy and reproducibility of intraoperative lymphatic mapping and sentinel lymphadenectomy, pioneered by Dr. Donald Morton at the John Wayne Cancer Center in Santa Monica, California [3]. This surgical technique has provided the surgeon with a precise tool that, when properly used, can stage for the presence or absence of a metastatic tumor down to a threshold of 10^5 to 10^6 cells with an accuracy of 95%.

The use of SLND has two inherent advantages over ELND. First, the indications for a complete lymph node dissection with selective lymph node dissection (SLND) are based upon a pathological documentation of nodal metastasis, whereas with ELND the decision for performing a complete node dissection is based upon the mathematical probability of a patient harboring occult nodal metastasis. Second, the SLND procedure provides the pathologist with a limited amount of lymph node tissue, which is most likely to contain metastases, and for which a more detailed examination with serial sectioning and immunohistochemical staining looking for micrometastases is better justified. The survival benefit of the ELND surgical trial described above provides an underpinning of data supporting the survival advantage of early surgical intervention to remove regional micrometastases; ELND should be considered with curative intent in the subgroups described above (i.e., intermediate thickness melanomas without ulceration) in those circumstances when SLND is not available, when a patient has already had a wide excision (which negates the accuracy of the mapping procedure), or if the mapping is not technically feasible. It is important for surgeons to minimize their false-negative rate when substituting SLND for ELND in those patients defined by this trial who might otherwise develop a later recurrence and have missed their opportunity for a curative intervention. In my opinion, the false-negative rate should not exceed 5%, especially in view of the recent evidence from the randomized ELND surgical trial demonstrating the benefit in nonulcerative melanomas of intermediate thickness.

The Melanoma Staging Committee of the American Joint Committee on Cancer (AJCC) has now proposed major revisions of the melanoma TNM and stage grouping criteria for melanoma [3]. These revisions delineate those factors that, in combination, can be used accurately for predicting patients at differing risk for harboring clinically occult metastases at regional and distant sites that should be taken into account when making management decisions regarding regional lymph nodes. Major revisions in melanoma staging include: (1) melanoma thickness and ulceration to be used in the T classification, (2) the number of metastatic lymph nodes rather than their gross dimensions and the delineation of microscopic vs. macroscopic nodal metastases to be used in the N classification, (3) an upstaging of all patients with stage I, II and III disease when a primary melanoma is ulcerated, and (4) a new convention for defining clinical and pathological staging so as to take into account the new staging information gained from intraoperative lymphatic mapping and sentinel node biopsy. The AJCC Melanoma Staging Committee concluded that it was important to separately identify patients with clinically occult (microscopic) from those with clinically apparent (macroscopic) nodal metastases in the staging classification. This is because of data demonstrating that patients with microscopic nodal involvement fare better compared to those who have a therapeutic node dissection for clinically evident nodal metastases.

There is also a very compelling rationale for pathological staging of the regional lymph nodes for patients prior to entry into adjuvant systemic therapy trials. Differences in 2-year and 5-year survival for patients with and without clinically occult nodal metastases can vary by as much as 20%–25%. Indeed, some of the problem in interpreting and comparing past clinical trials involving melanoma has been the inability to fully account for the pathological differences in nodal status in a heterogeneous group of T3 and T4 patients, some of whom had pathological assessment of their regional nodes while others had only clinical assessment.

In summary, decisions regarding node dissection for clinically occult disease are so much better today because of improved staging techniques and the technology associated with intraoperative lymphatic mapping and sentinel lymphadenectomy. Unquestionably, the SLND technique facilitates a more accurate pathological staging and, as a consequence, contributes to a significant "upstaging" of patients to stage III melanoma who previously would otherwise be designated as node-negative or stage I or II melanoma. It also creates a more homogeneous group of node-negative melanoma patients for entry into clinical trials. Such accurately staged melanoma patients at high risk for systemic micrometastases should be considered for clinical trials involving adjuvant systemic therapy. At long last, extensive efforts by surgeons using prospective surgical trials, developing technology advances with sentinel lymphadenectomy and collaborating to analyze prognostic factors have achieved a reasonable consensus about the management and staging of the regional lymph nodes in melanoma patients.

Nonsurgical Management of Melanoma

This chapter comprehensively describes the nonsurgical treatment options available for the physician treating high-risk melanoma patients after surgery.

At the outset, *it should be stated that there are no proven nonsurgical modalities that improve survival rates in any group of melanoma patients after surgery.* Therefore, high-risk patients after surgery should be encouraged to enter into an available prospective clinical trial testing the survival benefit of new systemic agents or radiation therapy. If an adjuvant therapy is used empirically, the patient should be informed that the potential benefit is unproven and that there are risks and attendant morbidity with such treatments. Just because a patient is at high risk for relapse does not necessarily mean that currently available systemic agents will benefit a patient in an adjuvant setting after surgery. For example, in a prospective randomized trial comparing DTIC chemotherapy to surgery alone in stage III patients, the patients on the DTIC treatment arm actually had a *worse* survival rate compared to the surgery-alone arm [4].

The most promising systemic agents at present include high doses of alpha-interferon, monoclonal antibodies and various vaccine preparations that are now being tested in clinical trials. The advantage of the vaccines or antibodies, of course, is that there is little or no attendant morbidity. On the other hand, there have been so many biological agents tested after "promising" results from nonrandomized trials that the treating physician should be wary of using them outside of a clinical trial until one or more of these agents have a consistently demonstrated survival advantage. Interferons and interleukins have been tested in high-quality adjuvant therapy trials and only alpha-interferon is still under active investigation. These agents have very high morbidity and cost, so the therapeutic benefit must be compelling and unequivocal. Witness the mixed results with the Intergroup alpha-interferon trials in the United States, one of which showed an improved overall survival for stage III melanoma patients while the sequel randomized trial using the same dose of interferon failed to demonstrate a survival advantage [5, 6]. There were extenuating circumstances, especially with the conduct of the second trial including different eligibility criteria and the ability to cross-over from the untreated to the interferon arm after relapse, so any conclusions about the effectiveness of adjuvant alpha-interferon cannot be made. Another randomized Intergroup trial with improvements in design and staging is now being conducted comparing high-dose alpha-interferon with a GM2 ganglioside melanoma vaccine.

With regard to adjuvant chemotherapy, there are no present regimens of proven value, although clinical trials are being conducted using biochemotherapy (e.g., with cisplatin, vinblastine, dacarbazine, interferon and interleukin). I agree that there is a limited role for regional perfusion using hyperthermia, L-PAM and possibly TNF. This approach has both cost and morbidity, so it should be applied only in circumstances to treat established, multiple in-transit metastases, satellites or extensive local recurrences. This is especially true when perfusion might provide palliation that would otherwise require amputation of an extremity due to extensive, debilitating and nonresectable disease. *There is no role for limb perfusion as an adjuvant therapy in high-risk patients.*

Adjuvant radiation therapy has been used for decades, especially after surgery for head and neck melanoma to reduce regional recurrence rates [7]. No randomized trial has been conducted, so it is impossible to prove any survival advantage. The ability to decrease regional failures with adjuvant electron beam hyperfractionated dose schedules is appropriate, since the morbidity is quite acceptable. I recommend adjuvant irradiation to my patients empirically after therapeutic lymphadenectomy in those circumstances where the estimated rate of regional relapse after surgery is estimated at 20% or greater. This would apply to patients who have six or more nodal metastases or where there are multiple nodes and gross extracapsular invasion. I also recommend this after complete surgical excision of *recurrent* regional lymph node metastases. When adjuvant radiation therapy is used in the cervical region, there is usually minimal morbidity, including lymphedema. One must be careful, however, when using this approach after radical lymphadenectomy of the axilla or groin. In these circumstances, it is important that the port size be confined to a boundary just outside the surgical dissection (as marked by surgical metal clips applied at surgery), so as to reduce the risk of obliterating important lymphatic collaterals with resultant debilitating lymphedema. I also recommend adjuvant radiation therapy after excision of metastatic melanoma to the brain, based upon our clinical experience [8].

In summary, surgical excision of metastatic melanoma remains the most effective treatment, both in terms of local/regional disease control, increasing cure rates and prolonging survival. Use of currently available adjuvant systemic therapy cannot be recommended as standard treatment and adjuvant radiation therapy might be used selectively based upon empirical data. It is vitally important for high-risk patients after melanoma surgery to be entered into high-quality clinical trials comparing systemic treatments to a surgical control arm, so that a better multidisciplinary approach can be deployed in the future.

References

1. Balch CM et al. (2000) Long-term results of a multi-institutional randomized trial comparing prognostic factors and surgical results for intermediate thickness melanomas (1.0 to 4.0 mm.). Ann Surg Oncol 7(2):87–97
2. Morton DL et al. (1992) Technical details of intraoperative lymphatic mapping for early stage melanoma. Arch Surg 127:392–399
3. Balch CM et al. (2000) A new American Joint Committee on Cancer staging system for cutaneous melanoma. Cancer 88(6):1484–1491
4. Hill GJ, Moss SE, Golumb FM, Grage TB, et al. (1981) DTIC and combination therapy for melanoma. Cancer 47:2557
5. Kirkwood JM, Strawderman MH, Ernstoff MS, Smith TJ, Borden EC, Blum RH (1996) Interferon alfa-2b adjuvant therapy of high-risk resected cutaneous melanoma: the Eastern Cooperative Oncology Group Trial EST 1684. J Clin Oncol 14:7–17
6. Kirkwood JM, Ibrahim V, Sondek M, et al. (1999) Preliminary analysis of the E1690 intergroup postoperative adjuvant trial of high- and low-dose IFN in high risk primary or lymph node metastatic melanoma. ASCO Proc 18:537a
7. Ang KK, Geara FB, Byers RM, Peters LJ (1998) Radiotherapy for melanoma. In: Balch CM, Houghton AN, Sober AJ, Soong S (eds) Cutaneous melanoma, 3rd edn. Quality Medical Publishers, St. Louis, pp 389–404
8. Skibber JM, Soong S-J, Austin L, Balch CM, Sawaya RE (1996) Cranial irradiation after surgical excision of brain metastases in melanoma patients. Ann Surg Oncol 3:118–123

Editorial Comment

In this chapter, Drs. Tyler and Seigler from Duke University present us with an enthusiastic overview of sentinel lymph node biopsy, Dr. Lev-Chelouche and Professor Klausner, from Tel Aviv, with an exhaustive review of nonsurgical modalities of treatment, and finally Dr. Balch - an established guru in the field - honors us with his balancing comments.

Dr. Balch as well as Drs. Tyler and Seigler are great proponents of sentinel lymph node biopsy in malignant melanoma. But not all submit to these views - there are those who claim that such practice should be confined to patients in clinical trials only. This is because there is no evidence as yet that completion node dissection (after positive sentinel node biopsy) improves survival and because even if a positive sentinel node biopsy could select patients for adjuvant therapy, the adjuvant therapy available is not effective in prolonging survival [1].

Reference

1. Meirion Thomas J, Patocskai EJ (2000) The argument against sentinel node biopsy for malignant melanoma. BMJ 321:3-4

CHAPTER 3

Primary Esophageal Motility Disorders

Investigations and Nonoperative Management

HUBERT J. STEIN · JÖRG THEISEN

Introduction

A disturbed propulsive activity or dyscoordination between peristalsis within the body of the esophagus and relaxation of the lower esophageal sphincter are the hallmarks of primary esophageal motility disorders resulting in nonobstructive dysphagia (i.e., dysphagia in the absence of structural abnormalities), regurgitation and/or noncardiac chest pain. These symptoms are, however, neither specific nor sensitive enough to establish a diagnosis. Rather, objective tests are required in order to guide therapy [1–3].

Based on stationary esophageal manometry a number of primary esophageal motility disorders are usually classified as separate disease entities [1]. These include achalasia, diffuse esophageal spasm, the so-called nutcracker esophagus, and nonspecific esophageal motor disorders. With the introduction of more physiological and prolonged esophageal motility recording techniques the clinical utility of stationary esophageal manometry and the classification of primary esophageal motor disorders has, however, been questioned [2].

Current controversies focus on the objective tests required for an adequate diagnosis and classification of the primary esophageal motor disorders and the efficacy of nonoperative therapy in comparison to the newly established techniques of minimally invasive surgical intervention.

Diagnostic Tests for Esophageal Motor Disorders

Several diagnostic tests are available to examine patients with suspected esophageal motor disorders. These include endoscopy, endoscopic ultrasonography, contrast radiography, stimulation tests, transit scintigraphy, stationary esophageal manometry, and ambulatory 24-h esophageal manometry. Their diagnostic accuracy and clinical value varies widely.

Upper gastrointestinal endoscopy with biopsy usually constitutes the first examination in a patient complaining of dysphagia or regurgitation. Although endoscopy with biopsy is superior to any other diagnostic test to identify structural abnormalities and epithelial alterations, it is a poor tool to identify motility disorders. Endoscopy in most instances thus only serves to exclude underlying disorders that may mimic esophageal motor abnormalities [2, 3].

Endoscopic ultrasound has been employed in patients with achalasia demonstrating a wall thickness in the area around the sphincter, but with a high rate of false-positive results [4]. Studies in patients with other motor disorders are scant. Endoscopic ultrasound is therefore currently not recommended as a routine tool in the diagnostic assessment of patients with motility disorders.

Contrast radiography of the esophagus is employed in many institutions as one of the first diagnostic techniques in patients with suspected esophageal motor disorders. Usually a video recording of at least five 10-cc swallows of barium is performed. To mimic a more realistic situation a barium-soaked hamburger bolus may be added, specifically in patients complaining of dysphagia for solids. Studies show a high sensitivity of video-esophagography in the evaluation of patients with achalasia, but sensitivity is low in patients with other forms of motor abnormalities [5].

Stimulation or provocative tests include the use of acid perfusion, administration of tensilon, or balloon distension to reproduce the patients' symptoms. Based on recent data from the literature and the authors' own experience, these tests are not very helpful since most of them have a low yield of symptom reproduction and the findings do not correlate with observations made during spontaneously occurring symptoms [2].

Scintigraphy with a fluid or semi-solid radiolabeled bolus allows the quantification and visualization of esophageal transport abnormalities. As is also the case with other stationary tests, scintigraphy lacks sensitivity and specificity for the diagnosis and classification of intermittently occurring esophageal motor disorders [2].

Stationary or standard esophageal manometry is widely accepted as the gold standard in the diagnosis and classification of esophageal motility disorders [1]. A typical pattern of motor abnormalities on a series of "wet swallows" on standard manometry has been the basis for the diagnosis of achalasia, diffuse esophageal spasm, "nutcracker esophagus" and nonspecific motor disorders. Recent studies show that stationary esophageal motility testing is particularly useful for evaluating patients with dysphagia but has little clinical utility in patients with noncardiac chest pain [6, 7]. This is because standard manometry is performed in a laboratory setting with the patient in the supine position and the analysis is normally based on five to ten water swallows only. Stationary manometry may thus miss intermittent motor abnormalities, particularly those occurring during meals only.

The technique of *ambulatory 24-h monitoring* of esophageal motor activity multiplies the number of esophageal motor events available for analysis. It thus provides an opportunity to assess esophageal motor function over a complete circadian cycle and correlate motor events with spontaneously occurring symptoms. This increases the accuracy and dependability of the measurement [8, 9]. The broad clinical application of this technology has provided new insights into esophageal motor function in health and disease under a variety of physiological conditions. Studies employing ambulatory motility monitoring show that patients with nonobstructive dysphagia show an increased prevalence of nonperistaltic and low amplitude contractions during meal periods. These contraction sequences are "ineffective" for bolus propulsion. In patients with noncardiac chest pain, ambulatory motility monitoring can document a direct correlation of abnormal esophageal motor activity with the symptom. Of particular interest is that ambulatory 24-h motility monitoring leads to a change in the diagnosis in a substantial portion of patients in whom one of the primary esophageal motor disorders has been diagnosed by standard manometry, contrast radiography or transit scintigraphy [2, 8, 9]. Whether this justifies the routine use of ambulatory 24-h esophageal manometry in every patient with symptoms suggesting an esophageal motor disorder remains controversial, particularly because of the high costs of ambulatory motility monitoring. When used selectively in patients in whom the primary investigation did not result in a satisfying diagnosis, ambulatory motility monitoring, however, appears to constitute a useful and cost-effective test [10].

Classification of Esophageal Motor Disorders

The data obtained by prolonged esophageal motility monitoring indicate that the classic categories of esophageal motor disorders are inappropriate. This appears to be due to the intermittent expression of esophageal motor abnormalities, which can be missed easily, or over-diagnosed in the nonphysiological setting of standard manometry and other stationary tests, but are detected with a higher degree of reliability when motor activity is monitored over 24 h in a variety of physiological conditions. Prolonged motility monitoring has shown that in asymptomatic volunteers the prevalence of "effective contractions," i.e., peristaltic contractions with sufficient amplitude to propel a bolus, increases with increasing states of consciousness, i.e., from sleep, to the upright, and meal periods. This is probably due to a modulatory effect of the central nervous system on esophageal motor activity. Patients with nonobstructive dysphagia lack this ability to increase the prevalence of effective contractions with increasing states of consciousness [9]. Clinical studies have shown that an analysis of the prevalence of effective contractions during meal periods on ambulatory esophageal motility monitoring allows to express the severity of esophageal body dysfunction on a linear scale (Fig. 1). In our opinion esophageal motility disorders should therefore be looked at as a spectrum of abnormalities, which reflects various stages of destruction of esophageal motor function rather than separate entities. The degree of regular function or dysfunction can be quantified by the prevalence of "effective" or "ineffective" contraction sequences during meal times. This approach obviates the need for the current categories of esophageal motor disorders and permits an objective assessment of nonsurgical and surgical therapy on esophageal body function [9].

Nonoperative Management of Primary Esophageal Motility Disorders

With the introduction of highly effective, minimally invasive surgical techniques the role of nonoperative treatment modalities has been challenged particularly in patients with achalasia. Nevertheless, a series of recent studies has shown that

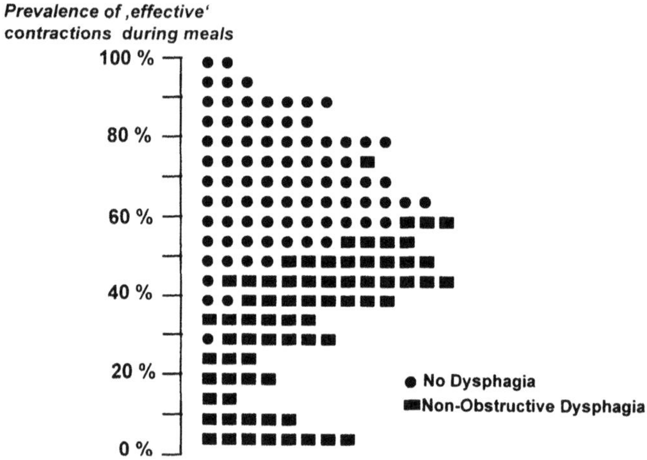

Fig. 1. Prevalence of "effective" esophageal body contractions, i.e., propulsive contraction sequences with a minimum amplitude >30 mmHg, during meal times as measured by ambulatory 24-h esophageal motility monitoring in asymptomatic subjects and patients with primary esophageal motor disorders and nonobstructive dysphagia

nonoperative therapeutic modalities remain the first-line treatment in most of the esophageal motor disorders. Controversies, however, still exist regarding the selection of the optimal nonoperative treatment modality, i.e., medical therapy, pneumatic dilatation, or botulinum toxin injection.

Achalasia

Calcium channel blockers and nitrates, once used as an initial treatment strategy for patients with *achalasia*, are now used only in patients who are not candidates for pneumatic dilation or surgery, and in patients who do not respond to botulinum toxin injections [11, 12]. Prospective randomized studies comparing pneumatic dilation with botulinum toxin injection in patients with achalasia demonstrated an equal early success in relieving dysphagia, but a significantly shorter long-term effect with botulinum injections [13, 14]. The most commonly used nonsurgical means of treating patients with achalasia is pneumatic dilation with the Rigiflex balloon (Boston Scientific, Boston, Mass., USA). This allows a graded approach for dilation with balloons ranging from 3 cm to 4 cm in size [15]. With this approach a durable symptom improvement can be achieved in up to 90% of patients, with most patients requiring only one dilatation session [12, 16]. These results have to be compared to surgical myotomy. Myotomy can now be performed laparoscopically with similar efficacy as the open procedure, but with markedly reduced morbidity and shorter hospital stay [17]. Studies comparing botulinum toxin injection therapy and laparoscopic myotomy showed that the surgical approach is superior to the injection with comparable complication rates [18]. Aggressive balloon dilation, however, is equally effective in relieving dysphagia as surgical myotomy [19]. The symptom of noncardiac chest pain in patients with achalasia cannot predictably be affected by any of the available treatment modalities [20, 21].

Diffuse Esophageal Spasm

There are only few clinical trials assessing the various treatment options in patients with *diffuse esophageal spasm*. In general, anticholinergics, nitrates and calcium channel antagonists have been used with varying results. The results of double-blind placebo-controlled studies in patients with diffuse esophageal spasm were disappointing as none of the tested nitrates or calcium channel antagonists showed a significant improvement of the clinical symptoms [22]. Single-case reports have suggested the use of anticholinergics as a promising approach, but randomized placebo-controlled investigations are lacking. Miller and co-workers [23] reported a prospective open-label trial on botulinum toxin injections in patients with diffuse esophageal spasm, suggesting that this treatment modality may reduce the patients' symptoms. Larger randomized placebo-controlled trials on botulinum toxin therapy in patients with diffuse esophageal spasm are still required to confirm these data.

Nutcracker Esophagus

Nutcracker esophagus is more often associated with noncardiac chest pain than with dysphagia. Propulsive esophageal peristalsis and esophageal transit are not affected in these patients. Although a dose-dependent depressive effect on esophageal contraction amplitude has been shown with calcium channel antagonists in these patients, double-blind placebo-controlled studies have not shown a significant improvement of the clinical symptoms [22, 24]. In contrast, the NO donor molsidomine has been shown to be effective on high contraction amplitudes and on symptom scores in patients with noncardiac chest pain [25]. These data, however, require confirmation in larger studies. For the anticholinergic agent cimetropium bromide a significant reduction of esophageal contraction amplitudes has been shown in patients with the hypercontractile esophagus [26]. Placebo-controlled investigations on cimetropium bromide effects on clinical symptoms are still missing. There have been reports that esophageal dilatation may relieve symptoms in patients with hypercontractile esophagus [22]. However, there is evidence that this effect can also be achieved by a "placebo dilatation." Medication with a weak sedative or antidepressant agents as well as behavioral therapy and biofeedback may also be useful in patients with nutcracker esophagus [22]. Again, controlled studies are lacking so far.

Nonspecific Esophageal Motility Disorders

The understanding of the pathophysiological mechanism and clinical role of the so-called *nonspecific esophageal motility disorders* is still limited. The patients present with a variety of abnormal manometric patterns, which do not meet the strict criteria of the classical primary esophageal motility disorders. In a randomized, double-blind placebo-controlled study the prokinetic agent cisapride was shown to be effective on delayed esophageal transit and the symptom score in these patients [27]. In some patients with nonspecific esophageal motor abnormalities an unrecognized gastroesophageal reflux disease may constitute the underlying disorder. Adequate acid suppression therapy has been successfully used in this subgroup of patients.

Conclusions

For the diagnosis of suspected esophageal motility disorders stationary esophageal manometry remains the first-line investigation after exclusion of a structural abnormality by endoscopy. If the diagnosis remains unclear, 24-h ambulatory manometry should be performed. Ambulatory manometry (in combination with esophageal pH monitoring) is currently the most accurate tool to quantify the efficacy of esophageal peristalsis during meal times and to prove or exclude a correlation of the patients' symptoms (dysphagia and chest pain) with esophageal motor events. In patients with achalasia balloon dilation or laparoscopic myotomy are equally effective therapeutic options, botulinum toxin injection of the lower esophageal sphincter should be reserved for patients who cannot undergo balloon dilation and are not surgical candidates. In patients with other primary motility disorders large and conclusive prospective treatment trials are usually lacking. Despite this lack of objective data, medical treatment with smooth muscle-relaxing, prokinetic or anticholinergic agents should be attempted first, followed by dilatation and/or botulinum toxin injection in those who do not respond. Surgical treatment has no proven role in these disorders.

References

1. Castell DO, Richter JE, Dalton CB (eds) (1987) Esophageal motility testing, Elsevier, New York
2. Stein HJ, DeMeester TR, Hinder RA (1992) Outpatient physiologic testing and surgical management of foregut motility disorders. Curr Probl Surg 29:415–555
3. Spechler SJ (1999) American gastroenterological association medical position statement on treatment of patients with dysphagia caused by benign disorders of the distal esophagus. Gastroenterology 117:229–233
4. Barthet M, Mambrini P, Audibert P, Boustiere C, Helbert T, Bertolino JG, Peyrot J, Salducci J, Grimaud JC (1998) Relationships between endosonographic appearance and clinical or manometric features in patients with achalasia. Eur J Gastroenterol Hepatol 10:559–564
5. Fuller L, Huprich JE, Theisen J, et al. (1999) Abnormal esophageal body function: radiographic-manometric correlation. Am Surg 65:911–914
6. DiMarino AJ Jr, Allen ML, Lynn RB, Zamani S (1998) Clinical value of esophageal motility testing. Dig Dis 16:198–204
7. Alrakawi A, Clouse RE (1998) The changing use of esophageal manometry in clinical practice. Am J Gastroenterol 93:2359–2362
8. Stein HJ, DeMeester TR, Eypasch EP, Klingman RP (1991) Ambulatory 24-hour esophageal manometry in the evaluation of esophageal motor disorders and non-cardiac chest pain. Surgery 110:753–763
9. Stein HJ, DeMeester TR (1993) Indications, technique, and clinical use of ambulatory 24-hour esophageal motility monitoring in a surgical practice. Ann Surg 217:128–137

10. Netzer P, Gut A, Heer R, Gries N, Pfister M, Halter F, Inauen W (1999) Five-year audit of ambulatory 24-hour esophageal pH-manometry in clinical practice. Scand J Gastroenterol 34:676–682
11. Bassotti G, Annese V (1999) Review article: pharmacological options in achalasia. Aliment Pharmacol Ther 13:1391–1396
12. Vaezi MF, Richter JE (1998) Current therapies for achalasia: comparison and efficacy. J Clin Gastroenterol 27:21–35
13. Muehldorfer SM, Schneider TH, Hochberger J, Martus P, Hahn EG, Ell C (1999) Esophageal achalasia: intrasphincteric injection of botulinum toxin A versus balloon dilation. Endoscopy 31:517–521
14. Vaezi MF, Richter JE, Wilcox CM, Schroeder PL, Birgisson S, Slaughter RL, Koehler RE, Baker ME (1999) Botulinum toxin versus pneumatic dilatation in the treatment of achalasia: a randomised trial. Gut 44:231–239
15. Gideon RM, Castell DO, Yarze J (1999) Prospective randomized comparison of pneumatic dilatation technique in patients with idiopathic achalasia. Dig Dis Sci 44:1853–1857
16. Katz PO, Gilbert J, Castell DO (1998) Pneumatic dilatation is effective long-term treatment for achalasia. Dig Dis Sci 43:1973–1977
17. Patti MG, Pellegrini CA, Horgan S, Arcerito M, Omelanczuk P, Tamburini A, Diener U, Eubanks TR, Way LW (1999) Minimally invasive surgery for achalasia: an 8-year experience with 168 patients. Ann Surg 230:587–593
18. Andrews CN, Anvari M, Dobranowski J (1999) Laparoscopic Heller's myotomy or botulinum toxin injection for management of esophageal achalasia. Patient choice and treatment outcomes. Surg Endosc 13:742–746
19. Felix VN, Cecconello I, Zilberstein B, Moraes-Filho JP, Pinotti HW, Carvalho E (1998) Achalasia: a prospective study comparing the results of dilatation and myotomy. Hepatogastroenterology 45:97–108
20. Stein HJ, DeMeester TR (1992) Therapy of non-cardiac chest pain: is there a role for surgery? Am J Med 92:122S–126S
21. Eckardt VF, Stauf B, Bernhard G (1999) Chest pain in achalasia: patient characteristics and clinical course. Gastroenterology 116:1300–1304
22. Storr M, Allescher H-D (1999) Esophageal pharmacology and treatment of primary motility disorders. Diseases Esoph 12 (in press)
23. Miller LS, Parkman HP, Schiano TD, et al. (1996) Treatment of symptomatic non-achalasia esophageal motor disorders with botulinum toxin injection at the lower esophageal sphincter. Dig Dis Sci 41:2025–2031
24. Richter JE, Dalton CB, Bradley LA, Castell DO (1987) Oral nifedipine in the treatment of noncardiac chest pain in patients with the nutcracker esophagus. Gastroenterology 93:21–28
25. Korda P, Barnert J, Schmidbaur W, Wienbeck M (1994) Effect of molsidomine on esophageal motility in patients with non-cardiac thoracic pain. Med Klin 89:73–74
26. Bassotti G, Gaburri M, Imbimbo BP, et al. (1988) Manometric evaluation of cimetropium bromide activity in patients with the nutcracker oesophagus. Scand J Gastroenterol 23:1079–1084
27. Song CW, Um SH, Kim CD, Ryu HS, Hyun JH, Choe JG (1997) Double-blind placebo-controlled study of cisapride in patients with nonspecific esophageal motility disorder accompanied by delayed esophageal transit. Scand J Gastroenterol 32:541–546

Surgical Perspectives

Robert Kalimi · Gary R. Gecelter

Esophageal motor disorders generally include achalasia, nutcracker esophagus, diffuse esophageal spasm and the so-called nonspecific esophageal motor disorders. Current controversies surrounding the surgical treatment of achalasia include:

- The role of surgery as first-line treatment
- The impact of preoperative balloon dilatation and botulinum toxin (BoTox) on subsequent surgery

- Thoracoscopic vs. laparoscopic approach
- The need for antireflux surgery following myotomy
- The role of myotomy before esophagectomy in the dilated esophagus

Achalasia

Overview

Achalasia is a manometrically well-defined entity that affects both the body of the esophagus and the lower esophageal sphincter. It is an incurable disease for which interventions provide palliation by means of improving subjective swallowing. In its early course, symptoms may be minimal and easily overcome by alterations in the rate of eating and in drinking liquids during meals to force the column of food through the poorly relaxing sphincter. As the disease progresses the esophageal body becomes dilated, elongated and then sigmoid-shaped, often with the lowest portion of esophagus dipping into the posterior costophrenic recess, creating a dependent reservoir from which the contents must rise through a step to enter the stomach. In untreated achalasia, mid-esophageal squamous carcinoma occurs in approximately 10% of patients [1]. Consequently, surgical options in the management of achalasia are dependent on the presenting stage of the disease, the age and health of the patient. This chapter will discuss these options and the issues that arise during their performance.

The Role of Surgery as First-Line Treatment for Achalasia

Prior to the introduction of minimally invasive surgery, forceful pneumatic dilatation was regarded as the appropriate first intervention after the diagnosis of achalasia was made. Heller myotomy was reserved for failed pneumatic dilatation, sometimes after multiple attempts. However, when compared directly in a series of 899 patients at the Mayo Clinic [2], myotomy provided 85% of patients with *good to excellent* early relief of dysphagia while forceful pneumatic dilatation afforded only 65% of patients a similar result. Perforation rate was also fourfold greater in the dilatation group (4% vs. 1%). Myotomy has also been demonstrated to better reduce lower esophageal sphincter resting pressure and has been associated with a longer duration of symptomatic relief [3]. In patients under the age of 40 years, typically with early disease, initial pneumatic dilatation was successful in less than 50% of patients and less than 70% successful after two or more attempts [4]. Based upon this age-related variability in the efficacy of pneumatic dilatation, the recommendation of myotomy as first-line treatment in the young patient began to emerge even before the laparoscopic operation became popular. In a review of 18 patients who choose BoTox as an initial treatment compared with 4 patients who chose laparoscopic Heller myotomy as the initial treatment, Andrews et al. reported that, although both procedures offered initial relief of symptoms, 78% of patients in the BoTox group required repeat injections, and 5 of the 18 patients opted to undergo a myotomy [5]. Although the laparoscopic approach requires special skills and training, given the benefits of minimally invasive surgery, it has been suggested that laparoscopic surgery of the gastroesophageal junction should be considered the new gold standard [6].

The Impact of Preoperative Balloon Dilatation and Botulinum Toxin on Subsequent Surgery

Medical management of achalasia, either by pneumatic dilatation or by BoTox injection, has been favored as a means of avoiding a surgical procedure. There is growing concern, however, that Heller myotomy following failed nonsurgical treatment is more difficult and is associated with a higher risk of intra-operative complications than the same operation performed as first-line treatment. This is based upon the concept that muscle disruption by forceful pneumatic dilatation or injection of BoTox through the submucosal plane initiates a fibrotic reaction that obscures the plane of dissection necessary to complete an adequate myotomy.

In a report of 21 patients who underwent laparoscopic Heller myotomy, two patients with previous pneumatic dilatation were complicated by intra-operative perforations [7]. In both patients the mucosal perforations were diagnosed intraoperatively and were sutured laparoscopically with no postoperative sequelae. Other studies also have implicated preoperative pneumatic dilatation as a cause of esophagogastric fibrosis and thus a risk factor for perforation [8, 9]. The authors in these studies concluded that preoperative pneumatic dilatation is not a contraindication to a laparoscopic approach but that it does increase the complexity of the surgery which may result in suboptimal results.

The effect of previous BoTox injection is believed to be more severe than dilatation as the toxin is injected across the submucosal plane on four quadrants of the gastroesophageal junction. In a review of 15 patients who underwent preoperative BoTox injections, 8 (53%) were noted to have a difficult dissection during a laparoscopic Heller myotomy, and 2 cases (13%) were complicated by perforation [10]. Moreover, Patti et al. separated the patients who initially responded to BoTox injections and those who did not, noting that initial responders had a more significant fibrotic reaction and experienced a 50% perforation rate (two of four patients) [9].

Although there are no prospective randomized studies that compare preoperative medical therapy to initial surgical therapy, the data provided in these studies suggest that a young patient with no surgical risk may benefit from initial surgical management rather than several preoperative attempts at pneumatic dilatation and/or BoTox injections. These nonsurgical modalities may be reserved for elderly patients and patients with contraindications to laparoscopic Heller myotomy.

Thoracoscopic Versus Laparoscopic Approach

Like open surgery, minimally invasive myotomy for achalasia can be performed either through the left chest or the abdomen. Both procedures have been reported with high short-term success rates [11]. Although the thoracoscopic procedure permits access to the mediastinal esophagus, it requires double lung ventilation as well as chest tube placement at the completion of the procedure. In addition, the performance of an antireflux procedure, which appears to be the current recommendation, is more easily accomplished through the abdomen.

In 1992 Pellegrini et al. documented an initial experience of 15 patients with achalasia treated via a thoracoscopic myotomy in which they reported effective results with low complications [12]. In 1999 the same group reported their cumulative series of 168 patients with achalasia undergoing minimally invasive surgery: 133 patients underwent a laparoscopic myotomy and 35 patients underwent left thoracoscopic myotomy. In this series laparoscopic myotomy plus partial fundoplication was associated with slightly better early symptomatic improvement (93% vs. 85% reporting *good to excellent* relief of dysphagia). They concluded that the laparoscopic approach more effectively relieved dysphagia, was associated with shorter hospital stay and was associated with less postoperative reflux. Consequently, they favor a laparoscopic approach with added partial fundoplication over their original preference for a thoracoscopic myotomy [9]. Others have similarly favored the transabdominal approach on the basis of decreased operating time, decreased rate of conversion to open procedure, and superior results in relieving dysphagia [13].

The Need for Antireflux Surgery Following Myotomy

The classical transthoracic approach to achalasia involves a longitudinal myotomy approximately 10 cm in length. With the laparoscopic approach the myotomy is generally extended only 4–5 cm superiorly from the anatomic gastroesophageal junction and 0.5–1 cm inferiorly onto the stomach. Where the oral length of the myotomy has been correlated with the degree of postoperative improvement in dysphagia, the length of extension onto the cardia of the stomach is believed to impact on the development of postoperative reflux. Proponents of long myotomy extending onto the stomach will generally advocate an accompanying partial fundoplication. Ellis et al. reported results of 68 patients who underwent a short esophagomyotomy (modified Heller myotomy) without an antireflux procedure. The length of the myotomy in this open procedure most closely resembles the laparoscopic operation done today. A median follow-up of 13.6 years (10–20 years) revealed a symptomatic improvement rate of 95.6% at 10 years, 85.8% at 15 years and 67.3% at 20 years [14]. It was felt that the clinical deterioration over time was a result of persistent or progressive disease of the esophageal body leading to poor emptying in some patients and the development of late reflux in others. In Patti's series, objective postoperative pH testing was conducted in 35 of 133 patients undergoing laparoscopic myotomy with partial fundoplication. Six (17%) had abnormal pH profiles of which only one was symptomatic. In contrast, 12 patients (11%) had persistent or recurrent dysphagia of which four were directly caused by complications of the partial fundoplication requiring re-operation.

In an era of potent acid-reducing medication the role of obligatory partial fundoplication may be difficult to justify especially when symptomatic reflux occurs in only 10%–15% of patients undergoing all forms of surgery [9, 15]. Further, objective pH evaluation in patients with gastroesophageal reflux disease undergoing posterior partial fundoplication revealed return of reflux in approximately 50% of cases at 2 years [16]. The current state of partial fundoplication is therefore one of a poor operation with its own risks that may not adequately treat the small subset of patients with reflux following esophagomyotomy. A prospective, blinded, multicenter trial is needed to address this pressing issue.

The Role of Myotomy Before Esophagectomy in the Dilated Esophagus

The megaesophagus (>6 cm diameter) is either straight or sigmoid. The sigmoid esophagus represents end-stage achalasia for which some surgeons believe myotomy is futile and for which esophagectomy provides the only definitive means of restoring adequate swallowing and avoiding the development of squamous carcinoma [17]. Even prior to the advent of minimally invasive surgery, others have proposed that myotomy should be attempted as an initial operative procedure in all patients with megaesophagus, reserving esophagectomy for those patients who do not experience significant improvement in swallowing [18]. Within the UCSF series were 30 patients with megaesophagus, 16 straight and 14 sigmoid, who underwent laparoscopic myotomy and D'Or anterior fundoplication. Surprisingly, 88% of straight and 93% of sigmoid cases reported good/excellent results. This lead to their conclusion that, even in the sigmoid esophagus, esophagectomy should be reserved only for patients with failed myotomy.

Surgery for Diffuse Esophageal Spasm and Nutcracker Esophagus

Calcium channel blockers usually represent first-line therapy for these rare causes of chest pain or dysphagia. Despite improving the manometric abnormalities, they are no better than placebo in alleviating symptoms [19]. Centers with experience in the surgical management of these conditions report significant improvement in 70%–90% of patients undergoing transthoracic long esophagomyotomy originally as an open procedure [20] and now thoracoscopically [21]. In diffuse esophageal spasm (DES), the manometric abnormality tends to be confined to the smooth muscle portion of the esophageal body and good results have been obtained through a left chest approach [22]. The manometric abnormality in nutcracker esophagus tends to involve the entire esophagus, thus requiring a right thoracic approach.

Conclusions

The surgical treatment of primary esophageal motor disorders has evolved significantly in the minimally invasive era because myotomy through the chest or abdomen is ideally suited to videoscopic approach. Laparoscopic myotomy is now the surgical standard in the treatment of achalasia with most surgeons adding either an anterior or posterior partial fundoplication. Myotomy tends to be more difficult, and associated with more complications when preceded by nonsurgical modalities, especially BoTox trans-sphincteric injection. Thoracoscopic long esophagomyotomy provides excellent quality-of-life improvement in patients with DES or nutcracker esophagus when performed by experienced surgeons.

References

1. Rosati R, Fumagalli U, Bonavino L, Segalin A, Montorsi M, Bena S, Peracchia A (1995) Laparoscopic approach to esophageal achalasia. Am J Surg 169:424
2. Okike N, Payne WS, Neufeld DM, et al. (1979) Esophagomyotomy versus forceful dilatation for achalasia of the esophagus: results in 899 patients. Ann Thorac Surg 28:119
3. Csendes A, Velasco N, Braghetto I, Henriquez A (1980) A prospective randomized study comparing forceful dilatation and esophagomyotomy in patients with achalasia of the esophagus. Gastroenterology 80:789
4. Parkman HP, Ogorek CP, Harris AD, Cohen S (1994) Nonoperative management of esophageal strictures following esophagomyotomy for achalasia. Dig Dis Sci 39:2102–2108
5. Andrews CN, Anvari M, Dobranowski J (1999) Laparoscopic Heller's myotomy or botulinum toxin injection for management of esophageal achalasia. Patient choice and treatment outcomes. Surg Endosc 13(8):742–746
6. Spivak H, Lelcuk S, Hunter JG (1999) Laparoscopic surgery of the gastroesophageal junction. World J Surg 23(4):356–367
7. Morino M, Rebecchi F, Festa V, Garrone C (1997) Preoperative pneumatic dilatation represents a risk factor for laparoscopic Heller myotomy. Surg Endosc 11(4):359–361
8. Beckingham IJ, Callanan M, Louw JA, Bornman PC (1999) Laparoscopic cardiomyotomy for achalasia after failed balloon dilatation. Surg Endosc 13(5):493–496
9. Patti MG, Feo CV, Arcerito M, De Pinto M, Tamburini A, Diener U, Gantert W, Way LW (1999) Effects of previous treatment on results of laparoscopic Heller myotomy for achalasia. Dig Dis Sci 44(11):2270–2276
10. Horgan S, Hudda K, Eubanks T, McAllister J, Pellegrini CA (1999) Does botulinum toxin injection make esophagomyotomy a more difficult operation? Surg Endosc 13(6):576–579
11. Wiechmann RJ, Ferguson MK, Naunheim KS, Hazelrigg SR, Mack MJ, Aronoff RJ, Weyant RJ, Santucci T, Macherey R, Landreneau RJ (1999) Video-assisted surgical management of achalasia of the esophagus. J Thorac Cardiovasc Surg 118(5):916–923
12. Pellegrini C, Wetter LA, Patti M, Leichter R, Mussan G, Mori T, Bernstein G, Way L (1992) Thoracoscopic esophagomyotomy. Initial experience with a new approach for the treatment of achalasia. Ann Surg 216(3):291–296, 296–299
13. Stewart KC, Finley RJ, Clifton JC, Graham AJ, Storseth C, Inculet R (1999) Thoracoscopic versus laparoscopic modified Heller Myotomy for achalasia: efficacy and safety in 87 patients. J Am Coll Surg 189(2):164–169, 169–170
14. Ellis FH Jr, Watkins E Jr, Gibb SP, Heatley GJ (1992) Ten to 20-year clinical results after short esophagomyotomy without an antireflux procedure (modified Heller operation) for esophageal achalasia. Eur J Cardiothorac Surg 6(2):86–89, 90
15. Wang PC, Sharp KW, Holzman MD, Clements RH, Holcomb GW, Richards WO (1998) The outcome of laparoscopic Heller myotomy without antireflux procedure in patients with achalasia. Am Surg 64(6):515–520
16. Jobe BA, Wallace J, Hansen PD, Swanstrom LL (1997) Evaluation of laparoscopic Toupet fundoplication as a primary repair for all patients with medically resistant gastroesophageal reflux. Surg Endosc 11:1080–1083
17. Orringer MB, Stirling MC (1989) Esophageal resection for achalasia: indications and results. Ann Thorac Surg 47(3):340–345
18. Waters PF, Pearson FG, Todd TR, Patterson GA, Goldberg M, Ginsberg RJ, Cooper JD, Ramirez J, Miller L (1988) Esophagectomy for complex benign esophageal disease. J Thorac Cardiovasc Surg 95(3):378–381
19. Richter JE, Dalton CB, Buice RG, Castell DO (1987) Oral nifedipine in the treatment of noncardiac chest pain in patients with the nutcracker esophagus. Gastroenterology 93:21–28
20. Ellis FH Jr (1992) Esophagomyotomy for noncardiac chest pain resulting from diffuse esophageal spasm and related disorders. Am J Med 92:129S–131S

21. Patti MG, Pellegrini CA, Arcerito M, Tong J, Mulvihill SF, Way LW (1995) Comparison of medical and minimally invasive surgical therapy for primary esophageal motor disorders. Arch Surg 130:609–615
22. Henderson RD, Ryder D, Marryatt G (1987) Extended esophageal myotomy and short total fundoplicaiton hernia repair in diffuse esophageal spasm: five-year review in 34 patients. Ann Thorac Surg 43:25–31

Invited Comment

Cedric G. Bremner

These two excellent reviews on primary motility disorders have highlighted practical approaches to diagnosis and treatment, which will assist the surgeon to manage those conditions more effectively. With the advent of less invasive laparoscopic and thoracoscopic procedures, the surgical approach has become more acceptable. The surgeons have to prove that these approaches are often preferable to medical care. This can only be done if there is a clear understanding of the underlying pathophysiology, and if the corrective procedure has been well designed and performed. An incorrect diagnosis or poor selection will inevitably result in an unacceptable outcome. The modern esophageal surgeon therefore must perform a complete and meticulous investigation of all patients.

Drs. Stein and Theisen suggest that esophageal motility disorders should be looked at as a spectrum of abnormalities which reflect various stages of destruction of esophageal motor function rather than separate entities. This may suggest that there is a common cause for the "spectrum," which is not the case. Certainly the prevalence of "effective" or "noneffective" contraction sequences during mealtimes may have clinical relevance. For example, contraction amplitudes do not increase in achalasia during mealtimes.

Esophageal responses to meals are either normal, hypotensive, hypertensive or incoordinate:

- Hypotensive responses are seen classically in scleroderma and achalasia, but also result from long-continued reflux esophagitis. Other less common causes are chronic alcoholism and diabetes.
- Hypertensive contractions in excess of 180 mmHg are named "nutcracker." Incoordinate contractions are seen classically in achalasia (simultaneous, mirror image responses). When simultaneous contractions occur in more than 30% of the ten swallows given during a stationary motility test, "diffuse esophageal spasm" is diagnosed. This diagnosis, in particular, is poorly designated and in such cases ambulatory motility may be of value.

I believe that it is still useful for the practicing esophagologist to have more specific terms to describe the manometric abnormalities.

Drs. Stein and Theisen include achalasia, diffuse esophageal spasm, nutcracker esophagus and nonspecific esophageal motor disorders in their classification. Ineffective esophageal motility (IEM) is a named motility disorder suggested by Leite

[1]. IEM is another diagnosis made when swallow responses are less than 30 mmHg in amplitude and when more than 30% of the responses are nonpropulsive. IEM will include scleroderma, diffuse esophageal spasm and end-stage reflux disease. A diagnosis of IEM may explain dysphagia in a patient who has normal endoscopy and upper gastrointestinal barium series.

Diagnostic Tests

Endoscopy should not be the first examination in a patient complaining of dysphagia. It is important in these patients to rule out a mechanical cause for dysphagia and to give a "road map" for further planning. The guidelines of the American Medical Association clearly state this point [2]. Video-esophagography is the first investigation performed at USC in patients with dysphagia [3]. An objective comparison of the videoesophagogram in the evaluation of esophageal motility disorders with stationary motility was made on 34 patients. The positive predictive value was 53%, specificity 79% and the negative predictive value 80%. Sensitivity was greatest in patients with achalasia (94%) and scleroderma (100%), and in patients presenting with dysphagia (89%). Sensitivity was poor for nonspecific esophageal motility disorders. Videoesophagogram is therefore relatively insensitive in detecting motility disorders, and useful in the detection of patients with esophageal dysfunction for which surgical treatment is beneficial.

Achalasia

This is the most common of the primary motility disorders, and the controversy of balloon dilatation vs. surgical myotomy continues. Surgical myotomy has repeatedly been shown to give better results than balloon dilatation, but because ballooning is less invasive and can be performed as an outpatient procedure, it is more acceptable as a primary procedure. The main controversy surrounding balloon dilatation is the end point of success. Should it be measured by symptom evaluation, lower esophageal sphincter pressure or esophageal emptying? There is a paucity of data to give guidance because objective evaluation following balloon dilatation is largely neglected. Vantrappen followed a protocol of progressive balloon dilatation until the lower esophageal sphincter pressure was adequately reduced [4]. At a pressure of less than 10 mmHg there is usually very little residual stasis in the esophagus. However, at this pressure, gastroesophageal reflux is more likely to occur. Balloon dilatation in young patients is not usually as successful as in older people, and the reason is unclear [5]. It should be contraindicated in patients under 30 years of age.

Many gastroenterologists use symptomatic assessment as the end point of success. However, a patient who is "better" may still have considerable esophageal stasis [6], and may learn to live with the residual symptoms. The goal of treatment should surely be to eliminate stasis. This is probably more important in the early achalasia in which the esophagus has not yet decompensated, so that it is not markedly dilated and still has swallow responses of a reasonable amplitude. Early treatment may result in recovery of peristalsis, and we have seen this in two patients. A long-term assessment of esophageal function and pH monitoring following pneumatic dilatation is desirable.

Laparoscopic myotomy is more acceptable to patients than open myotomy, and is the preferred route. The advantage over pneumatic dilatation is that an anti-reflux procedure can be added. Most surgeons will add a partial fundoplication procedure (Toupet or D'Or) because of the poor motility in the esophageal body. However, Donahue et al. [7] have reported on excellent results using a "floppy" Nissen fundoplication. Bonavina et al. [8] reported excellent results using the D'Or procedure, and because it does not require mobilization of the esophagus or a takedown of the short-gastrics it would seem to be the preferable approach. There is as yet no trial to suggest which is preferable.

"Vigorous" achalasia in which the swallow responses have an amplitude which falls into the normal range, or a hypercontractile range, should receive the same treatment as is given for achalasia without these responses. The abnormally high body responses are obviously secondary to the outflow obstruction at the sphincter, and balloon dilatation or myotomy will effectively change these responses [9]. It is possible that vigorous achalasia represents an early stage in the disease, and any treatment given should be aimed to relieve the esophagus of any obstruction, and so prevent decompensation. If effective treatment is given early enough, there is a possibility of a return of complete peristalsis in all segments of the body.

Outpatient balloon dilatation in older patients is a perfectly reasonable first approach, and is less costly with a low morbidity rate. The 20%–30% of failures can still have a laparoscopic procedure if necessary. Botulinum toxin injection should be reserved for a small group of achalasia patients who have a co-morbidity prohibiting surgery, or who have a short life expectancy. There is some experience which reports that myotomy is more difficult after these injections, and the duration of effective relief is limited to less than 9 months.

Diffuse Esophageal Spasm

This is probably the most difficult of the named motility disorders to treat. The reasons are that the pathogenesis is not understood, the diagnosis is often uncertain, the episodes of chest pain are intermittent and some cases even improve spontaneously. Ambulatory manometry may be of value, and in some cases endoscopic ultrasonography will show a thickened muscular layer. This thickening may suggest work hypertrophy in a muscle layer that has incoordinate contractions. A long myotomy should be undertaken only in very selective cases where the functional obstruction exceeds the propulsive activity. Eyspach and DeMeester [10] have suggested that at least 75% of the swallow responses should be simultaneous before myotomy should be considered. The nutcracker esophagus deserves a free trial of medical treatment as outlined by the authors. If the muscle is very thickened as seen on ultrasound, a long esophagomyotomy with a D'Or or Belsey Mark IV antireflux procedure is the treatment of choice.

Nonspecific Esophageal Motility Disorders

The response to a Nissen fundoplication is unaltered by the presence of a nonspecific esophageal motility disorder (NSEMD) [11], and if the indication for surgery exists, the motility abnormality is not a contraindication.

Ineffective Esophageal Motility

For several years a "tailored" approach to the surgical management of gastroesophageal reflux disease has been used. In the past, patients with swallow responses of less than 30 mmHg have been treated in some centers by a partial fundoplication (Toupet or D'Or), because of the theoretical concern that a full 360° fundoplication would cause dysphagia. This concern has not been proved, and in fact there is evidence to suggest that such patients will also benefit from a full 360° fundoplication [12]. Whether the short-term efficacy will be durable over time remains to be seen.

It is important to control all reflux in Barrett's esophagus, and the motility in long-segment Barrett's is often hypomotile. A floppy short-segment Nissen fundoplication performed over a 60F bougie is probably the best treatment in these patients, provided that peristalsis is preserved and the amplitudes of the responses are more than 25 mmHg. The short gastric vessels should be taken down and the hiatus closed adequately in all cases.

References

1. Leite LP, Johnston BT, Barrett J, Castell JA, Castell DO (1997) Ineffective esophageal motility (IEM). The primary finding patients with non-specific esophageal motor disorders. Dig Dis Sci 42:1859–1865
2. De Vault KR, Castell DO, and the Practice Parameters Committee of the American College of Gastroenterology (1999) Am J Gastroenterol 94(6):1434–1442
3. Fuller L, Huprich JE, Theisen J, Hagen JA, Crookes PF, DeMeester SR, Bremner CG, DeMeester TR, Peters JH (1999) Abnormal esophageal body function. Radiographic-manometric correlation. Am Surg 65(10):911–914
4. Vantrappen G, Hellemans J (1980) Treatment of achalasia and related motor disorders. Gastroenterology 79:144–154
5. Eckardt C, Aignherr C, Bernhard G (1992) Predictors of outcome in patients with achalasia treated by pneumatic dilatation. Gastroenterology 103:1732–1738
6. Lipschitz J, Bremner CG (1990) Achalasia. Assessment of results of pneumatic dilatation (PD) and oesophagomyotomy (HM). S Afr J Surg 28:118A
7. Donahue PE, Schlesinger PK, Sluss KF, Richter HM, Liu KJ, Rypins B, Nyhus LM (1994) Esophagocardiomyotomy – floppy Nissen fundoplication effectively treats achalasia without causing esophageal obstruction. Surgery 116(4):719–724
8. Bonavina L, Nosadini A, Bardini R, Baessato M, Peracchia A (1992) Primary treatment of esophageal achalasia. Long-term results of myotomy and D'Or fundoplication. Arch Surg 127:222–226
9. Parilla PP, Martinez De Haro LF, Escandell (1993) Short myotomy for vigorous achalasia. Br J Surg 80:1540–1542
10. Eypasch EP, De Meester TR, Klingman RR, Stein HJ (1992) Physiological assessment and surgical management of diffuse esophageal spasm. J Thorac Cardiovasc Surg 104(4):859–869

11. Bremner RM, DeMeester TR, Crookes PF, Costantini M, Hoeft SF, Peters JH, Hagen J (1994) The effect of symptoms and non-specific motility abnormalities on outcomes of surgical therapy for gastroesophageal reflux disease. J Thorac Cardiovasc Surg 107(5):1244–1249
12. Rydberg L, Ruth M, Abrahamson H, Lundell L (1999) Tailoring antireflux surgery. A randomized clinical trial. World J Surg 23(6):612–618

Editorial Comment

While issues related to achalasia are well studied and defined, the more rare esophageal motility disorders remain relatively obscure and controversial. Thus, for example, Drs. Stein and Theisen conclude their section with the notion that "surgical treatment has no proven role in these disorders," whereas Drs. Kalimi and Gecelter conclude that "long esophagomyotomy provides excellent quality of life improvement in patients with diffuse esophageal spasm or 'nutcracker esophagus' when performed by experienced surgeons." Dr. Bremner – who dedicated his entire professional life to the study of the esophagus – takes a middle of the road approach, recommending surgery in diffuse esophageal spasm "only in very selective cases."

Interestingly, Drs. Stein and Theisen suggest that esophageal motility disorders should be looked at as a spectrum of abnormalities rather than separate entities. Dr. Bremner, however, contends that current nomenclature is still useful in daily practice. Indeed, the manometric characteristics of the primary esophageal disorders are fairly distinct:

- *Achalasia* is due to a functional obstruction of the distal esophagus due to incomplete relaxation of the lower esophageal sphincter (LES). Histologically there is loss of ganglion cells in the myenteric plexus of Auerbach. Disordered esophageal motility follows with lack of progressive peristalsis. There is aperistalsis in the esophageal body and as the disease progresses the esophagus becomes massively dilated and tortuous.
- *Diffuse esophageal spasm* (DES) is characterized by simultaneous nonperistaltic contractions and causes substernal chest pain and/or dysphagia. It is primarily a disease of the esophageal body. In patients with advanced disease the radiographic appearance of tertiary contractions appears helical and has been termed "corkscrew esophagus."
- *Nutcracker esophagus* is a syndrome of high amplitude peristaltic waves. These patients usually complain of dysphagia in addition to chest pain. The identification of these patients is important, since according to DeMeester [1] esophageal myotomy is a therapeutic option for patients with dysphagia and DES, but is of questionable value in patients with chest pain secondary to nutcracker esophagus.

The major causes for secondary esophageal motility disorders are the collagen vascular diseases or systemic sclerosis, polymyositis, lupus, etc

We have to bear in mind the warning by Drs. Kalimi and Gecelter that laparoscopic myotomy for achalasia may be more difficult and hazardous after previous attempts at dilation or injections with botulinum toxin. Thus, the achalasia patient should be evaluated and treated from the start by a multi-specialty team including surgeons, capable of selecting and providing the best tailored therapy, rather than dilated or injected - in isolation - by gastroenterologists and referred to a surgeon only when everything fails.

Reference

1. DeMeester TR, Stein HJ (1992) Surgery for esophageal motor disorders. In: Castell DO (ed) The esophagus. Little Brown, Boston

CHAPTER 4

Benign Hepatic Lesions

Investigations and Nonoperative Management

IRVING S. BENJAMIN · SANJAY GUPTA

Benign lesions of the liver are increasingly diagnosed because of widespread use of noninvasive imaging for unrelated disorders and routine screening for metastatic disease. As most of these lesions are asymptomatic, it is imperative that they be diagnosed with maximum accuracy so that they may be safely observed. The commonest benign lesions, which cause a clinical dilemma, are hepatic cysts, hemangiomas, liver cell adenoma (LCA) and focal nodular hyperplasia (FNH). This chapter will address the issues shown in Table 1.

Diagnosis

Is Noninvasive Imaging Adequate for Most Lesions?

Distinction of *cystic* from *solid* lesions is usually straightforward. Cystic lesions on ultrasound (US) typically show a circular anechoic area with sharp smooth borders and posterior acoustic enhancement, and CT shows a smooth, thin-walled, nonenhancing, water-dense lesion. Atypical features such as septations, solid ele-

Table 1. Benign liver lesions - controversies

	Diagnosis
1	Is noninvasive imaging adequate for most lesions?
2	What is the role of angiography?
3	What is the role of biopsy?
	Cystic lesions
1	How simple is a "simple cyst"?
2	Do simple cysts need treatment?
3	Can cysts be cured by aspiration?
	Solid lesions
1	Adenoma, FNH, hemangioma and HCC - how to distinguish them?
2	Which liver cell adenomas are premalignant?
3	What is the optimum surveillance program for presumed benign liver lesions?

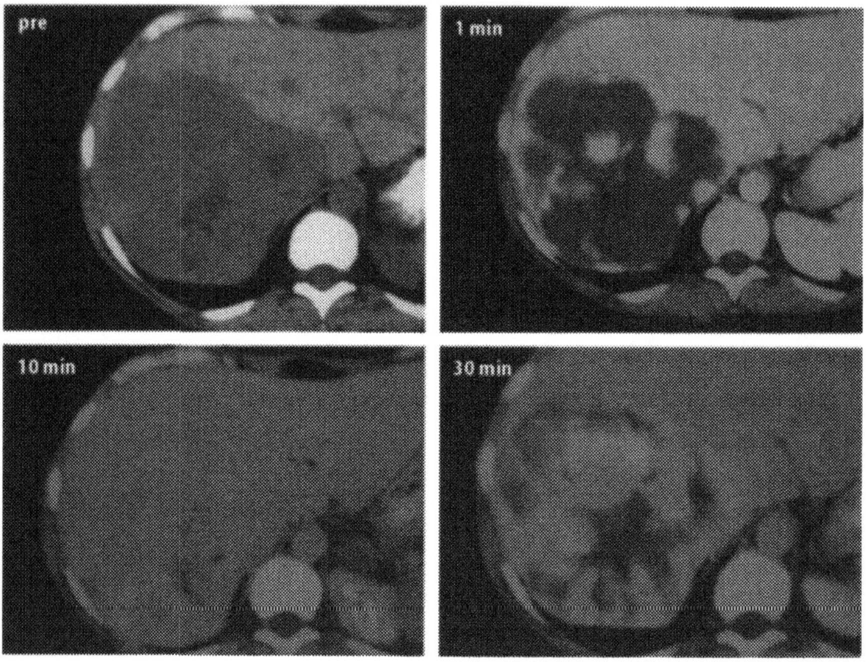

Fig. 1. Cavernous hemangioma of the liver: CT before and 1, 10, and 30 min after intravenous contrast injection, showing "creeping" globular peripheral enhancement

ments, daughter cysts and irregularity, thickening or calcification of the cyst wall suggest other disease processes and require careful investigation [1]. On MR simple cysts are usually hypointense on T1 weighting and hyperintense on T2 weighting. Hemorrhagic cysts are hyperintense on both T1 and T2 weighting.

In solid lesions *vascularity* is an important feature, best seen on dual or triple phase dynamic contrast enhanced CT scan, and few may therefore require direct angiography (see below). The characteristic feature of hemangiomas is "creeping" centripetal enhancement on delayed CT imaging (Fig. 1) [2]. Tc-99 m labeled RBC scan is much less commonly used nowadays. MR imaging with T2 weighting and dynamic contrast enhanced T1 weighting is perhaps the most sensitive and specific diagnostic modality [3, 4]. LCA and FNH exhibit varying degrees of vascularization, and while the appearances of each are *characteristic*, they are by no means *specific*. LCA has a rich arterial supply, and its propensity to outgrow this can result in hemorrhage, necrosis and rupture. The problem of distinguishing these two lesions is discussed further below.

US may add further information about *tissue characteristics*. Hemangiomas appear as a hyperechoic mass with large peripheral feeder(s). FNH may be isoechoic and easily missed on US. LCA is usually hyperechoic due to its high fat content.

What, then, can we conclude about noninvasive imaging? Most benign cystic lesions, and the larger hemangiomas, can be confidently diagnosed by a combination of these scanning methods (Fig. 2). There is, however, a considerable overlap

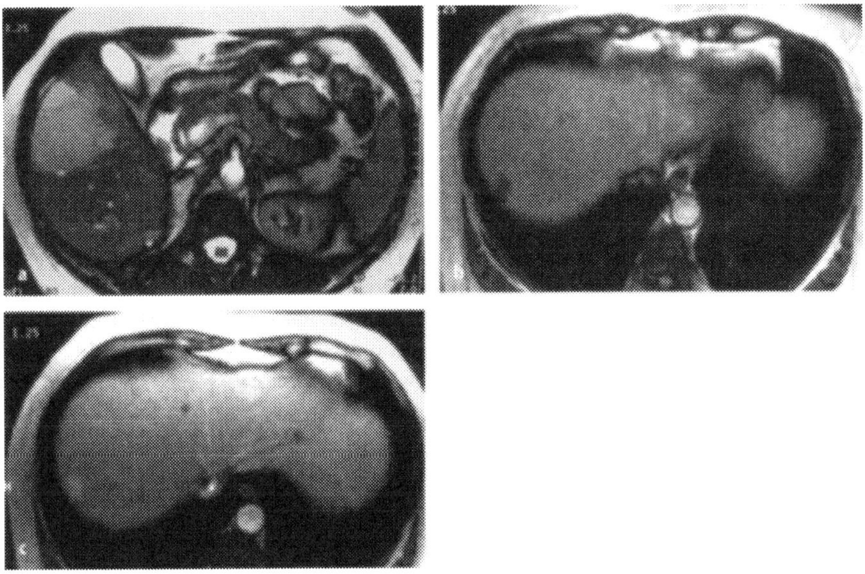

Fig. 2 a–c. Axial MRI scans in a woman who had previous resection of colon cancer. Lesions were found on scanning which were suggestive of metastases. Combination of US, CT and MRI characterized these as three simple cysts and three hemangiomas. **a** Gradient echo T2-weighted image showing the intense imaging of a simple cyst. **b** T1-weighted image before and **c** after gadolinium enhancement: a hemangioma is seen to enhance well, and on the second scan two nonenhancing simple cysts are seen. (Note in these scans the artefactual image of the aorta in the anterior part of the liver)

of appearances, perhaps especially in the case of FNH vs. LCA, and often there remains a lingering doubt about benign vs. malignant diagnosis. The next stage of refinement in imaging is often angiography, so this will be considered next.

What Is the Role of Angiography?

This technique is most helpful in the evaluation of hypervascular lesions in which there remains diagnostic uncertainty, or occasionally in lesions for which surgery is planned, as a preoperative "road map." Therapeutic angiography may sometimes be employed preoperatively in patients who present with life-threatening hemorrhage from a benign liver lesion, but embolization of large vascular lesions to render operation "safer" or easier is of very doubtful value.

The role of angiography in diagnosing hemangioma is limited, as the findings are usually sufficiently characteristic on noninvasive imaging [5]. Sometimes it is necessary to distinguish hemangiomas from secondary or primary liver cancers. Liver secondaries demonstrate neovascularity with only slight delay in the washout of contrast; hepatocellular carcinoma (HCC) on the other hand displays marked coarse vascularity, large arterial feeders with a-v shunting and visualisation of the portal vein during the arterial phase. Retention of iodized oil following intra-arterial injection is virtually diagnostic for HCC.

Angiographically LCA is still often difficult to distinguish from FNH or HCC. The findings of each, though characteristic, are nonspecific [6–9], and it may still be necessary to proceed to a formal tissue diagnosis if there is still doubt.

What Is the Role of Biopsy?

Biopsy techniques include fine needle aspiration for cytology (FNAC) and core needle biopsy guided by CT or US or by direct targeting at laparoscopy. Aspiration of cystic lesions for cytology when cystadenocarcinoma is suspected may be of value, though false negatives abound. Biopsy of lesions with a strong suspicion of hemangioma is rarely necessary, and of doubtful safety. The important problem therefore lies in distinguishing amongst LCA, FNH and HCC, and the issues are those of accuracy and safety. Core biopsies will generally have a higher diagnostic yield than FNAC, and a recent radiological review places the diagnostic accuracy between 65% and 100% [10]. Ha et al. reported 88% specific diagnosis with 14-gauge Trucut needle compared to 39% for 20-gauge aspiration needle for benign focal disease [11]. Combining the two may be especially useful in diagnosing HCC, with accuracy rising up to 97.9% [12, 13]. Though useful for HCC, FNAC is unlikely to distinguish between LCA and FNH.

Most accounts report a complication rate of less than 2%, and a mortality rate of 0.3% or less [14]. Hemorrhage is the commonest complication and it appears that platelet count is more important than PT in procedure related bleeding [15]. The presence of ascites does not alter the complication rate [16]. The authors do not advocate preliminary biopsy in lesions thought to be malignant and suitable for resection: there are many cases of tumor implantation in the needle track [17]. FNAC or laparoscopically guided biopsy may be safer, but the latter is more invasive.

When should we not perform a biopsy? Firstly, if there is a strong suspicion of malignancy, good indications for surgical excision of the lesion, and the risk of formal excision is low, e.g., in peripheral rather than central masses. Secondly, in highly vascular lesions, especially if situated at the liver capsule. Thirdly, if there would be no significant difference in the management plan: if follow-up by conservative management and repeat scans is considered appropriate, the academic curiosity to distinguish between FNH and LCA does not constitute an indication for biopsy!

Cystic Lesions

How Simple Are Simple Cysts?

In one large series, only 17% of cysts were reported to be symptomatic [18], and most were diagnosed on imaging for symptoms due to unrelated disorders. Serial scans performed over years reveal no change or growth in the majority of cases [19]. Symptomatic cysts appear to be seen more often in females and usually come to attention in the fifth through seventh decades, perhaps indicating the long duration required to become large enough to produce symptoms. Common presentations in symptomatic patients include abdominal mass (55%), hepatomegaly (40%), pain (33%) and jaundice (9%) [19]. Impaired liver function is extremely uncommon. Rarely simple cysts may first present with complications such as intracystic bleeding, producing acute onset of upper abdominal pain [20]. Pain may less commonly signify rupture or infection. Rarely has compression of the IVC [21], obstructive jaundice [20, 22–24], portal hypertension due to portal vein compression [25], hepatic venous outflow occlusion with Budd-Chiari syndrome [26] and carcinoma of the cyst lining [27] been reported. Torsion of a pedunculated cyst presenting as an acute abdomen has also been reported [28].

Do Simple Cysts Need Treatment?

As the complication rate remains extremely low, uncomplicated *asymptomatic* cysts require no active treatment. Serial scans may be reassuring both for the surgeon and the patient. The real controversy lies in the management of symptomatic liver cysts. It is vital to exclude other causes of symptoms: one series [29] excluded up to a third of patients with liver cysts for this reason. Moreover, not all interventions for cysts are curative: Gigot et al. [30] reported recurrence of symptoms after surgery in 23% of patients. Strict selection therefore cannot be overemphasized. The usual symptom which leads to treatment is chronic, dull right hypochondrial or epigastric pain with local fullness, and cysts less than 5 cm are unlikely to produce these symptoms. However, size alone is not an indication for therapeutic intervention. The symptomatic effect of percutaneous cyst aspiration may be a helpful guide, and may both improve patient selection and serve as a predictor of the long-term success of surgical decompression. Thus while treatment for symptomatic cysts is indicated, the risk of treatment must not exceed the small risk of the disease: mere technical feasibility of a procedure does not justify its performance [31, 32]. This applies equally to minimally invasive techniques such as laparoscopic fenestration.

Similar observations may be made with reference to polycystic liver disease (PLD). Symptomatic PLD with single or multiple dominant lesions are more likely to benefit from decompression procedures compared to diffuse small cysts replacing the liver parenchyma.

Can Cysts Be Cured by Aspiration?

Cyst aspiration alone [33–38] has often produced unsatisfactory long-term results, because there is a high recurrence rate unless the functioning secretory lining epithelium is ablated or permanent drainage is achieved. Aspiration with sclerotherapy seems more promising [36–42]. Historically results with formaldehyde sclerotherapy were plagued with high relapse rates [43, 44] and concern about hepatotoxicity [45]. After sclerotherapy with 95% alcohol, most of the epithelial lining cells were found to be fixed and nonviable in 1–3 min after con-

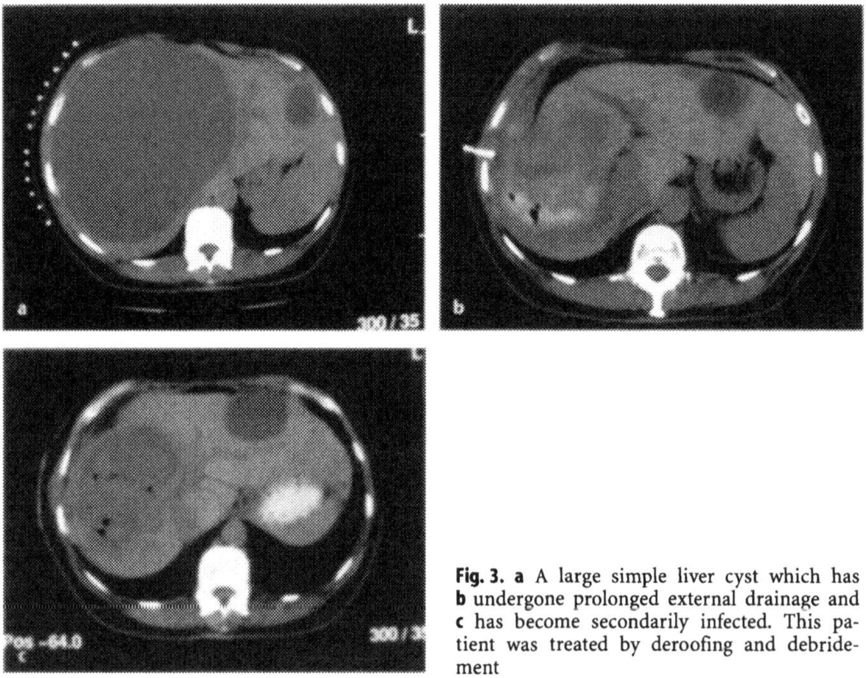

Fig. 3. **a** A large simple liver cyst which has **b** undergone prolonged external drainage and **c** has become secondarily infected. This patient was treated by deroofing and debridement

tact, although it required 4–12 h for the alcohol to penetrate the cyst capsule [39]. Andersson et al. reported cyst and symptomatic regression in eight out of nine patients with a mean cyst size of 10 cm and a median follow-up of 18 months following ethanol sclerotherapy [37], and similar results have been reported by others in smaller series [36, 39]. This method may be less suitable for very large cysts, because the volume required for good epithelial contact may be excessive. Repeated performance carries some risk of infection (Fig. 3) [35]. Endoscopic retrograde cholangiopancreatography or injection of contrast medium, to rule out communication with the biliary tree or extravasation outside the cyst, should preferably be performed before sclerotherapy. Since it is minimally invasive, ethanol sclerotherapy could perhaps be the first line of therapy, and initial symptomatic relief may help in selecting patients for surgical intervention should there be a recurrence.

Solid Lesions

LCA, FNH, Hemangioma and HCC: How To Distinguish Them?

The clinical problem of (usually) a young woman with an incidental finding of a solid liver mass is one which confronts us often, and one which both invokes enormous anxiety and consumes much investigative effort. The practical issue is whether a lesion thus discovered can be positively identified (a) as nonmalignant and (b) as car-

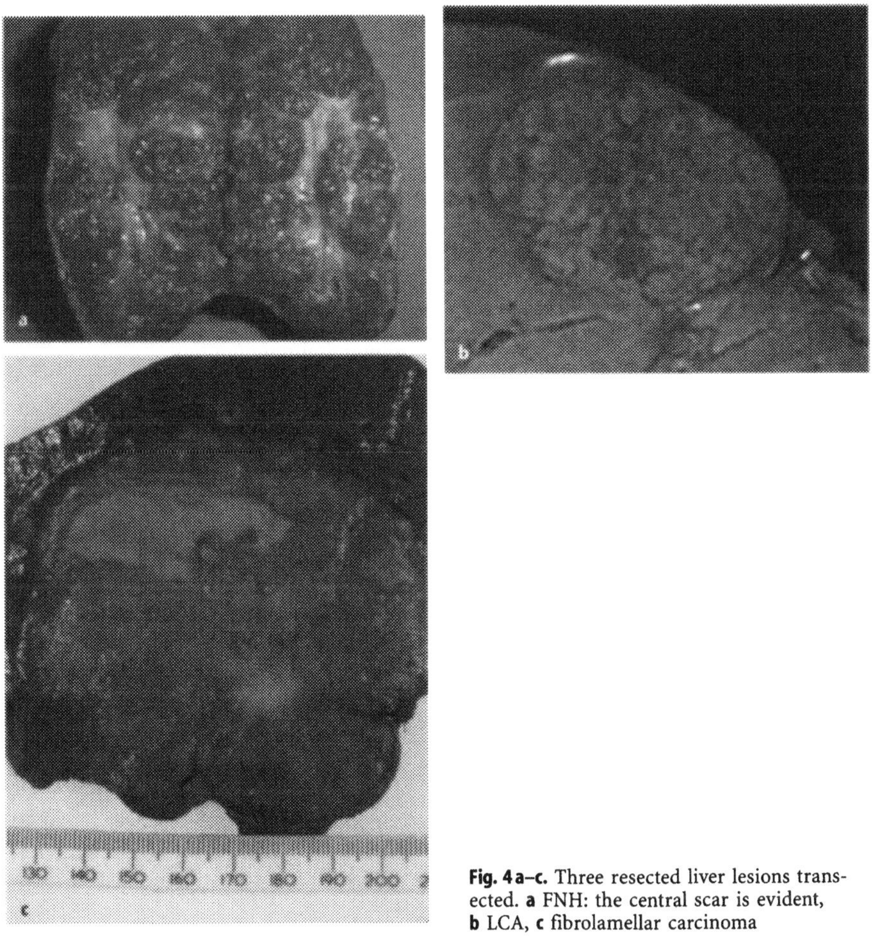

Fig. 4a–c. Three resected liver lesions transected. **a** FNH: the central scar is evident, **b** LCA, **c** fibrolamellar carcinoma

rying a low risk of future malignant potential. There is no one test (short of excision) which will allow this distinction with certainty, and we must often rely on multiple investigations and a reasonable balance of probabilities (Fig. 4).

Hemangiomas do not constitute as great a problem, and their characteristics have been discussed above. Some of the main features of LCA and FNH are compared in Table 2.

The US appearances of LCA and FNH are highly nonspecific. LCA is more prone to internal hemorrhage and this may leave the appearance of resolving hematoma. A linear hyperechoic band within the lesion suggestive of a central scar may be seen in up to 20% of FNH [46]. Color doppler may demonstrate hypervascularity and subcapsular feeding vessels in LCA, and increased vascular flow within the scar in FNH.

CT scan findings are highly dependent on the phase of examination, so that every patient should undergo contrast enhanced triple phase imaging on a helical

Table 2. Liver cell adenoma (*LCA*) vs. focal nodular hyperplasia (*FNH*)

	LCA	FNH
US	Hyperechoic (high fat content) areas of hemorrhage	Hyper-, iso- (may be missed altogether), or hypoechoic Hyperechoic central scar in 20% [46]
CT pre-contrast	Hypodense, patchy	Hypo- or isodense [9, 46–48] Central stellate scar
CT post-contrast	Arterial enhancement	Arterial enhancement
MR	Very variable – hyperintense T1 and T2	Hypointense T1, hyperintense T2
HIDA	Mostly "cold"	Mostly "hot"
Tc-99 m	80% "cold"	80% "hot"
Angiography	Hypervascular – peripheral vessels	Hypervascular – spoke-wheel pattern

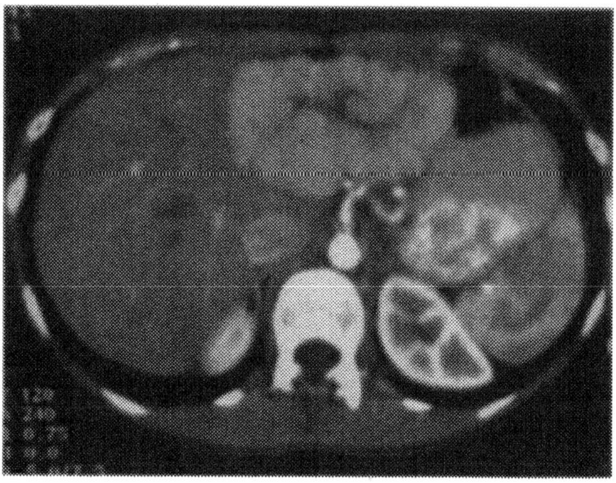

Fig. 5. FNH shown on a contrast-enhanced CT. Note the hypervascular lesion and the hypodense central scar (same case as Fig. 4a)

scanner. A high fat content renders LCA hypodense on plain CT scan, and as with US there may be the picture of a resolving hematoma. FNH is usually hypo- or isodense on unenhanced CT [9, 46–48]. The hypodense central scar, although characteristic, is appreciable in one-third of cases only (Fig. 5) [46].

In the arterial phase LCA may show early peripheral enhancement with a centripetal pattern due to subcapsular feeding vessels, returning to iso-hypodensity in portal phase [49]. FNH usually enhances in the hepatic arterial phase, and becomes isodense in the portal phase with a relatively hyperdense central scar.

On the whole, MR findings of LCA are variable and nonspecific and it is therefore difficult to distinguish LCA from HCC on imaging alone. LCA is a hyperintense lesion on T1 and T2 weighting with a heterogeneous appearance. Expert hepatic radiological evaluation is essential to interpret the range of findings in these cases [50–55].

Tc-99 m sulphur colloid scans show a cold lesion in 80% of LCA, though a small percentage may show some uptake because of good vascularity of Kupffer cells [56]. Similarly, hepatobiliary scan may demonstrate an uptake without any excretion as the lesion is devoid of biliary radicles. Contrary to LCA, 80% of FNH demonstrate an increased uptake of Tc-99 m sulphur colloid.

Having used all available modalities, there is still often doubt about the diagnosis. The images will provide anatomical guidance, and allow some assessment of operative risk, since central lesions will demand a more extensive operative procedure and so tend to suggest a more conservative approach than that for peripheral lesions. In the final analysis it is the risk of malignancy which will dictate the management policy.

Which LCAs Are Premalignant?

LCA is a rare lesion with only a few hundred cases reported over the last three decades. While malignant transformation of LCA is perhaps an equally rare phenomenon [57], the exact risk remains unquantified [58]. To the best of our knowledge, less than ten reports of a benign diagnosis followed up to a convincing malignant transformation have been reported in the literature [57, 59–62]. In a large collected review by Foster and Berman [57], only 5 out of 39 (13%) unresected LCA patients revealed malignant transformation with an average time interval of 4.5 years (range 2–7 years). Whether this represents a coincidence or a logical progression to be expected if the tumors were not resected remains debatable. Two-thirds of 22 patients with unresected or incompletely resected LCA in this series showed decrease in size on follow-up studies, while the remainder were unchanged. The factors relevant for regression were indeterminate. None of the patients developed rupture and few patients within this group developed any symptoms. Another recent study from Rotterdam [63] reported malignant transformation in two out of eight (25%) patients with unresected proven LCA over a median follow-up of 39 months (range 2–6 years). The disease was stable in three patients and regressed in the remaining three patients. As liver resection has become safer and more widely practiced, the risk of resection may now be less than the risk of malignant transformation.

What criteria should then be adopted for the management of proven LCA? If a conservative approach is to be pursued, this must include active long-term follow-up with regular scans. Certainly no sex steroids should be administered. The association of LCA and HCC with the use of oral contraceptive medication (OCM) is also well accepted [64, 65], although the association may be independent of any association of adenoma to carcinoma. Shrinkage of LCA following cessation of oestrogenic and androgenic hormone therapy is widely reported [60–62, 66] but the risk of subsequent malignant change, though small, remains unaltered [57, 58]. Many surgeons would now advocate resection of all LCAs which are larger than 4 cm, or are symptomatic, or in which the diagnosis is in doubt. The threshold for resection will depend on these factors as well as assessment of the operative risks, taking account of the fitness of the patient and the magnitude of the surgery required.

What Is the Optimum Surveillance Program for Presumed Benign Liver Lesion?

No definite recommendations exist for the optimum surveillance of benign liver lesions. LCA remains the most significant of these lesions because of its propensity to malignant transformation. Hemangiomas on the contrary are extremely benign lesions with no evidence of malignant transformation even on long-term follow-up [67, 68]. FNH may occupy an intermediate position, with a relatively low (but not absent) risk of malignant change. For LCA, serial hepatic ultrasound evaluation at 6- to 12-month intervals is perhaps a reasonable plan. Further tests should be performed if these show a serial change. Alpha fetoprotein at best is an inconsistent marker of malignant transformation in an LCA [69] and normal levels certainly do not exclude a malignancy.

References

1. Hattner RS, Engelstad BL (1983) Diagnostic imaging and quantitative physiological function using radionuclide techniques in gastrointestinal disease. In: Sleisinger MH, Fordtran JS (eds) Gastrointestinal disease. Saunders, Toronto, p 1667
2. Leslie DF, Johnson CD, Johnson CM, et al. (1995) Distinction between cavernous haemangioma of the liver and hepatic metastases on CT: value of contrast enhancement patterns. Am J Roentgenol 164:625–629
3. Birnbaum BA, Weinreb JC, Megibow AJ, et al. (1990) Definitive diagnosis of hepatic hemangiomas: MR imaging versus Tc-99m-labeled red blood cell SPECT. Radiology 176:95–101
4. Mergo PJ, Ros PR (1998) Benign lesions of the liver. Radiol Clin North Am 36:319–331
5. Johnson CM, Sheedy PF, Stanson AW, et al. (1985) Computed tomography and angiography of cavernous haemangiomas of the liver. Radiology 138:115–121
6. Casarella WJ, Knowles DM, Wolffe M, et al. (1978) Hyperplasia and liver cell adenoma: radiologic and pathologic differentiation. AJR 131:393–402
7. Goldstein HM, Neiman HL, Mena E, et al. (1974) Angiographic findings in benign liver cell tumours. Radiology 110:339–343
8. Welch TJ, Sheedy PF, Johnson IT, et al. (1985) Focal nodular hyperplasia and hepatic adenoma: comparision of angiography, CT, US and scintigraphy. Radiology 156:593–595
9. Rogers JV, Mack LA, Freeny PC, et al. (1981) Hepatic focal nodular hyperplasia: angiography, CT, sonography and scintigraphy. Am J Roenrgenol 137:983–990
10. Bellavia R, Haaga JR, Herbener T (1998) Liver biopsy. In: Gazelle GS, Saini S, Mueller PR (eds) Hepatobiliary and pancreatic radiology-imaging and intervention. Thieme, New York, pp 400–416
11. Ha HK, Sachs PB, Haaga JR, et al. (1991) CT guided liver biopsy: an update. Clin Imaging 15:99–104
12. Buscarini L, Fornari F, Bolondi L, et al. (1990) Ultrasound guided fine needle biopsy of focal liver lesions. Techniques, diagnostic accuracy and complications: a retrospective study of 2091 biopsies. J Hepatol 11:344–348
13. Fornari F, Buscarini L (1992) Ultrasonically guided fine needle biopsy of gastrointestinal organs: indications, results and complications. Dig Dis 10:121–133
14. Gilmore IT, Burroughs A, Murray-Lyon IM, Williams R, Jenkins D, Hopkins A (1995) Indications, methods and outcomes of percutaneous liver biopsy in England and Wales: an audit by the British Society of Gastroenterology and the Royal College of Physicians of London. Gut 36:437–441
15. Gazelle GS, Haaga JR, Rowlands DY (1992) Effect of needle gauge, level of anticoagulation and target organ on bleeding associated with aspiration biopsy. Radiology 183:509–513
16. Murphy FB, Barefield KP, Steinberg HV, Bernardino ME (1988) CT or sonography guided biopsy of the liver in the presence of ascites: frequency of complications. Am J Roentgenol 151:485–486
17. Quaghebeur G, Thompson JN, Blumgart LH, Benjamin IS (1991) Implantation of hepatocellular carcinoma after percutaneous needle biopsy. J Roy Coll Surg Edin 36:127

18. San Felippo PM, Beahrs OH, Weiland LH (1974) Cystic disease of the liver. Ann Surg 179:922–925
19. Benhamou JP, Menu Y (1994) Nonparasitic cystic disease of the liver and intrahepatic biliary tree. In: Blumgart LH (ed) Surgery of the liver and biliary tract, 2nd edn. Churchill Livingstone, London, pp 1197–1210
20. Moreaux J, Bloch P (1971) Les kystes biliaires solitaires du foie. Archives Francaises des Maladies de l'Appareil Digestif 60:203–224
21. Frisell J, Rojdmark S, Arvidsson H, Lundh G (1979) Compression of the inferior caval vein – a rare complication of a large non-parasitic liver cyst. Acta Med Scand 205:541–542
22. Santman FW, Thijs LG, Van der Veen EA, Den Otter G, Block P (1977) Intermittent jaundice: a rare complication of solitary nonparasitic liver cyst. Gastroenterology 72:325–328
23. Clinkscales NB, Trigg LP, Poklepovic J (1985) Obstructive jaundice secondary to benign hepatic cyst. Radiology 154:643–644
24. Cappell MS (1988) Obstructive jaundice from benign, nonparasitic hepatic cysts: identification of risk factors and percutaneous aspiration for diagnosis and treatment. Am J Gastroenterol 83:93–96
25 Lebon J, Bourgeon R, Claude R (1955) Kyste solitaire du foie. Archives Francaises des Maladies de l'Appareil Digestif 44:1274–1277
26. Johnstone AJ, Turnbull LW, Allan PL, Garden OJ (1993) Cholangitis and Budd-Chiari syndrome as complications of simple cystic liver disease – a case report. HPB Surg 6:223–228
27. Americks J, Appleman H, Frey C (1972) Malignant nonparasitic cyst of the liver. Ann Surg 172:713–716
28. Sood SC, Watson A (1974) Solitary cyst of liver presenting as an abdominal emergency. Postgrad Med J 50:48
29. Morino M, De Giuli M, Festa V, Garrone C (1994) Laparoscopic management of symptomatic nonparasitic cysts of the liver: indications and results. Ann Surg 219:157–164
30. Gigot JF, Legrand M, Hubens G, et al. (1996) Laparoscopic treatment of nonparasitic liver cysts: adequate selection of patients and surgical technique. World J Surg 20:556–561
31. Sanchez H, Gagner M, Rossi R, et al. (1991) Surgical management of nonparasitic cystic liver disease. Am J Surg 161:113–119
32. Fernandez M, Cacioppo JC, Davis RP, Nora P (1984) Management of solitary nonparasitic liver cyst. Am Surg 50:205–208
33. Rashed A, May RE, Williamson RCN (1982) The management of large congenital liver cysts. Postgrad Med J 58:536
34. Roemer CE, Ferrucci JT Jr, Mueller PR, et al. (1981) Hepatic cysts: diagnosis and therapy by sonographic needle aspiration. Am J Roentgenol 136:1065
35. Saini S, Mueller PR, Ferrucci JT Jr, et al. (1983) Percutaneous aspiration of hepatic cysts does not provide definitive therapy. Am J Roentgenol 141:559
36. Kakizaki K, Yamauchi H, Teshima S (1998) Symptomatic liver cyst: special reference to surgical management. HPB Surg 5:192–195
37. Andersson R, Jeppsson B, Lunderquist A, Bengmark S (1989) Alcohol sclerotherapy of nonparasitic cysts of the liver. Br J Surg 76:254–255
38. Henne-Bruns D, Klomp HJ, Kremer B (1990) Nonparasitic liver cysts and polycystic liver disease: results of surgical treatment. Hepatogastroenterology 40:1–5
39. Bean WJ, Rodan BA (1985) Hepatic cysts: treatment with alcohol. Am J Roentgenol 144:237
40. Furata T, Yoshida Y, Saku M, et al. (1990) Treatment of symptomatic nonparasitic liver cysts: surgical treatment versus alcohol injection therapy. HPB Surg 2:269
41. Kairaluoma MI, Leinonen A, Stohlberg M, et al. (1989) Percutaneous aspiration and alcohol sclerotherapy for symptomatic hepatic cysts: an alternative to surgical intervention. Ann Surg 210:208
42. Montorsi M, Torzilli G, Fumagalli U, et al. (1994) Percutaneous alcohol sclerotherapy of simple hepatic cysts: results from a multi-centric survey in Italy. HPB Surg 8:89
43. Rosenberg GV (1956) Solitary non-parasitic cysts of the liver. Am J Surg 91:441–444
44. Coffey RJ, Fitzmaurice MTA (1959) Non-parasitic hepatocystic disease: a report of 9 cases. Ann Surg 25:301–305
45. Longmire WP (1965) Hepatic surgery. Trauma, tumors and cysts. Ann Surg 161:1–14
46. Shamsi K, De Schepper A, Degryse H, Deckers F (1993) Focal nodular hyperplasia of the liver: radiologic findings. Abdominal Imaging 18:32–38
47. Shirkhoda A, Farah MC, Bernacki E, et al. (1994) Hepatic focal nodular hyperplasia: CT and sonographic spectrum. Abdominal Imaging 19:34–38
48. Paulson EK, McClennon JS, Washington K, et al. (1994) Hepatic adenoma: MR characteristics and correlation with pathologic findings. Am J Roentgenol 163:113–116

49. Mathieu D, Bruneton JN, Drouillard J, et al. (1986) Hepatic adenomas and focal nodular hyperplasia: dynamic CT study. Radiology 160:53–58
50. Chung KY, Mayo-Smith WW, Saini S, et al. (1995) Hepatocellular adenoma: MR imaging features with pathologic correlation. Am J Roentgenol 165:303–308
51. Lee M, Humm B, Saini S (1991) Focal nodular hyperplasia of the liver: MR findings in 35 proved cases. Am J Roentgenol 56:317–320
52. Virgin V, Flejou J, Arrive L, et al. (1992) Focal nodular hyperplasia of the liver MR imaging and pathological correlation in 37 patients. Radiology 184:699–703
53. Buelow PC, Pantongrag-Brown L, Buck JL, et al. (1996) Focal nodular hyperplasia of the liver: imaging-pathological correlation. Radiographics 16:369–388
54. Rummeny E, Weissleder R, Sironi S, et al. (1989) Central scars in primary liver tumors: MR features, specificity and pathologic correlation. Radiology 171:323–326
55. Mahfouz A, Hamm B, Tapitz M, Wolf K (1993) Hypervascular liver lesions. Differentiation of focal nodular hyperplasia from malignant tumours with dynamic gadolinium enhanced MR imaging. Radiology 186:133–138
56. Lubbers PR, Ross PR, Goodman ZD, Ishak KG (1987) Accumulation of technitium-99 m sulphur colloid by hepatocellular adenoma: scintigraphic-pathologic correlation. Am J Roentgenol 148:1105–1108
57. Foster JH, Berman MM (1994) The malignant transformation of liver cell adenomas. Arch Surg 129:712–717
58. Nagorney DM (1996) Are hepatic adenomas premalignant? HPB Surg 10:59–63
59. Leese T, Farges O, Bismuth H (1988) Liver cell adenomas: a 12-year surgical experience from a specialist hepato-biliary unit. Ann Surg 208:558–564
60. Tesluk H, Lawrie J (1981) Hepatocellular adenoma: its transformation to carcinoma in a user of oral contraceptives. Arch Pathol Lab Med 105:296–299
61. Gordon SC, Reddy KR, Livingstone AS, et al. (1986) Resolution of a contraceptive-steroid-induced hepatic adenoma with subsequent evolution into hepatocellular carcinoma. Ann Intern Med 105:547–549
62. Gyorffy EJ, Bredfeldt JE, Black WC (1989) Transformation of hepatic cell adenoma to hepatocellular carcinoma due to oral contraceptive use. Ann Intern Med 110:489–490
63. de Wilt JH, de Man RA, Lameris JS, et al. (1998) Hepatocellular adenoma in 20 patients; recommendations for treatment. Nederlands Tijdschrift voor Geneeskunde 142:2459–2463
64. Edmondson HA, Henderson B, Benton B (1976) Liver cell adenomas associated with use of oral contraceptives. N Engl J Med 294:47S, 0–472
65. Henderson BE, Preston-Martin S, Edmondson HA, et al. (1983) Hepatocellular carcinoma and oral contraceptives. Br J Cancer 48:437–440
66. Iwatsuki S, Todo S, Starzl TE (1990) Excisional therapy for benign hepatic lesions. Surg Gynecol Obstet 171:240–246
67. Weimann A, Ringe B, Klempnauer J, et al. (1997) Benign liver tumours: differential diagnosis and indications for surgery. World J Surg 21:983–990
68. Kerlin P, Davis GL, McGill DB, et al. (1983) Hepatic adenoma and focal nodular hyperplasia: clinical, pathological and radiologic features. Gastroenterology 84:994–1002
69. Foster JH, Berman MM (1994) The malignant transformation of liver cell adenomas. Arch Surg 129:712–717

Surgical Management

Jonathan Koea · Yuman Fong

Introduction

Benign liver lesions represent a management and therapeutic challenge for the hepatobiliary surgeon. They are the most common group of lesions affecting the liver and, with the increased use of radiological intervention, many more hepatic abnormalities are being identified and referred for surgical consultation. In addition, their management is often less clearly defined than that for malignancies as knowledge of the natural history of benign lesions, in spite of their frequency, is limited. This chapter reviews the controversies in the management of the three most common benign soft tissue lesions (hepatic adenoma, solitary hepatic cysts and giant hemangioma) in the liver as all three disorders are not infrequently encountered by hepatobiliary surgeons.

Controversies

- Is the lesion premalignant?
- Is the risk of intraperitoneal rupture significant?
- What is the natural history of the untreated condition - is it necessary to treat?
- What is the optimal treatment strategy - surgical resection vs. nonresectional methods?

Hepatic Adenomas

Liver cell adenomas are an uncommon problem characteristically affecting young women of childbearing age. The clinical suspicion that these lesions are premalignant has led to the recommendation that all adenomas be resected to prevent the development of cancer [1]. However, the resection of multiple adenomas may pose significant risk to the patient's life and it is currently unclear what constitutes the optimum treatment for multifocal disease. Recommendations for treatment range from observation only to total hepatectomy and orthotopic liver transplantation.

Is This Lesion Premalignant?

The risk of malignant transformation of a hepatic adenoma in patients without diffuse metabolic disease is not known. A review of the literature demonstrates only eight reports of clearly documented malignant transformation within a hepatic cell adenoma (Table 3). The paucity of reports of malignant transformation does indicate that this is a rare problem. For select patients with multifocal disease with medical or technical contraindications to surgery a policy of careful observation may be justified. However, because malignant transformation may not be easily detected, we still recommend resection of all adenomas if no contraindication exists. In a significant proportion of patients who develop carcinoma, serum α-fetoprotein levels are normal (Table 3), which makes close observation for malignant change problematic. This situation is further confounded by the fact that the definition between a benign adenoma and well-differentiated hepatocellular carcinoma is often contentious and pathologists may disagree on the diagnostic criteria for both tumors. A negative percutaneous needle aspiration biopsy is difficult to interpret due to possible sampling errors as adenomas can harbor small foci of differentiated carcinoma [8]. In addition, some benign adenomas - particularly those associated with the use of anabolic steroids [1, 5] - may exhibit cellular atypia.

Table 3. Summary of published reports clearly documenting malignant transformation in a hepatic adenoma

Reference	Sex/age	Number of adenomas	Interval (years)	*a*FP level	Resectable	Outcome
Tesluk [2]	F/34	Solitary	3	–	Yes	Postop death
Gordon [3]	F/36	Solitary	7	Normal	Yes	NED 6 years
Leese [1]	M/13	Multiple	5	High	Transplant	NED 1 year
Gyorffy [4]	F/53	Multiple	2	High	No	DOD 7 months
Foster [5]	F/56	Multiple	5	Increased	No	DOD 5 months
Ferrel [6]	F/29	Solitary	–	Normal	Yes	NED 1 year
Perret [7]	F/24	Solitary	–	Normal	Yes	NED 1 year
Weiman [8]	NS	Solitary	Increased	Normal	Yes	NED 1 year

*a*FP, *a* fetoprotein; DOD, dead of disease; NED, no evidence of disease.

Similarly no clear relationship has been established between the size of a hepatic adenoma and the risk of developing cancer [3].

The exact effect of estrogens and pregnancy on the tumorigenic potential of hepatic adenomas remains to be clarified. However, estrogens may potentiate the effects of carcinogens in experimental animals [9] and growth of adenomas has been noted in patients receiving estrogen containing medications [10]. However, none of 16 women who became pregnant after removal of their adenomas had a known recurrence [10]. Long-term follow-up of these patients following complete resection of their adenomas has never demonstrated any evidence of either recurrent adenoma or carcinoma [5]. Hepatocellular carcinoma has developed in at least two patients following regression of adenoma after cessation of the oral contraceptive [2].

Is the Risk of Intraperitoneal Rupture Significant?

Rupture of an adenoma with associated intra-abdominal hemorrhage is a relatively rare event, which however carries a mortality of up to 70% [11]. Increased risk of adenoma rupture is associated with estrogenic stimulation. Rooks et al. [10] reported rupture in five of six women who were pregnant or within 6 weeks postpartum at the time of diagnosis of the adenoma. Rapid growth and rupture of adenoma also appears more likely to occur in women who use oral contraceptives than in women who do not use estrogen-containing medications [10]. In contrast, less than 30% of nonpregnant women had evidence of rupture as a clinical presentation. In almost all cases of intraperitoneal rupture there is a symptomatic prodrome in previously asymptomatic lesions [12].

The risk of bleeding within adenomas is at least partly related to the size and site of the lesion. Ribero et al. [11] found that the majority of adenomas greater than 4 cm in diameter had evidence of bleeding either within the lesion or into the peritoneal cavity. However, massive intraperitoneal hemorrhage has been reported with very small lesions [10] and the relationship between increasing size and the risk of rupture is not constant [10, 11]. In addition, the site of the adenoma also influences the risk of rupture with peripherally placed tumors most likely to result in intraperitoneal hemorrhage. In contrast, central lesions are more likely to be associated with self-limiting intratumoral bleeding without hemoperitoneum [8].

What Is the Natural History of the Untreated Condition: Is It Necessary to Treat?

There is little information available in the literature on the natural history of unresected lesions. Most reports are in resected patients and follow-up is often short. In ten patients in whom the tumor was biopsied or partially resected prior to a follow-up of between 7 months and 11 years [1, 10, 13–17], tumor size decreased in seven (in five following the cessation of oral contraceptives, and in two patients following hepatic artery embolization or ligation). There was no change in tumor size in the three untreated patients. None of the adenomas increased in size and no patient developed intra-abdominal hemorrhage or carcinoma during the follow-up period. In addition, there are reports of 13 patients with multiple adenomas who were followed for between 3 months and 11 years [14, 16, 18–23]. These tumors decreased in size during follow-up in seven patients (three of whom had stopped taking the oral contraceptive) and were unchanged in four patients. In one patient there was an increase in tumor size after 3 years of observation, which required resection. None of these 12 patients experienced rupture or carcinomatous transformation.

Our current recommendation for the management of adenomas is to resect all solitary lesions in patients with no contraindications to surgery or multifocal lesions if they are technically approachable, particularly lesions associated with elevations in α-fetoprotein or symptoms. Resection should be considered in patients taking estrogen-containing medications such as fertility drugs or in whom pregnancy is likely due to the risk of growth stimulation, intraperitoneal hemorrhage and malignant change regardless of size or symptomatology. Others have advocated a policy of observation with regular ultrasound and α-fetoprotein determinations and the avoidance of estrogen-containing medication in asymptomatic patients with an adenoma less than 4 cm in diameter.

What Is the Optimal Treatment Strategy? Formal Surgical Resection Versus Enucleation

Operative techniques available to the surgeon are anatomical resection or lesional enucleation. Hepatic resection has been the traditional "gold standard" of treatment for adenomas. This has been accompanied by complication rates of up to 33% and deaths, though rare, have occurred due to intraoperative blood loss even in recent series [8]. In addition, resection may not be curative as there has been at least one widespread recurrence of adenomas in a patient following trisegmentectomy for multiple lesions [24].

Eckhauser [25] described the technique of enucleation as applied to adenomas and concluded that it provided a safe alternative to conventional segmental resection, although anatomical resection is probably safer for large central lesions. To date there have been no documented recurrences after enucleation in women with solitary lesions who discontinue the oral contraceptive. In addition, this procedure is safe and accompanied by minimal blood loss and reasonable tumor clearance. Even with formal hepatic resection it is not necessary to take a margin of normal hepatic tissue. Liver transplantation for large lesions has also been described and has been suggested in patients with large unresectable lesions involving both lobes as prophylaxis against rupture or malignant transformation [26], although this is rarely indicated.

The application of laparoscopic technology to liver resection, particularly small superficial lesions, has provided suitably trained surgeons with a minimally invasive technique with which to treat these lesions [27]. In a woman of child-bearing age who wishes to take oral contraceptives or begin a family, laparoscopic resection may provide an oncologically safe and minimally invasive method of resecting these lesions and alleviating patient and physician anxiety.

Giant Hemangioma

Cavernous hemangiomas are found in 2% of patients undergoing autopsy [11] and are the most common benign tumors of the liver. Historically, most lesions were reported in symptomatic patients and this encouraged the liberal application of surgical resection. However, the demographics of presentation has changed as the incidental finding of liver hemangioma has increased and as more patients undergo radiological imaging of the upper abdomen. This has resulted in a parallel increase in surgical referrals for this condition. There is general agreement that small lesions require no intervention once a secure diagnosis is made; however, the management of giant hemangiomas (defined as those larger than 4 cm in diameter) is thought to behave differently from smaller lesions with a tendency to enlarge and rupture [28].

Is This Lesion Premalignant?

Malignant transformation of a hemangioma is unheard of. Trastek et al. [28] followed 36 patients with sequential CT scans for between 1 and 15 years and recorded no cases of malignant degeneration. However, Lise et al. [29] have reported a mistakenly diagnosed hemangioma on preoperative imaging in one patient who, following resection, was found to have an angiosarcoma – emphasizing the importance of an accurate secure diagnosis in the management of this condition. Other lesions confused with hemangiomas include hemangioendotheliomas. Since biopsy of hemangioma is associated with a significant risk of hemorrhage requiring surgical intervention [28], this diagnosis should rely on tagged red cell scans [8] and the typical appearance on ultrasound, CT scan and MRI [11]. Occasionally direct angiography will be necessary.

Is the Risk of Intraperitoneal Rupture Significant?

There are a number of reports of spontaneous hemorrhage from cavernous hemangioma which were often fatal. Shumaker [30] estimated the risk of rupture at nearly 20% in 1942. However, Henson et al. [31] found no rupture in 35 patients and Adam et al. [32] reported spontaneous rupture in only 1 of 106 patients. Farges et al. [33] reported a total of 28 cases of rupture in the medical literature since 1898. There are, however, anecdotal reports of rupture associated with forced valsalva, pregnancy or following increased growth on estrogen therapy [28, 34]. Given the incidence of hemangiomas found at autopsy and the bias for reporting symptomatic patients, the risk of spontaneous hemorrhage must therefore be very small. Farges et al. [33] have also reported two patients with large hemangioma and Kassabach-Merrit syndrome which resulted in spontaneous hemorrhage. Both rupture and pain can occur in small lesions [33] and probably represent areas of intralesional thrombosis and necrosis complicated by capsular rupture. However, these complications are most frequently seen in lesions larger than 4 cm in diameter.

What Is the Natural History of the Untreated Condition? Is It Necessary to Treat?

Pietrabissa et al. [35] followed 20 patients with giant hemangiomas with clinical examination and ultrasound for between 16 and 72 months. In this period no patient developed symptoms or rupture. Most lesions remained unchanged in size but a small increase in diameter ($\leq$0.5 cm) was observed in three patients. These investigators also noted two rapidly growing lesions, both of which had an initial diameter of less than 10 cm. No specific feature at the time of initial presentation such as age, hormonal treatment or associated pathology could be identified retrospectively in these two patients to allow differentiation from those with stable hemangiomas. Similarly, Lise et al. [29] found mild enlargement of untreated hemangiomas on sequential ultrasound scans in only 3 of 26 patients, none of whom developed symptoms. Trastek [28] has followed 36 patients with giant hemangioma for up to 15 years. During follow-up no patient died, no tumor bled and no patient experienced an increase in symptoms or altered quality of life due to their hemangioma. No patient that was observed has subsequently been required to undergo surgical resection for any reason. On sequential CT scans, three of these lesions have decreased in size while four have increased. These investigators also made the observation that enlargement is probably due to ectasia rather than further neoplastic growth, and infiltrative growth does not occur. Consequently enlargement of a lesion during a period of observation is unlikely to compromise later resection as the interface between tumor and normal liver is unchanged by expansion. Farges [33] reported that symptoms have diminished or become minimal in 21 of 25 patients who were initially symptomatic but were managed with observation only. Pain proved to be related to the tumor itself in a little over half of the cases (42% of patients presenting with pain were found to have other disorders responsible) and 25% (two of eight patients) carefully selected for resection had persisting pain following uncomplicated resection [33].

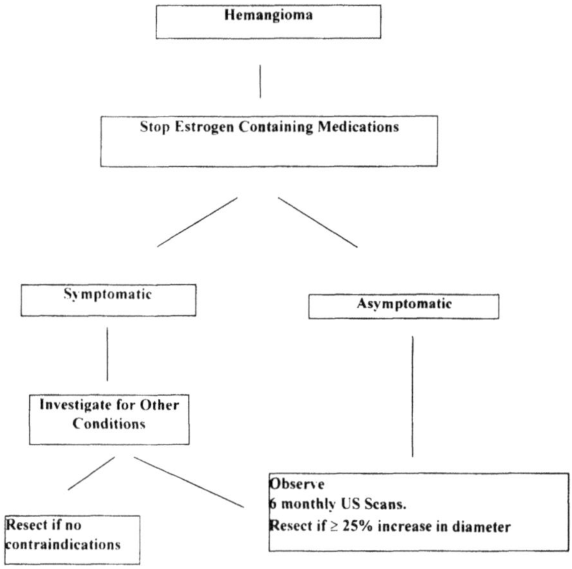

Fig. 6. Management algorithm for hepatic hemangioma

Seven of nine patients in the series of Pietrabissa et al. [35] with a lesion exceeding 10 cm in diameter presented with symptoms and were resected compared with only 2 of 37 patients with hemangioma between 4.0 and 5.9 cm. These authors concluded that symptoms were more likely to be associated with very large hemangiomas. It has also been suggested that lesions of greater than 10 cm in diameter have a greater potential for internal bleeding, growth and rupture [36], which would provide justification for the prophylactic removal of asymptomatic large lesions. However, Pietrabissa et al. [35] noted rapid enlargement in two lesions whose initial diameter was less than 10 cm and minor size changes in most lesions with an initial diameter between 4.0 and 7.9 cm. The pattern of growth on follow-up CT scan or ultrasound can be used to decide which asymptomatic patient may benefit from surgery. An increase of 25% in diameter within a period of 6 months should provide the threshold for surgical intervention [35].

Current recommendations for therapy would be to observe asymptomatic lesions of any size with serial ultrasound examinations. Patients should be counseled against intake of estrogen-containing medications and pregnancy should be avoided. An increase in size of hemangioma of 25% or greater during observation should be an indication for either enucleation, anatomical resection or transplantation depending on size and distribution within the liver. Symptomatic patients should be thoroughly investigated for other disorders and considered for resection. The rare patient with Kasabach-Merritt syndrome should be considered for early operation (Fig. 6). For patients who are unsuitable for surgical intervention, external beam radiation may be a useful measure.

What Is the Optimal Treatment Strategy? Surgical Resection Versus Nonresectional Methods?

The management of giant hemangioma should be based on the balance between the estimated operative risk and the outcome achieved with surgical resection. Trastek [28] has reported one patient treated with external beam radiation therapy which was followed by a marked reduction in the size of the hemangioma. The risks with this therapy are minimal as the usual dose is low and is well tolerated by the adjacent liver. Systemic steroid therapy has also been used with some success in infants; however, the effectiveness of steroids in adults is unknown [28].

Two surgical techniques have been utilized in the management of hemangioma: formal resection and lesional enucleation. Since the growth of a hemangioma causes only compression of the surrounding hepatic parenchyma, there is usually a relatively avascular connective tissue plane surrounding the lesion. Enucleation in this plane with temporary inflow occlusion allows safe removal of giant hemangiomas with minimal blood loss and preservation of all normal liver tissue [37]. The reported mortality for elective liver resection for hemangioma is low (0%–4%) when performed by experienced surgical teams [33]. However, recurrence following surgical resection has been reported and has resulted in reoperation [34]. Transplantation has been successfully performed in very selected cases with large diffuse lesions associated with the Kasabach-Merritt syndrome [33].

Solitary Hepatic Cyst

Simple hepatic cysts are uncommon. Their overall prevalence is 0.1% to 2.5% of abdominal ultrasound examinations [38]. Usually they are asymptomatic and are more common in females than males [38]. Simple cysts are lined by biliary columnar epithelium and usually contain clear or straw-colored fluid which can become dark after intracystic bleeding. Communication with the bile ducts is unusual. Most commonly they are located in the right lobe and are considered to be embryological malformations.

Is This Lesion Premalignant?

Contrary to other cystic diseases of the liver such as Caroli's disease and choledochal cysts, malignancy is rare in simple cysts [39, 40]. Reports of tumors arising in preexisting simple cysts have been disparate and include mucoepidermoid carcinoma [41], multi-focal papillary cystadenocarcinoma [42], and squamous cell carcinoma [43]. The rarity indicates that these may be coincidental associations rather than complications. However, the observation of cystadenoma and cystadenocarcinoma in association with hamartomatous bile ducts does suggest that there is a causal link between the two [42].

Is the Risk of Intraperitoneal Rupture Significant?

All benign cysts are subject to a variety of complications. Bleeding into or infection of the cyst contents may result in pain. Enlargement of cysts does occur without obvious cause and can lead to abdominal distension [39], obstructive jaundice or intraperitoneal rupture [44, 45]. Rupture has been only rarely reported and is usually associated with trauma rather than spontaneous.

What Is the Natural History of the Untreated Condition? Is It Necessary to Treat?

The majority of simple cysts are asymptomatic. However, complications are more frequent in cysts greater than 8 cm in diameter [46]. Periodic monitoring with ultrasound is prudent since growth in the absence of symptoms may mandate surgical intervention because of possible complications or concern regarding cystic neoplasm [46]. Growth probably occurs as evidenced by reports of simple cysts that contain several liters of fluid [47] and presentation with either abdominal wall ulceration [48] or dyspareunia [49].

For large symptomatic cysts either open or laparoscopic fenestration represents the optimal management strategy. Although sclerosis using percutaneous alcohol injection has been reported, the risk of biliary sclerosis from such treatment exists and can be catastrophic (Fig. 7).

What Is the Optimal Treatment Strategy: Surgical Fenestration Versus Nonresectional Methods

Ergun et al. [50] reported the first intervention with percutaneous cyst aspiration in a jaundiced patient. However, recurrence rates of up to 100% have been reported following simple aspiration. Bean and Rodan [51] reported the use of alco-

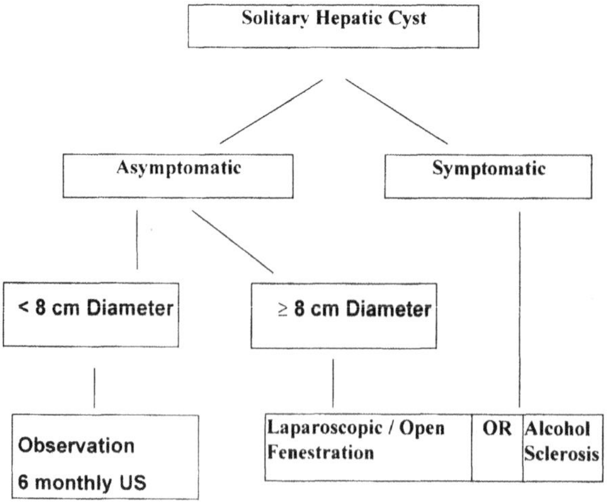

Fig. 7. Management algorithm for solitary simple hepatic cysts

hol to sclerose six symptomatic cysts in 1985 and several subsequent reports have shown this to be an effective form of therapy. Absolute alcohol is instilled with a percutaneous catheter placed under radiological guidance. Usually 25% of the cyst volume of alcohol is instilled for a 10- to 20-min dwell time and this is successful in over 95% of cases. For very large cysts, an indwelling catheter has been used for multiple therapies over a 24-h period. Common side effects are transient pain and a low-grade fever [47]. Moderate alcohol intoxication has occurred and blood alcohol levels correlate with the total volume of alcohol used. Recently minocycline and doxycycline have also been reported as effective sclerosants [52]. There is no clear consensus on the techniques used. However, a wide bore catheter is thought to be safer than a narrow one as the latter increases the time for drainage with concomitant increased risk for infection, bleeding, and systemic absorption of the sclerosant [53]. Cholangiography should also be performed prior to sclerosant injection to exclude a communication between the cyst and biliary tree [54]. The initial results with this technique are promising although the published follow-up is short. Sclerosis does not appear to compromise the prospects of subsequent fenestration should cyst recurrence develop. However, the primary concern is that any communication of the cyst with the biliary tree will result in biliary sclerosis.

Surgical fenestration of cysts without drainage of the residual cavity is recommended if surgery is thought indicated [55]. In Toronto, 17 of 22 patients treated with this method had excellent results with no complications. In comparison, four of the remaining five patients treated with either external or Roux-en-Y drainage suffered septic complications [46]. The development of laparoscopic cyst fenestration provides the hepatobiliary surgeon with a less invasive method of accomplishing these goals [56] and must be regarded as the treatment of choice. However, it must be emphasized that benign, asymptomatic, simple cysts of any size do not require treatment of any type.

References

1. Leese T, Farges O, Bismuth H (1988) Liver cell adenomas: a 12-year surgical experience from a specialist hepato-biliary unit. Ann Surg 208:558–564
2. Tesluk H, Lawrie J (1981) Hepatocellular adenoma: its transformation to carcinoma in a user of oral contraceptives. Arch Pathol Lab Med 105:296–299
3. Gordon SC, Reddy KR, Livingstone AS, Jeffers LJ, Schiff ER (1986) Resolution of a contraceptive-steroid-induced hepatic adenoma with subsequent evolution into a hepatocellular carcinoma. Ann Intern Med 105:547–549
4. Gyorffy EJ, Bredfeldt JE, Black WC (1989) Transformation of hepatic cell adenoma to hepatocellular carcinoma due to oral contraceptive use. Ann Intern Med 110:489–490
5. Foster JH, Berman MM (1994) The malignant transformation of liver cell adenomas. Arch Surg 129:712–717
6. Ferrel LD (1993) Hepatocellular carcinoma arising in a focus of multilobular adenoma: a case report. Am J Surg Pathol 17:525–529
7. Perret AG, Mosnier JF, Porcheron J, Cuilleron M, Berthoux P, Boucheron S, Audigier JC (1996) Role of oral contraceptive in the growth of a multilobular adenoma associated with hepatocellular carcinoma in a young woman. J Hepatol 25:976–979
8. Weiman A, Ringe B, Klempnauer J, Lamesch P, Gratz KF, Prokop M, Maschek H, Tusch G, Pichlmayr R (1997) Benign liver tumors: differential diagnosis and indications for surgery. World J Surg 21:983–991
9. Gindhart TD (1978) Liver tumors and oral contraceptives: pathology and pathogenesis. Ann Clin Lab Sci 8:443–446

10. Rooks JB, Ory HW, Ishak KG, et al. (1979) Epidemiology of hepatocellular adenoma: the role of oral contraceptive use. JAMA 242:644–648
11. Ribero A, Burgart LJ, Nagorney D, Gores GJ (1998) Management of liver adenomatosis: results with a conservative surgical approach. Liver Transplant Surg 4:388–398
12. Kent DR, Nissen ED, Nissen SE, Ziehm DJ (1978) Effect of pregnancy on liver tumor associated with oral contraceptives. Obstet Gynecol 51:148–151
13. Anderson PH, Packer JT (1976) Hepatic adenoma: observations after estrogen withdrawal. Arch Surg 111:898–900
14. Chan CK, Detmer DE (1977) Proper management of hepatic adenoma associated with oral contraceptives. Surg Gynecol Obstet 144:703–706
15. Edmondson HA, Reynolds TB, Henderson B, Benton B (1977) Regression of liver cell adenomas associated with oral contraceptives. Ann Intern Med 86:180–182
16. Neuberger J, Nunnerly HB, Davis M, Portmann B, Laws JW, Williams R (1980) Oral-contraceptive-associated liver tumors: occurrence of malignancy and difficulties in diagnosis. Lancet 1:273–276
17. Tao L-C (1991) Oral contraceptive-associated liver cell adenoma and hepatocellular carcinoma: cytomorphology and mechanism of malignant transformation. Cancer 68:341–347
18. Bein NN, Goldsmith HS (1977) Recurrent massive hemorrhage from benign hepatic tumors secondary to oral contraceptives. Br J Surg 64:433–435
19. Benedict KT, Chen PS, Janower ML, Farmelant MH, Howard JT, McDermott W (1979) Contraceptive associated hepatic tumor. Am J Roentgenol 132:452
20. Flejou J-F, Barge J, Menu Y, et al. (1985) Liver adenomatosis: an entity distinct from liver adenoma? Gastroenterology 89:1132–1138
21. Marks WH, Thompson N, Appleman H (1988) Failure of hepatic adenomas (HCA) to regress after discontinuance of oral contraceptives: an association with focal nodular hyperplasia (FNH) and uterine leiomyoma. Ann Surg 208:190–195
22. Ramseur WL, Cooper MR (1978) Asymptomatic liver cell adenomas: another case of resolution after discontinuation of oral contraceptive use. JAMA 239:1647–1648
23. Propst A, Propst T, Waldenberger P, Vogel W, Judmaier G (1995) A case of hepatocellular adenomatosis with a follow-up of 11 years. Am J Gastroenterol 90:1345–1346
24. Caballes RL, Caballes RA (1999) Multiple hepatocellular adenomas in a patient with a history of oral contraception. Int J Gynecol Obstet 64:177–180
25. Eckhauser FE, Knol JA, Raper SE, Thompson NW (1994) Enucleation combined with hepatic vascular exclusion is a safe and effective alternative to hepatic resection for liver cell adenoma. Am Surg 60:466–471
26. Mueller J, Keeffe EB, Esquivel CO (1995) Liver transplantation for treatment of giant hepatocellular adenomas. Liver Transplant Surg 1:99–102
27. Ferzli G, David A, Kiel T (1995) Laparoscopic resection of a large hepatic tumor. Surg Endosc 9:733–735
28. Trastek VF, van Heerden JA, Sheedi PF II, Adson MA (1983) Cavernous hemangiomas of the liver: resect or observe. Am J Surg 145:49–53
29. Lise M, Feltrin G, Da Pian PP, Miotto D, Pilati PL, Rubaltelli L, Zane D (1992) Giant cavernous hemangiomas: diagnosis and surgical strategies. World J Surg 16:516–520
30. Shumaker HB (1942) Hemangioma of the liver. Discussion of symptomatology and report of a patient treated by operation. Surgery 11:209–222
31. Henson SW, Gray HK, Dockerty MB (1956) Benign tumors of the liver. Surg Gynecol Obstet 103:327–331
32. Adam YG, Huvos AG, Fortner JG (1970) Giant hemangiomas of the liver. Ann Surg 172:239–245
33. Farges O, Daradkeh S, Bismuth H (1995) Cavernous hemangioma of the liver: are there any indications for resection. World J Surg 19:19–24
34. Conter RL, Longmire WP Jr (1988) Recurrent hemangiomas. Possible association with estrogen therapy. Ann Surg 207:115–119
35. Pietrabissa, Giulianotti P, Campatelli A, Di Candio G, Farina F, Signori S, Mosca F (1996) Management and follow-up of 78 giant haemangiomas of the liver. Br J Surg 83:915–918
36. Iwatsuki S, Todo S, Starzl TE (1990) Excisional therapy for benign hepatic lesions. Surg Gynecol Obstet 171:240–246
37. Bauer HU, Dennison AR, Mouton W, Stain SC (1992) Enucleation of giant hemangiomas of the liver. Technical and pathologic aspects of a neglected procedure. Ann Surg 216:673–676
38. Gaines PA, Sampson MA (1989) Prevalence and characterization of simple hepatic cysts by ultrasound examination. Br J Radiol 62:335–337

39. Roisman I, Barak V, Fields S, Bloom R, Manny J (1989) Solitary nonparasitic cyst of the liver: a rare cause of abdominal distension. Am J Gastroeneterol 84:1095–1099
40. Bloustein PA (1977) Association of carcinoma with congenital cystic conditions of the liver and bile ducts. Am J Gastroenterol 67:40–46
41. Hayashi I, Tomoda H, Tanimoto M, et al. (1987) Mucoepidermoid carcinoma arising from a preexisting cyst of the liver. J Surg Oncol 36:122–125
42. Rehulova E, Dite P, et al. (1981) Multifocal carcinoma arising from a congenital cyst of the liver and kidneys. Cesk Patol 17:198–203
43. Lynch MJ, McLeod MK, Weatherbee L, Gilsdorf JR, Guice KS, Eckhauser FE (1988) Squamous cell carcinoma of the liver arising from a solitary benign hepatic cyst. Am J Gastroenterol 83:426–431
44. Ayyash K, Haddad J (1988) Spontaneous rupture of a solitary hepatic nonparasitic cyst of the liver. Acta Chir Scand 154:241–243
45. Lotz GW, Stahlschmidt M (1989) Intra-abdominal bleeding after rupture of hepatic cyst. South Med J 82:667
46. Taylor BR, Langer B (1998) Current surgical management of hepatic cystic disease. Adv Surg 31:127–148
47. Kairaluoma MI, Leinonen A, Stahlberg M, et al. (1989) Percutaneous aspiration and alcohol sclerotherapy for symptomatic hepatic cysts: an alternative to surgical intervention. Ann Surg 208–215
48. Minton JP, Kinsey DL (1961) Surgical management of a recurrent solitary multilocular nonparasitic cyst of the liver. Am J Surg 102:710–712
49. Jennings WK (1939) Solitary nonparasitic cyst of the liver. Surgery 6:507–510
50. Ergun H, Wolf BH, Hissong SL (1980) Obstructive jaundice caused by polycystic liver disease. Radiology 136:435–436
51. Bean WJ, Rodan BA (1985) Hepatic cysts: treatment with alcohol. Am J Radiol 144:237–241
52. Hagiwara H, Kasahara A, Hayashi N, et al. (1992) Successful treatment of a hepatic cyst by one-shot instillation of minocycline chloride. Gastroenterology 103:675–677
53. Tokunaga K, Teplick SK, Banerjee B (1994) Simple hepatic cysts. First case of percutaneous drainage and sclerosis with doxycycline, with review of the literature. Dig Dis Sci 39:209–214
54. Forbes A, Murray-Lyon IM (1991) Cystic disease of the liver and biliary tract. Gut [Suppl] 1:S116–S122
55. Huguier M, Paquet JC, Roland J, Houry S, Lacaine F (1990) Biliary cysts of the liver. Dig Surg 7:93–97
56. Marvik R, Myrvold HE, Johnson G, et al. (1993) Laparoscopic ultrasonography and the treatment of hepatic cysts. Surg Laparosc Endosc 3:172–174

Invited Comment

O. James Garden

Benign hepatic lesions are not uncommon and generally give rise to problems of management due to difficulties in differentiating them from primary and secondary malignant hepatic tumors. Although the benign hepatic lesions are generally asymptomatic, they may declare themselves because of a mass effect or as a consequence of necrosis, thrombosis, hemorrhage or rupture. In such circumstances, the principal focus of management is not on whether such lesions should be treated but rather by which form of intervention.

Whilst the contributors from London and New York have been right to focus specifically on the nonoperative and surgical management of benign cystic and solid lesions, the difficulty of establishing a firm diagnosis by noninvasive means should not be underestimated. Routine liver function tests are invariably within normal limits in patients with benign hepatic pathology. Symptomatic benign lesions may be associated with increases in serum levels of liver analytes although elevation in tumor markers and the development of paraneoplastic syndromes are rarely observed with benign pathology. Whilst it is possible to characterize hepatic lesions using a variety of imaging tests, currently ultrasonography and computed tomography are pivotal in establishing a diagnosis. Nonetheless, as Benjamin and Gupta have indicated, magnetic resonance imaging may noninvasively characterize such lesions and have largely rendered obsolete angiography and isotope imaging. Concerns do remain over the safety of percutaneous tissue biopsy both in terms of the procedure precipitating hemorrhage and also due to the potential risk of dissemination of tumor cells. When faced with the anxious patient who wishes absolute reassurance regarding the nature of the hepatic lesion, it has to be accepted that a definitive diagnosis may not be certain until the lesion has been excised. For the frailer, elderly patient unfit for surgical intervention, a tissue diagnosis may provide reassurance and assist in determining prognosis.

Cysts

Nonparasitic cystic disease of the liver can be categorized into "simple" and "polycystic" variants. Simple cysts are also referred to as benign hepatic cysts, biliary cysts, congenital hepatic cysts, unilocular cysts of the liver and solitary cysts of the liver, although this latter categorization is inappropriate since simple cysts are invariably multiple. The importance of excluding a diagnosis of cystadenoma has previously been emphasized, although this lesion represents rare pathology, which has only been encountered on three occasions in our own unit over a 12-year period – when over 50 patients have undergone surgical intervention for symptomatic cystic disease of the liver. In such patients, excision of the entire cyst is mandatory to eliminate the risk of subsequent malignant transformation.

In our experience, percutaneous aspiration with or without sclerotherapy has little to offer the symptomatic patient and the advent of laparoscopic deroofing or fenestration is a more satisfactory approach [1]. Whilst we have embraced this new technology in the management of simple cysts, longer term follow-up of our own population does suggest that a minimally invasive approach may not always allow a sufficiently radical fenestration to prevent recurrence [2]. Similarly, simple deroofing of large centrally or posteriorly placed cysts at laparoscopic or open surgery may allow reconstitution of the cyst. In such patients we would now advocate the more radical approach of resection, which does not often entail substantial sacrifice of functioning hepatic parenchyma [2].

For patients with symptomatic polycystic liver disease, it is difficult to accept that a laparoscopic approach is likely to be successful. For the few patients with an obviously symptomatic dominant cyst, laparoscopic deroofing may have a limited role but experience with open surgery has long suggested that liver resection rather than limited cyst fenestration is likely to result in a better long-term outcome for the patient [3]. In our own series, reintervention following laparoscopic intervention for polycystic disease was invariable [2]. It is appreciated, however, that hepatic resection in such patients is fraught with difficulty. The vascular anatomy is distorted and postoperative ascites may be problematic. Although hepatic replacement may be considered in a few patients, this may seem an aggressive option for patients with normal liver function [4]. Furthermore, immunosuppressive therapy may have an adverse effect on those patients with renal involvement by polycystic disease. A combined liver and kidney transplant may be appropriate therapy for the patient with symptomatic polycystic disease and renal failure.

Solid Lesions

The management of benign solid lesions of the liver does pose some difficulties in management. However, the acceptance by all the authors that intervention is required for symptomatic patients with a suspected adenoma larger than 4 cm or when there is diagnostic doubt, leaves little scope for observation alone [5]. Whilst there is acceptance that the rarer adenoma is at risk of rupture, it has been difficult to quantify the risk of malignant transformation in such lesions [6, 7]. There are limitations with diagnostic needle biopsy and it may still be difficult to distinguish the histological features of a well-differentiated hepatoma from an adenoma following resection. Despite the one cited case of misdiagnosis, it seems that modern imaging techniques can safely differentiate hemangioma from other malignant vascular lesions. It would seem prudent to excise symptomatic lesions but an aggressive surgical approach for lesions measuring more than 4 cm in maximal diameter may not be appropriate for the asymptomatic patient with a recently diagnosed hemangioma. The difficulty of attributing symptoms to the hemangioma is evidenced by the occasional persistence of symptoms after resection [8]. Radiological surveillance may suffice in the patient who has been reassured of the benign nature of the lesion since life-threatening hemorrhage from such lesions is rare.

Conclusions

The management of both cystic and solid lesions of the liver will continue to challenge the clinician. Developments in radiological imaging have increased the detection of such lesions but at the same time have assisted by enabling these to be better characterized by noninvasive means. Whilst surgical intervention can be contemplated for the symptomatic patient, operation in the asymptomatic patient may be inappropriate unless the risk of complication can be well defined. When dealing with the individual patient, however, it may be difficult not to be pressurized into an operative approach when there remains doubt regarding the natural history of the hepatic lesion.

References

1. Klingler PJ, Gadenstatter M, Schmid T, et al. (1997) Treatment of hepatic cysts in the laparoscopic era. Br J Surg 84:438–444
2. Martin IJ, McKinley AJ, Currie EJ, et al. (1998) Tailoring the management of nonparasitic liver cysts. Ann Surg 228:167–172
3. Que F, Nagorney DM, Gross JB Jr, Torres VE (1995) Liver resection and cyst fenestration in the treatment of severe polycystic liver disease. Gastroenterology 108:487–494

4. Starzl TE, Reyes J, Tzakis A, et al. (1990) Liver transplantation for polycystic liver disease. Arch Surg 125:575–577
5. Nagorney DM (1995) Benign hepatic tumors: focal nodular hyperplasia and hepatocellular adenoma. World J Surg 19:13–18
6. Weimann A, Ringe B, Klempnauer J, et al. (1997) Benign liver tumors: differential diagnosis and indications for surgery. World J Surg 21:983–991
7. Belghiti J, Paterson D, Panis Y, et al. (1993) Resection of presumed benign liver tumours. Br J Surg 80:380–383
8. Farges O, Daradkeh S, Bismuth H (1995) Cavernous hemangiomas of the liver: are there any indications for resection? World J Surg 19:19–24

Editorial Comment

After reading the contributions by the leading hepatic surgeons from London, New York and Edinburgh it is clear that the vast majority of patients with benign lesions of the liver can be treated conservatively and re-assured, after appropriate noninvasive diagnostic work-up. Even if it is a cliché, let us repeat here: do not treat the image on CT, but the whole patient.

CHAPTER 5

Cholelithiasis

Chronic Cholecystitis

Samuel Eldar · Ibrahim Matter

Introduction

Gallstones are a major cause of morbidity. Over the past two decades, extensive progress has been achieved in the understanding, diagnosis, and treatment of gallstones and gallbladder disease. Long-lived studies such as oral cholecystography and intravenous cholangiography have been replaced by ultrasonography of the gallbladder, HIDA scintigraphy, and endoscopic retrograde cholangiopancreatography (ERCP) of the bile ducts. The decades-long supremacy of open surgical cholecystectomy for gallstones and gallbladder disease was challenged by gallstone-dissolution techniques and shock-wave lithotripsy and has now been replaced by laparoscopic cholecystectomy. With the modern approach new questions arise regarding the pathogenesis and risk factors of cholelithiasis, the management of incidental and asymptomatic gallstones, the correct order of procedures when choledocholithiasis is suspected, and the indications for intraoperative cholangiography.

Risk Factors in the Pathogenesis of Cholelithiasis

The general epidemiology of gallstone formation relates primarily to cholesterol and mixed stones, which comprise about 75% of the total of gallstones. Pigment stone formation has hardly been studied. Risk factors that have been established to be associated with pigment stones include age, chronic hemolytic states, biliary tract infection, cirrhosis, and alcoholism [1, 2]. Risk factors associated with cholesterol and mixed stones have been extensively reported. While some of the risk factors are no longer believed to be controversial, others are still under discussion. To the former group belong progressive age [3–6], female gender [3–5], geographic location (gallstone prevalence appears to be highest in the Scandinavian countries, northern Europe [4, 7], and Chile [8], and lowest in sub-Sahara Africa [9]), race and ethnicity (gallstone prevalence is over 70% in Pima women over age 25) [10]. Gallstones are common in various American Indian groups [11, 12] and particularly low among African blacks [13]. Parity, obesity [6], rapid and excessive weight loss [14, 15], parenteral nutrition [16], and Crohn's disease [17] are also known risk factors for stone formation.

Controversial risk factors with regards to cholelithiasis are family history [5, 18], diabetes mellitus [19, 20], lower socioeconomic status [21, 22], alcohol use that prevents cholelithiasis [23, 24], smoking [25, 26], use of oral contraceptives and estrogen replacement therapy [27, 28]. Conflicting evidence exists also with regards to the relation of serum cholesterol and serum triglyceride levels to cholelithiasis [25, 29–31]. Although extensively studied, the influence of fasting and dieting on the risk of gallstone formation has not yet been established [32, 33]. Several studies indicate that consumption of large amounts of sugar may increase the risk of cholelithiasis [33], while in vegetarians gallstone prevalence may be low [34]. No proven dietary recommendations are yet available to prevent gallstone formation. Regarding medications, clofibrate was clearly found to be associated with cholelithiasis [35]. Other lipid-lowering medications such as cholestyramine and nicotinic acid showed a similar tendency but yet of no statistical significance [35–37]. Controversial findings exist regarding the association of thiazide diuretics and acute cholecystitis [38, 39]. Studies in animal models and in humans suggest that aspirin may prevent cholelithiasis [40, 41].

Natural History of Asymptomatic and Mildly Symptomatic Gallstones

Friedman, discussing these particular groups, noted how difficult it was, firstly, to define the groups, and then, to follow them [42]. Comfort et al. from the Mayo Clinic were the first to report on asymptomatic gallstones [43]. They followed 112 patients with asymptomatic gallstones that were diagnosed during laparotomy for other intra-abdominal pathologies. Within a follow-up period of 10–20 years, 19% of the patients developed biliary colic, yielding an average annual rate of 1.4%. Lund described in 1960, 70 women and 25 men from Copenhagen, Denmark, who were followed for asymptomatic or for slightly symptomatic gallstones for 5–20 years [44]. The average annual rate for the development of severe symptoms or complications such as acute cholecystitis, jaundice or pancreatitis was 6% in women and 3% in men. These and other related studies [45–47] indicate that in patients with asymptomatic gallstones, biliary colic, acute cholecystitis, jaundice, or pancreatitis will develop in about 1%–2% per year, and after 20 years, two-thirds of patients will still be free of biliary complaints. When patients with mild complaints were studied, mainly in the form of dyspepsia and biliary colic, it was noted that complications developed at a rate slightly higher than that of asymptomatic patients, reaching 1%–3% per year [46–49]. Under these circumstances, after 20 years, about 54% of patients will still be free of complaints.

In view of this, the clinical approach depends on the primary leading assumption: considering that most of the patients develop symptoms before complications set in, it is justified to wait with surgery until complaints begin. If, on the other hand, we assume that complications may set in without preceding symptoms, and that their consequences may be hazardous, then it is justified to consider prophylactic cholecystectomy in asymptomatic patients. Patino and Quintero recently proposed criteria for prophylatic cholecystectomy. These included: life expectancy of more than 20 years, women younger than 60 years with calculi, concomitant diabetes mellitus, calculi smaller than 3 mm or larger than 2 cm, radiopaque calculi, polyps in the gallbladder, a nonfunctioning gallbladder, porcelain gallbladder, and individuals in geographic regions with a high prevalence of gallbladder cancer [50].

Treatment Modalities

In the late 1980s and early 1990s, a number of therapeutic techniques were investigated in an attempt to improve the approach to cholelithiasis. Beside the traditional open cholecystectomy, a variety of new surgical methods such as open minicholecystectomy and laparoscopic cholecystectomy were introduced. Additional procedures investigated included laparoscopic lithotripsy, oral bile acid therapy (BAT), extracorporeal shock-wave lithotripsy (ESWL), percutaneous transhepatic contact dissolution, percutaneous extraction [(cholecystolithotomy; percutaneous cholecystolithotomy (PCCL)], and transduodenal endoscopic contact dissolution.

Oral bile acid therapy (BAT) consists of the administration of ursodeoxycholic acid (at a dose of 8–13 mg/kg per day) and chenodeoxycholic acid (at a dose of 7 mg/kg per day), which desaturate the bile and dissolve cholesterol stones. Although the ability of the technique to dissolve gallstones was noted already in 1936 [51], it was introduced as treatment for cholelithiasis in the early 1970s [52]. The effectiveness of therapy depends on a number of preconditions which are classified as superoptimal (when the stones are 5 mm or smaller in diameter, when they are entirely cholesterol-stones, when the gallbladder is functioning, when the patient is non-obese, and when the symptoms are mild), optimal (when the stones are 10 mm or smaller in diameter and radiolucent), and acceptable (when the stones are 20 mm or smaller) [53]. The more selective the conditions, the better the chances for dissolving the stones, but the smaller the group of patients that will benefit from the therapy. The cure rate with BAT is 90% and 60% under superoptimal and optimal criteria, respectively, but applicable for only 3% and 12% of patients with gallstones, respectively. When patients with acceptable criteria are added, the optimal cure-rate may reach only 40% and the recurrent stone formation is about 50% [53]. The effectiveness of BAT therapy to prevent gallstone reformation under superoptimal, optimal, and acceptable criteria was calculated to be 45%, 27%, and 10%, respectively [53]. A lipid-lowering drug that competitively inhibits the enzyme 3-hydroxymethyl-glutaryl CoA reductase has been shown to reduce the cholesterol saturation index in bile. Together with ursodeoxycholic acid it is believed to accelerate the dissolution of cholesterol gallstones or prevent recurrence [54]. In terms of complications, BAT is safe. Side effects such as diarrhea, hepatotoxicity, and increase in low-density lipoprotein were believed to follow the use of chenodeoxycholic acid and to be eliminated with the introduction of ursodeoxycholic acid [55].

Extracorporeal shock-wave lithotripsy (ESWL) was introduced for gallstone therapy in 1986 by a group from Munich [56]. As with BAT therapy, the cure rate with ESWL depends upon patient selection criteria; a single, radiolucent stone of a diameter of 20 mm or smaller in a functioning gallbladder provides optimal criteria, while stones up to 30 mm in diameter, up to three in number, with a calcified rim of less than 3 mm, and in a functioning gallbladder present acceptable criteria for therapy [53]. While optimal criteria are met by only 7% of gallstone patients and their cure rate reaches 95%, acceptable criteria are met by 9% of the patients and their cure rate is 75%. However, about 84% of the patients with gallstones do not meet any of the selection criteria and remain ineligible for ESWL therapy [53]. The effectiveness of ESWL therapy to prevent gallstone reformation is about 77% with single stones and 38% with up to three stones [53]. ESWL was reported to be associated with a total complication rate of 9.6%. 6.8% of the complications were mild and included cholestasis, transient hematuria, and mild pancreatitis, and 2.8% were more serious, demanding further surgery [57]. Oral treatment with stone-dissolving drugs needs to be continued. Any remaining fragments of stones can act as a nidus for recurrent stones.

Percutaneous transhepatic contact dissolution was introduced by Thistle et al. in 1989 [58]. Using methyl *tert*-butyl ether (MTBE) in direct contact with gallbladder stones, they achieved in part a complete and in part an incomplete dissolution of the stones. Transduodenal endoscopic contact dissolution was attempted by Edison et al. due to the invasive nature of the transhepatic catheterization [59]. Using first ESWL for patients with multiple stones and then MTBE for direct dissolution, complete or partial stone-dissolution was achieved in about 77% of the cases. Percutaneous cholecystolithotomy (PCCL) is an invasive interventional radiologic procedure for the clearance of gallbladder stones, with a success rate that exceeds 90% [60].

The disadvantages of these techniques are that they require strict criteria for therapy, their applicability is low, their treatment duration extends over months to years, their performance demands a fair amount of patient endurance, they are associated with a high recurrence rate of gallstones, and more appealing therapeutic alternatives are present.

Laparoscopic Cholecystectomy

In recent years, laparoscopic cholecystectomy has become the standard treatment for gallbladder stones. Originally, the technique was associated with significant major biliary injuries and a fair degree of conversion to open cholecystectomy, but has stabilized in recent years, reaching a main bile duct injury rate of about 0.5% or less and a conversion rate of about 2% [61, 62]. Although the technique is already common practice around the world, slight controversies still exist regarding clinical and technical aspects of the procedure:

Symptomatology

Controversy surrounds the symptomatology of gallbladder disease. The common concept is that symptomatic cholelithiasis leads to the diagnosis of chronic cholecystitis, and laparoscopic cholecystectomy results in the relief of complaints. Practically, however, the flow of events is more complicated. Similar to the experience in the era of open cholecystectomy [63, 64], about 25%–30% of the patients, diagnosed as having cholelithiasis and chronic cholecystitis, are not relieved of their symptoms by laparoscopic cholecystectomy [65]. In a minority of patients, despite typical symptoms, no gallbladder stones are detected, and a diagnosis of biliary dyskinesia [66, 67], or chronic acalculous cholecystitis [68, 69], is made. The diagnosis is supported by functional cholescintigraphy, demonstrating a reduced gallbladder ejection fraction (<35%) in response to intravenous administration of cholecystokinin [66]. However, in most of the cases, cholecystectomy does result in the relief of symptoms.

The Pneumoperitoneum

Another controversy relates to the introduction of the Veress needle and insertion of trocars, and the possibility of injuries associated with them. Vascular and bowel injuries during laparoscopic cholecystectomy have been widely reported, with approximately half being caused by blind puncture with the Veress needle or the trocar [70–72]. Moreover, a number of aorto-iliac injuries which resulted in deaths have been noted [73]. Despite the fact that the blind access technique is the method of choice recommended by the American Association of Gynecological Laparoscopists [74] and adopted by most general surgeons, open access methods have been advocated by others [75, 76]. The open access technique is believed to avoid injuries on one hand, but to be time-consuming on the other. The facts, however, remain controversial. It appears that the open access method is not a guarantee against access-related bowel injury [77]. In a review of more than 9,000 patients, 15 injuries were access related. Four of these occurred during the use of the blind technique and 11 during the use of an open access method [78]. In terms of operating time, the open access technique was reported to be shorter than blind access in two comparative studies [79, 80]. This was achieved by early high flow insufflation of the peritoneal cavity, once the 10-mm trocar was inserted, as compared with the low flow of the Veress needle, and by obtaining quick fascial closure by tying the already-placed purse string sutures around the trocar port.

Intra-abdominal Pressure

Concern was raised over possible harmful effects of high intra-abdominal pressures. By comparing carbon dioxide pneumoperitoneum with the gasless, mechanical abdominal wall lift method in a randomized study, it was found that pulmonary compliance was greater and arterial pressures were lower in the abdominal lift method. End-tidal carbon dioxide concentrations were significantly higher following conventional pneumoperitoneum, and patients of this group experienced longer postoperative drowsiness, and a higher incidence of nausea, vomiting and shoulder-tip pain [81]. Venous stasis, caused by elevated intra-abdominal pressure, is another cause of concern. Doppler ultrasonography revealed that the combination of pneumoperitoneum and a head-up position reduced significantly the flow through the common femoral vein [82]. The flow could be normalized again by intermittent sequential compression of the calves during the operation.

Recently, the effect of laparoscopy and CO_2 pneumoperitoneum on bacteremia and bacterial translocation was studied experimentally. In one report discussing peritonitis in an animal model, it was noted that laparoscopy increased the incidence of positive blood cultures, but did not change the incidence of endotoxemia or that of intraabdominal abscesses [83]. In another recent study, 1 h after the inoculation of *Escherichia coli* intraperitoneally and insufflating the abdominal cavity with CO_2, bacteremia occurred and 6 h later, bacteria translocated to the lungs and the kidneys [84]. The mechanism of this translocation is not yet clear.

Number of Trocars

Schwartzman et al., who suggest performing laparoscopic cholecystectomy via only three ports, challenge the standard four-trocars technique. This reduction in the number of ports is believed to reduce the incidence of incisional hernias, to improve the cosmetic results, and to lower the operative costs. It is practical in about 85% of the cases, while in the remaining 15%, a fourth cannula may be unavoidable [85]. Recently, Ramachandran and Arora modified the approach even further, suggesting a two-port laparoscopic cholecystectomy. According to their technique, the procedure is performed via supraumbilical and mid-epigastric access-ports, with the help of percutaneously placed three-traction sutures, passing through the gallbladder wall and used for its manipulation [86].

"Lost" Gallstones

The rate of spillage of bile and stones varies between 10% and 40% [87]. Originally, this mishap seemed to be of no significant clinical concern, so that based on this, and supported by some animal studies [88, 89], most surgeons believed that free intraperitoneal gallstones were harmless. However, with the accumulation of clinical data, more and more complications are reported to be associated with the spillage of gallstones. These reports include intra-abdominal abscesses, wound infections, cutaneous sinuses, fistula formation, fibrosis, adhesions, and small bowel obstruction [90–95]. There is still limited information regarding the complication rate of intra-abdominal lost stones. In a recent retrospective study, analyzing 10,174 laparoscopic cholecystectomies performed in 82 surgical institutions in Switzerland over a 3-year period, it was noted that iatrogenic gallbladder perforation occurred in 6%, and serious postoperative complications due to this mishap occurred in 0.08% [96]. Based on their experience and on a review by Memon et al. [97], we now tend to pay more attention to the perforated gallbladder, using gallbladder bags more frequently, thereby controlling the spillage of gallstones better. When spillage does occur, we now make greater efforts to retrieve the lost stones. Large and medium-sized stones are manually extracted, while smaller stones are irrigated and sucked out.

Cholangiography

The controversy regarding the routine or selective use of intraoperative cholangiography during laparoscopic cholecystectomy is still unsettled. The fact that unsuspected common bile duct stones are present in about 10%–15% of cases undergoing laparoscopic cholecystectomy is the main argument for routine intraoperative cholangiography [98, 99]. But data revealing no more than 6% of unsuspected common bile stones in patients undergoing laparoscopic cholecystectomy, and data stressing the time consumed and the extra costs associated with intraoperative cholangiography are all in favour of selective use of the procedure [100, 101]. Two additional studies are available, one reporting that only 0.8% of patients who did not have intraoperative cholangiography went on to develop symptoms [102], and another discussing selective cholangiography [103], concluding that routine intraoperative cholangiography was not indicated during laparoscopic cholecystectomy in the presence of an efficient and safe ERCP service. Another argument for the performance of intraoperative cholangiography is the detection of anatomical abnormalities. In one prospective study, pathologies of this kind were observed in 19% [104]. In another review, however, 67.6% of bile duct injuries occurred despite the performance of intraoperative cholangiography. The fact that six of seven severe injuries did not have intraoperative cholangiography may suggest that intraoperative cholangiography might have been effective in avoiding the more severe injuries [78].

The tendency in most of the centers is now to perform selective intraoperative cholangiography during laparoscopic cholecystectomy. This technique, however, is part of a more complicated and inter-related approach that takes into consideration the preoperative and postoperative ERCPs as well. In its wider context, it will be discussed next.

Associated Choledocholithiasis

ERCP and intraoperative cholangiography are useful adjuncts to laparoscopic cholecystectomy. Their precise individual and inter-related roles in the era of laparoscopic surgery have not yet been established. ERCP performed preoperatively or postoperatively and intraoperative cholangiography are first-line modalities for assessing the common bile duct (CBD) for the presence of stones, as a first stage, and for clearing them, as a second stage. Early in the laparoscopic era, preoperative ERCP was the preferred approach for assessing and treating CBD stones. It was routinely utilized, so that most of the endoscopic cholangiograms were normal [105]. The consequent risks and costs of the routine preoperative ERCP initiated a more selective approach to the procedure. The selection of criteria for preoperative ERCP was and is still the subject of numerous studies [106–109]. The criteria studied include factors such as jaundice, biliary pancreatitis, the presence of small gallstones, dilatation of the bile ducts, and the visualization of CBD stones on US or CT scans. The specificity of these criteria is improved by their stricter use [109], on the one hand, and by the use of the logistic regression analysis [107, 108], on the other hand, reaching diagnostic yields of 56% [109] to 94% [107].

Supporters of this preoperative approach underline the advantage of the timing of the procedure, so that in case the ERCP fails, surgery can still be adjusted.

Intraoperative laparoscopic cholangiography addresses the problem of preoperative excessive and unnecessary ERCP procedures, but pays the price in giving up any preoperative extraction of CBD stones by ERCP. The CBD stones that are detected demand laparoscopic extraction or conversion to explore the CBD, or alternatively, their clearing by postoperative ERCP. While in the majority of the cases conversion and CBD exploration is common practice, the tendency seems to be moving towards laparoscopic extraction [110]. This total laparoscopic approach is reported to be successful, cost effective, and safe, but demands skill and experience, special training, and the availability of sophisticated equipment [111]. Postoperative ERCP is the ideal answer for the excessive preoperative use of this procedure. Usually, at this late stage, if symptoms and signs suggesting CBD stones are present, their diagnostic yield is very high. By the same token, it is important to note that if the procedure fails, an additional operation may be indicated.

A number of facts dictate our approach to assess CBD stones:

- Intraoperative laparoscopic cholangiography is the safest method for assessing the CBD.
- Preoperative ERCP, intraoperative cholangiography, and postoperative ERCP as parts of a CBD clearing technique are associated with comparable success and complication rates of 85%–100% and 10%–12%, respectively [111].
- When preoperative ERCP fails, there is still time for adjustment of the following operation, but when postoperative ERCP fails, another operation may be indicated.

Based on these facts, preoperative ERCP is indicated if there is a high degree of suspicion for common duct stones, or when there is uncertainty regarding the diagnosis. Our criteria for a high degree of suspicion include: bilirubin elevated over 5 mg%, alkaline phosphatase about twice its upper normal range, markedly dilated CBD on sonography, and CBD stones visualized on sonography or CT scan. Intraoperative cholangiography is a useful tool for clarifying anatomical variations during the laparoscopic procedure, and for the diagnosis of choledocholithiasis with a low suspicion rate (based on bilirubin <5 mg%, moderately elevated alkaline phosphatase, biliary pancreatitis, slight dilatation of the bile ducts). ERCP is indicated postoperatively for retained CBD stones (suspected by the previously mentioned criteria) and for the evaluation and therapy of biliary injuries, particularly following laparoscopy.

CT and MRI [112] cholangiography, virtual CT cholangiopancreatoscopy [113], laparoscopic [114] and endoscopic [115] ultrasound are new studies and procedures in evolution that may change our future approach. For the time being it is premature to discuss their role.

Cholelithiasis and Cancer

Cholelithiasis, gallbladder disease, and cholecystectomy are associated with cancer in a number of aspects. Cholelithiasis and various forms of chronic cholecystitis are believed to be directly associated with the pathogenesis of gallbladder cancer. In patients with gallbladder carcinoma, the incidence of cholelithiasis varies from 70% to 90%, and that of porcelain gallbladders reaches about 60% [116, 117]. Also, Mirizzi syndrome was reported to be associated with gallbladder carcinoma [118].

There are only a few reports that discuss the incidence of gallbladder cancer in patients with cholelithiasis. In one study it occurred in 10 of 3,208 patients [119], and in another study it occurred in 5 of 2,583 patients with gallstones [120]. According to the last study, the risk for gallbladder cancer was increased threefold over that of the general population.

Conflicting reports suggest and deny correlation between cholecystectomy and cancer of the large bowel [121–123], and between cholelithiasis and colorectal cancer [124]. Uncertain and still controversial associations between cholelithiasis and other cancers concern cholangiocarcinoma [125–127] and pancreatic carcinoma [126, 128]. Other studies emphasize correlations between cholecystectomy and increased risk of pancreatic cancer, extrahepatic bile duct cancer [127], and cancer of the ampulla of Vater [129]. The association between cholelithiasis and an increased risk for colonic cancer was further supported by reports of increased concentrations of primary and secondary bile acids in patients with colorectal cancer [130]. In a number of studies, cholecystectomy was associated with a slightly increased risk of proximal colonic cancer in women [131]. Johansen et al. noted borderline association between gallstones and cancers of the colon, pancreas, and small intestine in the general population, as well as breast cancer in women [132].

An unrecognized gallbladder cancer presents a special problem for laparoscopic cholecystectomy. In advanced cases of chronic cholecystitis and extensive fibrosis, gallbladder cancer may be masked and unrecognized during the laparoscopic procedure. Manipulations during the laparoscopic approach may facilitate neoplastic dissemination, causing cancer implantation at the trocar site, on one hand, and peritoneal metastatic spread, on the other hand. A number of studies have already raised and discussed these particular problems [133–136], and based on them, it is now recommended to avoid laparoscopic surgery whenever gallbladder cancer is suspected and to proceed with open cholecystectomy. The suspicion of gallbladder cancer is usually based on US and/or intraoperative findings of gallbladder polyps or of a thickened and infiltrated gallbladder wall. When the diagnosis is made intraoperatively, the gallbladder should be extracted within a bag and the exsufflation should be performed while the trocars are still in place, so that the wounds are maximally protected. Following laparoscopic surgery and a diagnosis of gallbladder cancer, radiation to the gallbladder bed and to the trocar sites should be considered, or alternatively, the sites should be excised [135, 136].

References

1. Trotman BW (1983) Pigment gallstone disease. Semin Liver Dis 3:112–119
2. Schwesinger WH, Kurtin WE, Levine BA, et al. (1985) Cirrhosis and alcoholism as pathogenetic factors in pigment gallstone formation. Ann Surg 201:319–322
3. Barbara L, Sama C, Labate AMM, et al. (1987) A population study on the prevalence of gallstone disease: the Sirmione study. Hepatology 7:913–917
4. Glambek I, Kvaale G, Arnesjo B, et al. (1987) Prevalence of gallstones in a Norwegian population. Scand J Gastroenterol 22:1089–1094
5. Rome Group for the Epidemiology and Prevention of Cholelithiasis (GREPCO) (1984) Prevalence of gallstone disease in an Italian adult female population. Am J Epidemiol 119:796–805
6. Bernstein RA, Werner LH, Rimm AA (1973) Relationship of gallbladder disease to parity, obesity, and age. Health Serv Rep 88:925–936
7. Mellstrom D, Asztely M, Svanvik J (1988) Gallstones and previous cholecystectomy in 77 to 78 year old women in an urban population in Sweden. Scand J Gastroenterol 23:1241–1244
8. Medina E, Pascual JP, Medina R (1983) Frecuencia de la litiasis biliar en Chile. Rev Med Chile 111:668–675
9. Adedeji A, Akande B, Olumide F (1986) The changing pattern of cholelithiasis in Lagos. Scand J Gastroenterol 21:63–66
10. Sampliner RE, Bennett PH, Comess LJ, et al. (1970) Gallbladder disease in Pima Indians. Demonstration of high prevalence and early onset by cholecystography. N Engl J Med 283:1358–1364
11. Thistle JL, Eckhart KL Jr, Nensel RE, et al. (1971) Prevalence of gallbladder disease among Chippewa Indians. Mayo Clin Proc 46:603–608
12. Williams CN, Johnston JL, Weldon KLM (1977) Prevalence of gallstones and gallbladder disease in Canadian Micmac Indian women. Can Med Assoc J 117:758–760
13. Sichieri R, Everhart JE, Roth HP (1990) Low incidence of hospitalization with gallbladder disease among blacks in the United States. Am J Epidemiol 131:826–835
14. Deitel M, Petrov I (1987) Incidence of symptomatic gallstones after bariatric operations. Surg Gynecol Obstet 164:549–552
15. Liddle RA, Goldstein RB, Saxton J (1989) Gallstone formation during weight-reduction dieting. Arch Intern Med 149:1750–1753
16. Messing B, Bories C, Kunstlinger F, et al. (1983) Does total parenteral nutrition induce gallbladder sludge formation and lithiasis? Gastroenterology 84:1012–1019
17. Whorwell PJ, Hawkins R, Dewbury K, et al. (1984) Ultrasound survey of gallstones and other hepatobiliary disorders in patients with Crohn's disease. Dig Dis Sci 29:930–933
18. Gilat T, Feldman C, Halpern Z, et al. (1983) An increased familial frequency of gallstones. Gastroenterology 84:242–246
19. Honore LH (1980) The lack of a positive association between symptomatic cholesterol cholelithiasis and clinical diabetes mellitus: a retrospective study. J Chronic Dis 33:465–469
20. Haffner SM, Diehl AK, Mitchell BD, et al. (1990) Increased prevalence of clinical gallbladder disease in subjects with non-insulin-dependent diabetes mellitus. Am J Epidemiol 132:327–335
21. Diehl AK, Rosenthal M, Hazuda HP, et al. (1985) Socioeconomic status and the prevalence of clinical gallbladder disease. J Chronic Dis 38:1019–1026
22. Jorgensen T (1988) Gallstones in a Danish population: familial occurrence and social factors. J Biosoc Sci 20:111–120
23. Schwesinger WE, Kurtin WE, Johnson R (1988) Alcohol protects against cholesterol gallstone formation. Ann Surg 207:641–646
24. Rome Group for Epidemiology and Prevention of Cholelithiasis (GREPCO) (1988) The epidemiology of gallstone disease in Rome, Italy. Part II. Factors associated with the disease. Hepatology 8:907–913
25. Friedman GD, Kannel WB, Dawber TR (1966) The epidemiology of gallbladder disease: observations in the Framingham Study. J Chronic Dis 19:273–292
26. Jorgensen T (1989) Gallstones in a Danish population. Relation to weight, physical activity, smoking, coffee consumption, and diabetes mellitus. Gut 30:528–534
27. Boston Collaborative Drug Surveillance Program (1974) Surgically confirmed gallbladder disease, venous thromboembolism, and breast tumors in relation to postmenopausal estrogen therapy. N Engl J Med 290:15–19
28. Kakar F, Weiss NS, Strite SA (1988) Non-contraceptive estrogen use and the risk of gallstone disease in women. Am J Public Health 78:564–566

29. Diehl AK, Haffner SM, Hazuda HP, et al. (1985) Coronary risk factors and clinical gallbladder disease. J Chronic Dis 38:1019–1026
30. Scragg RKR, Calvert GD, Oliver JR (1984) Plasma lipids and insulin in gall stone disease: a case-control study. Br Med J 289:521–525
31. Jorgensen T (1989) Gallstones and plasma lipids in a Danish population. Scand J Gastroenterol 24:916–922
32. Low-Beer TS (1985) Nutrition and cholesterol gallstones. Proc Nutr Soc 44:127–143
33. Jorgensen T, Jorgensen LM (1989) Gallstones and diet in a Danish population. Scand J Gastroenterol 24:821–826
34. Pixley F, Wilson D, McPherson K, et al. (1985) Effect of vegetarianism on development of gall stones in women. Br Med J 291:11–12
35. Coronary Drug Project Research Group (1977) Gallbladder disease as a side effect of drugs influencing lipid metabolism. Experience in the Coronary Drug Project. N Engl J Med 296:1185–1190
36. Lipid Research Clinics Program (1984) The Lipid Research Clinics Coronary Primary Prevention Trial results. I. Reduction in incidence of coronary heart disease. JAMA 251:351–364
37. Frick MH, Elo O, Haapa K, et al. (1987) Helsinki Heart Study: primary-prevention trial with gemfibrozil in middle-aged men with dyslipidemia. Safety of treatment, ranges in risk factors, and incidence of coronary heart disease. N Engl J Med 317:1237–1245
38. Rosenberg L, Shapiro S, Slone D, et al. (1980) Thiazides and acute cholecystitis. N Engl J Med 303:546–548
39. Porter JB, Jick H, Dinan BJ (1981) Acute cholecystitis and thiazides. N Engl J Med 304:954–955
40. Lee SP, Carey MC, LaMont JT (1981) Aspirin prevention of cholesterol gallstone formation in prairie dogs. Science 211:1429–1431
41. Broomfield PH, Chopra R, Sheinbaum RC, et al. (1988) Effects of ursodeoxycholic acid and aspirin on the formation of lithogenic bile and gallstones during loss of weight. N Engl J Med 319:1567–1572
42. Friedman GD (1993) Natural history of asymptomatic and symptomatic gallstones. Am J Surg 165:399–404
43. Comfort MW, Gray HK, Wilson JM (1948) The silent gallstone: a ten to twenty year follow-up study of 112 cases. Ann Surg 128:931–937
44. Lund J (1960) Surgical indications in cholelithiasis: prophylactic cholecystectomy elucidated on the basis of long-term follow up on 526 nonoperated cases. Ann Surg 151:153–161
45. Gracie WA, Ransohoff DF (1982) The natural history of silent gallstones: the innocent gallstone is not a myth. N Engl J Med 307:798–800
46. McSherry CK, Ferstenberg H, Calhoun WF, et al. (1987) The natural history of diagnosed gallstone disease in symptomatic and asymptomatic patients. Ann Surg 202:59–63
47. Friedman GD, Raviola CA, Fireman B (1989) Prognosis of gallstones with mild or no symptoms: 25 years of follow-up in a health maintenance organization. J Clin Epidemiol 42:127–136
48. Wenckert A, Robertson B (1966) The natural course of gallstone disease: eleven year review of 781 nonoperated cases. Gastroenterology 50:376–381
49. Newman HF, Northup JD, Rosenblum M, Abrams H (1968) Complications of cholelithiasis. Am J Gastroenterol 50:476–496
50. Patino JF, Quintero GA (1998) Asymptomatic cholelithiasis revisited. World J Surg 22:1119–1124
51. Rewbridge AG (1937) The disappearance of gallstone shadows following the prolonged administration of bile salts. Surgery 1:395–400
52. Danzinger R, Hofmann AF, Schoenfield LJ, Thistle JL (1972) Dissolution of cholesterol gallstones by chenodeoxycholic acid. N Engl J Med 286:1–8
53. Strasberg SM, Clavien PA (1992) Cholecystolithiasis: lithotherapy for the 1990s. Hepatology 16:820–839
54. Bateson MC (1990) Simvastatin and ursodeoxycholic acid for rapid gallstone dissolution. Lancet 336:1196
55. Roehrkasse R, Fromm H, Malavolti M, et al. (1986) Gallstone dissolution treatment with a combination of chenodeoxycholic and ursodeoxycholic acids: studies on safety, efficacy and effects of high lithogenicity, bile acid pool and serum lipids. Dig Dis Sci 31:1032–1040
56. Sauerbruch T, Delius B, Paumgartner G, et al. (1986) Fragmentation of gallstones by extracorporeal shock waves. N Engl J Med 314:818–822
57. Sackmann M, Pauletzki J, Sauerbruch T, et al. (1991) The Munich gallbladder lithotripsy study: results of the first 5 years with 711 patients. Ann Intern Med 114:290–296

58. Thistle JL, May GR, Bender CE, et al. (1989) Dissolution of cholesterol gallbladder stones by methyl tert-butyl ether administered by percutaneous transhepatic catheter. N Engl J Med 320:633–639
59. Edison SA, Maier M, Kohler B, et al. (1993) Direct dissolution of gallstones with methyl tert-butyl ether by endoscopic cannulation of the gallbladder. Am J Gastroenterol 88:1242–1248
60. Goodacre B, vanSonnenberg E, D'Agostino H, Sanchez R (1991) Interventional radiology in gallstone disease. Gastroenterol Clin North Am 20:209–227
61. MacFadyen BV Jr, Vecchio R, Ricardo AE, Mathis CR (1998) Bile duct injury after laparoscopic cholecystectomy. The United States experience. Surg Endosc 12:315–321
62. Matthews BD, Williams GB (1999) Laparoscopic cholecystectomy in an academic hospital: evaluation of changes in perioperative outcomes. JSLS (Society of Laparoendoscopic Surgeons) 3:9–17
63. Gunn A, Keddie N (1972) Some clinical observations on patients with gallstones. Lancet 2:239–241
64. Gilliland TM, Traverso LW (1990) Modern standards for comparison of cholecystectomy with alternative treatments for symptomatic cholelithiasis with emphasis on long-term relief of symptoms. Surg Gynecol Obstet 170:39–44
65. Gui GP, Cheruvu CV, West N, et al. (1998) Is cholecystectomy effective treatment for symptomatic gallstones? Clinical outcome after long-term follow-up. Ann R Coll Surg Engl 80:25–32
66. Klieger PS, O'Mara RE (1998) The clinical utility of quantitative cholescintigraphy: the significance of gallbladder dysfunction. Clin Nucl Med 23:278–282
67. Goncalves RM, Harris JA, Rivera DE (1998) Biliary dyskinesia: natural history and surgical results. Am Surg 64:493–497
68. Jones DB, Soper NJ, Brewer JD, et al. (1996) Chronic acalculous cholecystitis: laparoscopic treatment. Surg Lap Endosc Percut Tech 6:114–122
69. Adams DB, Tarnasky PR, Hawes RH, et al. (1998) Outcome after laparoscopic cholecystectomy for chronic acalculous cholecystitis. Am Surg 64:1–5
70. Baadsgaard SE, Bille S, Egeblad K (1989) Major vascular injury during gynecologic laparoscopy. Acta Obstet Gynecol Scand 68:283–285
71. Macintyre IMC, Wilson RG (1993) Laparoscopic cholecystectomy. Br J Surg 80:552–559
72. Deziel D, Millikan K, Economou SG, et al. (1993) Complications of laparoscopic cholecystectomy: a national survey of 4292 hospitals and an analysis of 77,604 cases. Am J Surg 165:9–14
73. Peterson HB, Greenspan JR, Ory WH (1982) Death after puncture of the aorta during laparoscopic sterilisation. Am J Obstet Gynecol 59:133–134
74. Philips JW, Hulka JF, Peterson HB (1984) American Association of Gynecologic Laparoscopists' 1982 membership survey. J Reprod Med 29:592–594
75. Macintyre IMC, Wilson RG (1993) Laparoscopic cholecystectomy. Br J Surg 80:552–559
76. Lafullarde T, Van Hee R, Gys T (1999) A safe and simple method for routine open access in laparoscopic procedures. Surg Endosc 13:769–772
77. Soper NJ, Stockmann PT, Dunnegan DL, Ashley SW (1992) Laparoscopic cholecystectomy. The new 'gold standard'? Arch Surg 127:917–923
78. Wherry DC, Marohn MR, Malanoski MP, et al. (1996) An external audit of laparoscopic cholecystectomy in the steady state performed in medical treatment facilities of the Department of Defence. Ann Surg 224:145–154
79. Ballem RV, Rudomanski J (1993) Techniques of pneumoperitoneum. Surg Laparosc Endosc 3:42–43
80. Sigma HH, Fried GM, Garzon J, et al. (1993) Risk of blind versus open approach to celiotomy for laparoscopic surgery. Surg Laparosc Endosc 3:296–299
81. Lindgren L, Koivusalo AM, Kellokumpu I (1995) Conventional pneumoperitoneum compared with abdominal wall lift for laparoscopic cholecystectomy. Br J Anaesth 75:567–572
82. Millard JA, Hill BB, Cook PS, et al. (1993) Intermittent sequential pneumatic compression in prevention of venous stasis associated with pneumoperitoneum during laparoscopic cholecystectomy. Arch Surg 128:914–918
83. Jakobi A, Ordemann J, Boehm B, et al. (1997) Does laparoscopy increase bacteremia and endotoxemia in a peritonitis model? Surg Endosc 1:235–238
84. Özmen MM, Cöl C, Aksoy AM, et al. (1999) Effect of CO_2 insufflation on bacteremia and bacterial translocation in an animal model of peritonitis. Surg Endosc 13:801–803
85. Schwartzman A, Cirocco WC, Alfonso AE (1995) Minimizing trochar site herniation in laparoscopic cholecystectomy. J Laparoendosc Surg 5:157–161
86. Ramachandran CS, Arora V (1998) Two-port laparoscopic cholecystectomy: an innovative new method for gallbladder removal. J Laparoendosc Adv Surg Tech A 8:303–308

87. Harvey MH, Pardoe H (1994) Retrieval of spilled stones during laparoscopic cholecystectomy. Br J Hosp Med 52:439–442
88. Cline RW, Poulos E, Clifford EJ (1994) An assessment of potential complications caused by intraperitoneal gallstones. Am Surg 60:303–305
89. Welch N, Hinder RA, Fitzgibbons RJ Jr, Rouse JW (1991) Gallstones in the peritoneal cavity: a clinical and experimental study. Surg Laparosc Endosc 1:246–247
90. Johnston S, O'Malley K, McEntee G, et al. (1994) The need to retrieve the dropped stone during laparoscopic cholecystectomy. Am J Surg 167:608–610
91. Golub R, Nwogu C, Cantu R, Stein H (1994) Gallstone shrapnel contamination during laparoscopic cholecystectomy. Surg Endosc 8:898–900
92. Tschmelitsch J, Glaser K, Klingler A, et al. (1993) Late complication caused by stone spillage during laparoscopic cholecystectomy. Lancet 342:369
93. Cacdac RG, Lakra YP (1993) Abdominal wall sinus tract secondary to gallstones: a complication of laparoscopic cholecystectomy. J Laparoendosc Surg 3:509–511
94. Campbell WB, McGarity WC (1992) An unusual complication of laparoscopic cholecystectomy. Am Surg 58:641–642
95. Huynh T, Mercer D (1996) Early postoperative small bowel obstruction caused by spilled gallstones during laparoscopic cholecystectomy. Surgery 119:352–353
96. Schäfer M, Suter C, Klaiber Ch, et al. (1998) Spilled gallstones after laparoscopic cholecystectomy: a relevant problem? A retrospective analysis of 10,174 laparoscopic cholecystectomies. Surg Endosc 12:305–309
97. Memon MA, Deeik RK, Maffi TR, Fitzgibbons Jr (1999) The outcome of unretrieved gallstones in the peritoneal cavity during laparoscopic cholecystectomy. Surg Endosc 13:848–857
98. Martin DF, Tweedle DEF (1987) Endoscopic management of common duct stones without cholecystectomy. Br J Surg 74:209–211
99. Gibney EJ (1990) Asymptomatic gallstones. Br J Surg 77:368–372
100. Morris JB, Margolis R, Rosato EF (1993) Safe laparoscopic cholecystectomy without intraoperative cholangiography. Surg Laparosc Endosc 3:17–20
101. Barkun JS, Fried GM, Barkun AN, et al. (1993) Cholecystectomy without operative cholangiography. Implications for common bile duct injury and retained common bile duct stones. Ann Surg 218:371–377
102. Grace PA, Qureshi A, Burke P, et al. (1993) Selective cholangiography in laparoscopic cholecystectomy. Br J Surg 80:244–246
103. Madhavan KK, Macintyre IM, Wilson RG, et al. (1995) Role of intraoperative cholangiography in laparoscopic cholecystectomy. Br J Surg 82:249–252
104. Kullman E, Borch K, Lindstrom E, et al. (1996) Value of routine intraoperative cholangiography in detecting aberrant bile ducts and bile duct injuries during laparoscopic cholecystectomy. Br J Surg 83:171–175
105. Neuhaus H, Hoffmann W, Feussner H, et al. (1992) Prospective evaluation of the utility and safety of endoscopic retrograde cholangiography (ERC) before laparoscopic cholecystectomy. Gastrointest Endosc 38:257
106. Surick B, Washington M, Ghazi A (1993) Endoscopic retrograde cholangiopancreatography in conjunction with laparoscopic cholecystectomy. Surg Endosc 7:387–391
107. Barkin AN, Barkun JS, Fried GM, et al. (1994) Useful predictors of bile duct stones in patients undergoing laparoscopic cholecystectomy. Ann Surg 220:32–39
108. Robertson GSM, Jagger C, Johnson PRV, et al. (1996) Selection criteria for preoperative endoscopic retrograde cholangiopancreatography in the laparoscopic era. Arch Surg 131:89–94
109. Tham TCK, Lichtenstein DR, Vandervoort J, et al. (1998) Role of endoscopic retrograde cholangiopancreatographyfor suspected choledocholithiasis in patients undergoing laparoscopic cholecystectomy. Gastrointest Endosc 47:50–56
110. Liberman MA, Phillips EH, Carroll BJ, et al. (1996) Cost-effective management of complicated choledocholithiasis: laparoscopic transcystic duct exploration of endoscopic sphincterotomy. J Am Coll Surg 182:488–494
111. Geron N, Reshef R, Shiller M, et al. (1999) The role of endoscopic retrograde cholangiopancreatography in the laparoscopic era. Surg Endosc 13:452–456
112. Guibaud L, Bret PM, Reihold C, et al. (1995) Bile duct obstruction and choledocholithiasis diagnosis with MRI cholangiography. AJR 197:109–115
113. Prassopoulos P, Raptopoulos V (1998) Development of virtual CT cholangiopancreatoscopy. Radiology 209:570–574
114. Santambrogio R, Montorsi M, Bianchi P, et al. (1997) Common bile duct exploration and laparoscopic cholecystectomy: role of intraoperative ultrasonography. J Am Coll Surg 185:40–48

115. Palazzo L, Girollet PP, Salmeron M, et al. (1995) Value of endoscopic ultrasonography in the diagnosis of common bile duct stones: comparison with surgical exploration and ERCP. Gastrointest Endosc 42:225–231
116. Arnaud JP, Graf P, Granfort JL, et al. (1979) Primary carcinoma of the gallbladder: review of 25 cases. Am J Surg 138:403
117. Polk HC (1966) Carcinoma of the calcified gallbladder. Gastroenterology 50:582
118. Redaelli CA, Buchler MW, Schilling MK, et al. (1997) High coincidence of Mirizz syndrome and gallbladder carcinoma. Surgery 121:58–63
119. Malet PF, Soloway RD (1992) Diseases of the gallbladder and bile ducts. In: Wyngaarden JB, Smith LH Jr, Bennett JC (eds) Cecil textbook of medicine,19th edn. Saunders, Philadelphia, pp 804–816
120. Maringhini A, Moreau JA, Melton LJ, et al. (1987) Gallstones, gallbladder cancer, and other gastrointestinal malignancies: an epidemiologic study in Rochester, Minnesota. Ann Intern Med 107:30–35
121. Friedman GD (1988) Cancer of the large bowel after cholecystectomy. Biomed Pharmacother 42:369–372
122. Adami HO, Meirik O, Gustavsson S, et al. (1983) Colorectal cancer after cholecystectomy: absence of risk increase within 11–14 years. Gastroenterology 85:859–865
123. Friedman GD, Goldhaber MK, Quesenberry CP Jr (1987) Cholecystectomy and large bowel cancer. Lancet 1:906–908
124. Jorgensen T, Rafaelsen S (1992) Gallstones and colorectal cancer: there is a relationship, but it is hardly due to cholecystectomy. Dis Colon Rectum 35:24–28
125. Kaczynski J, Hansson G, Wallerstedt S (1996) Incidence of primary liver cancer and aetiological aspects: a study of a defined population from a low-endemicity area. Br J Cancer 73:128–132
126. Bansal P, Sonnenberg A (1996) Comorbid occurrence of cholelithiasis and gastrointestinal cancer. Eur J Gastroenterol Hepatol 8:985–988
127. Khan ZR, Neugut AI, Ahsan H, Chabot JA (1999) Risk factors for biliary tract cancers. Am J Gastroenterol 94:149–152
128. Gullo L, Pezzilli R, Morselli-Labate AM (1996) Risk of pancreatic cancer associated with cholelithiasis, cholecystectomy, or gastrectomy. Italian Pancreatic Cancer Study Group. Dig Dis Sci 41:1065–1068
129. Chow WH, Johansen C, Gridley G, et al. (1999) Gallstones, cholecystectomy and risk of cancer of the liver, biliary tract and pancreas. Br J Cancer 79:640–644
130. Tocchi A, Basso L, Costa G, et al. (1996) Is there a causal connection between bile acids and colorectal cancer? Surg Today 26:101–104
131. Rahman MI, Gibson-Shreve LD, Yuan Z, Morris HA (1996) Selection from current literature: cholelithiasis, cholecystectomy and the risk of colorectal cancer. Fam Pract 13:483–487
132. Johansen C, Chow WH, Jorgensen T, et al. (1996) Risk of colorectal cancer and other cancers in patients with gall stones. Gut 39:439–443
133. Cotlar AM, Mueller CR, Pettit JW, et al. (1996) Trocar site seeding of inapparent gallbladder carcinoma during laparoscopic cholecystectomy. J Laparoendosc Surg 6:35–45
134. Shirai Y, Ohtani T, Hatakeyama K (1998) Laparoscopic cholecystectomy may disseminate gallbladder carcinoma. Hepatogastroenterology 45:81–82
135. Nduka CC, Monson JRT, Menzies-Gow N, Darzi A (1994) Abdominal wall metastases following laparoscopy. Br J Surg 81:648–652
136. Contini S, Dalla Valle R, Zinicola R (1999) Unexpected gallbladder cancer after laparoscopic cholecystectomy. Surg Endosc 13:264–267

Acute Cholecystitis

Ulf Haglund · Ib Rasmussen

The following controversies will be discussed herein:
- Intraoperative cholangiogram
- Type of surgical procedure and timing of surgery in acute cholecystitis
- Acute cholecystitis and pregnancy
- Acute cholecystitis and diabetes mellitus
- Acute cholecystitis in high-risk patients

Intraoperative Cholangiogram

The intraoperative cholangiogram was initially introduced as a means to detect common bile duct stones [1]. Many surgeons now find efforts to detect such stones to be unnecessary in the large subpopulation of patients in which the likelihood of missing common bile duct stones is quite small (patients with normal laboratory tests, without a history of jaundice or pancreatitis and younger than 65 years) in the elective as well as in the acute situation. Missed stones that later give rise to symptoms can today be handled with ERC, papillotomy and stone extraction, thus preventing a re-operation. Today, most cholecystectomies are done laparoscopically. In this procedure the dissection in the triangle of Calot is often less extensive than it used to be in an open procedure and the ductal anatomy is not always quite clearly demonstrated [2]. This may be especially true when operating for acute cholecystitis. The question is therefore whether an intraoperative cholangiogram should be included in the routine during a laparoscopic cholecystectomy to verify the anatomy before transection of the cystic duct thereby preventing common bile duct injuries. Such injuries, recently classified as "a health and financial disaster" [3] have increased in frequency (0.6%–1.3%) since the laparoscopic procedure was introduced [4–6], which calls for some action. On the other hand, as early as in the era of open cholecystectomies it was demonstrated that performing an intraoperative cholangiogram is per se not a guarantee of prevention of bile duct injury – the surgeon has to wait for the results and accept that an abnormal radiogram indicates that something might be seriously wrong [7]. Today's equipment with direct-time visualization using fluoroscopy and possibilities for transferring the radiogram at the same time to a radiologist's monitor for discussion should effectively prevent such unfortunate misunderstandings during investigation. Performing an intraoperative cholangiogram laparoscopically could be technically difficult and is therefore sometimes time consuming. This has been used as an argument not to perform laparoscopic cholangiograms routinely. On the other hand, if not used as a routine, it is quite uncertain whether a satisfactory cholangiogram could be performed when it is considered necessary since it demands some training for a high success rate.

The NIH Consensus Report [8] states that the "opinion is divided about the necessity of intraoperative cholangiography," but agrees that "identification of ductal anatomy prior to excision of the gallbladder" is necessary. This statement is to some extent contradictory to the advice given by Hunter [2] if not combined with an intraoperative cholangiogram. The Consensus document also states that the ability to perform an intraoperative cholangiogram should be available in all centers. The review by Kullman et al. [9] illustrates the diversity of opinions regarding routine cholangiography in laparoscopic cholecystectomy and the usefulness of this technique to detect anatomical aberrations without causing injury. A recent report by Fletcher et al. [6] demonstrates a high incidence of ductal injuries (1.33%) for laparoscopic cholecystectomy, higher than for open (0.67%). The risk for a bile duct injury was highest in complex cases (including acute cholecystitis, acute pancreatitis and cholangitis) and, moreover, they were able to demonstrate that the risk for bile duct injury was significantly reduced in patients having intraoperative cholangiography (odds ratio 0.41 vs. 1.9, respectively). They concluded that laparoscopic surgery had a twofold higher risk for major complications but intraoperative cholangiography had a protective effect.

Since the ductal anatomy can be very difficult to assess laparoscopically in patients with acute cholecystitis, it follows from the above that an intraoperative cholangiogram is then especially indicated. However, it could be more technically difficult to perform. To minimize technical obstacles in the instances it is needed, routine intraoperative cholangiograms are recommended.

Type of Surgical Procedure and Timing of Surgery in Acute Cholecystitis

About 90% of all cholecystectomies are done laparoscopically [10]. To some extent this is due to patient as well as doctor preference, a strong feeling that it is a really superior procedure, but there are no high quality randomized controlled trials to support this. In the early period after the introduction of laparoscopic cholecystectomy acute cholecystitis was considered a relative contraindication. It had become generally accepted in the prelaparoscopic era that it was an advantage to get the inflamed gallbladder out early during the disease. An acute operation, i.e., within 7 days from onset of symptoms, was demonstrated to be more convenient for the patient and probably more cost effective since a second hospitalization and recovery period were eliminated [11]. However, with the introduction of laparoscopic cholecystectomy as the standard procedure in elective patients, many surgeons took a conservative attitude to patients with acute cholecystitis, i.e., wait for the inflammation to heal and perform an elective laparoscopic procedure. This most often means surgery 8–12 weeks following the onset of cholecystitis. However, with time and more technical skills, acute cholecystitis was no longer considered a relative contraindication to laparoscopic surgery. Laparoscopic cholecystectomy for acute cholecystitis is still considered a more technically demanding procedure and it requires longer operating time than elective surgery. However, only a few studies have evaluated laparoscopic surgery in acute cholecystitis.

In a study from Israel, patients undergoing laparoscopic surgery for acute cholecystitis were followed prospectively to study the factors associated with complications and conversion to open surgery [12]. The study includes 130 patients; 37 (28%) needed to have their surgical procedure converted. The conversion rate was significantly higher in acute gangrenous cholecystitis (49%) than for uncomplicated acute cholecystitis (4.5%). The complication rate was significantly lower for patients having surgery within 96 h of onset of symptoms compared with those having a delay of surgery for a period longer than 96 h. The complication rate was higher in the converted group. Age over 65 years, previous history of biliary disease, a nonpalpable gallbladder, and a white blood cell count (WBC) of more than 13,000/cc were independently associated with a high conversion rate. Male patients, finding of large bile stones, serum bilirubin over 0.8 mg/dl, and a WBC of more than 13,000/cc were independently associated with high complication rates following laparoscopic surgery with or without conversion [12]. Eldar et al. conclude that laparoscopic surgery for acute cholecystitis can be performed safely and should be performed within 96 h of the onset of the disease.

Recently, a Finnish group with significant experience in laparoscopic surgery published a randomized trial on laparoscopic vs. open early surgery for acute gangrenous cholecystitis [13]. With 31 and 32 patients in both treatment arms, these authors could demonstrate that laparoscopic surgery is feasible. Laparoscopic surgery had a conversion rate of 16% in this series, most often due to difficulties in making the ductal anatomy clear. The postoperative complications were more frequent following open surgery. Hospital stay and postoperative sick leave were shorter in the laparoscopic group. The authors conclude that laparoscopic surgery for acute cholecystitis is technically demanding even in experienced hands but it is safe and effective, and it does not raise the complication rate. A moderately high conversion rate should be accepted.

Two prospective randomized trials on early vs. delayed laparoscopic surgery for acute cholecystitis have recently been published by independent groups from Hong Kong [14, 15]. These authors evaluated early (within 72 h from onset or 24 h from randomization, respectively) vs. delayed (8–12 and 6–8 weeks after onset, respectively) laparoscopic surgery. The study of Lo and coworkers included 45 patients in the early and 41 in the delayed group. Eight of the latter failed to respond to conservative treatment and had laparoscopic surgery at a median of 63 h from admission. These patients had the longest operation time (188 min). The early group had a longer operation time than the delayed group (135 vs. 90 min). Eleven percent in the early and 23% in the delayed group were converted and among the latter there was no difference between those requiring an emergency intervention following failed conservative treatment (conversion rate 25%) and the remainder. Thirteen percent in the early and 29% in the delayed group had postoperative complications. In the study of Lai et al. [15], 53 patients were randomized to early and 51 to delayed laparoscopic surgery. Of the latter, eight failed conservative treatment and had laparoscopic surgery (two conversions; no postoperative complications). Five patients in the delayed group defaulted surgery and, thus, 38 patients had delayed surgery. The conversion rate among them was 24% compared with 21% in the early group. Failure to perform a proper dissection was the most common cause for conversion. Operating time was 122 min in the early and 106 min in the delayed group. Postoperative complications were found in 9% and 8%, respectively. In neither study was there any bile duct injury or postoperative death. The length of hospital stay was shorter in the early group in both studies. Based on their reports it could be concluded that early laparoscopic surgery for acute cholecystitis is safe and should be the preferred approach by surgeons. Delayed surgery following conservative treatment does not offer any benefits except in marginally shorter operating time, but there are risks and inconvenience for patients.

Acute Cholecystitis and Pregnancy

Acute cholecystitis is a condition seldom encountered during pregnancy. Therefore, the reported experience is relatively limited and the safest management remains controversial. It has been estimated that one to eight of every 10,000 pregnancies would require cholecystectomy [16, 17]. Due to the relative lack of patients no prospective, randomized, controlled trials comparing the different management modalities have been published. Therefore, only retrospective case reports and series are available to give some insight into the relative risks and benefits of the different treatments. Medical treatment of acute cholecystitis may be prolonged and result in recurrent admissions, whereas surgical management endangers the mother and fetus due to the risks of surgery and anesthesia particularly during the first trimester [18–20].

In the majority of patients, conservative management of cholecystitis is successful [21] but subsequent repeated attacks may require surgery [22]. Cholecystectomy may result in prematurity, spontaneous abortion, perinatal mortality and maternal morbidity and mortality [23]. The treatment of choice for uncomplicated acute cholecystitis during pregnancy has, therefore, been nonoperative, with elective cholecystectomy done after childbirth [16, 24–27]. Cholecystectomy during pregnancy is considered indicated in patients with repeated acute cholecystitis or insufficient response to conservative treatment [19, 27–29]. Moreover, most authors advocate conservative treatment during the first and third trimester because of the relatively high reported incidence of fetal morbidity and mortality [18, 20, 27, 30–34].

It is probably the severity of the disease and not the surgical procedure itself that is the most important factor in determining fetal and maternal morbidity and mortality. Open cholecystectomy in patients with uncomplicated disease does not appear to increase maternal mortality, and fetal risk can be kept under 5% [20, 30]. In two recent reports of open cholecystectomy during pregnancy, no maternal or fetal morbidity or mortality was reported [27, 32].

Pregnancy has previously been a contraindication to laparoscopic cholecystectomy due to the medical concerns caused by the unknown effects of a prolonged carbon dioxide pneumoperitoneum on the fetus [35] and to the risk of uterine damage in the third semester [8]. However, since 1993 more than 100 laparoscopic cholecystectomies in pregnant patients have been reported [36, 37]. The incidence of fetal and maternal morbidity and mortality has been below 5%. Most of the procedures have been performed in the second trimester. One study argued against laparoscopic cholecystectomy in pregnancy because of the high incidence of spontaneous abortion [38]. The authors theorize that the fetal losses could be due to acidosis caused by carbon dioxide pneumoperitoneum.

Percutaneous cholecystostomy under local anesthesia may provide a safe and effective alternative for the palliation of acute cholecystitis in pregnancy until a cholecystectomy can be performed after delivery [39, 40], but has not yet gained a broad acceptance.

In conclusion, conservative treatment and subsequent cholecystectomy after delivery may be the option for most pregnant patients with acute cholecystitis. For patients with complicated, recurrent or nonresolving acute cholecystitis, surgical treatment is recommended. Percutaneous cholecystostomy could be an alternative in difficult situations. The maternal and fetal morbidity and mortality rates following laparoscopic cholecystectomy during pregnancy are comparable with those of open cholecystectomy and thus laparoscopic cholecystectomy is indicated also in pregnant patients.

Laparoscopic cholecystectomy in pregnant patients with acute cholecystitis should, if possible, be performed in the second trimester of gestation after organogenesis is complete and prior to the uterine fundus reaching a height that interferes with the operative field. To prevent inadvertent injury to the uterus, an open insertion of the initial port or alternative sites of insertion in the right upper quadrant should be used. Hyperventilating and close monitoring of the end-tidal carbon dioxide should be used to prevent fetal acidosis. Perioperative consultation with obstetricians is highly advisable, as is perioperative monitoring of fetal heart tones [41]. The issue of whether to use tocolytic agents routinely in these patients is still debated as are the effects, if any, of prolonged carbon dioxide pneumoperitoneum on fetal physiology.

Acute Cholecystitis and Diabetes Mellitus

The management of gallstones in diabetic patients has been considered problematic. Earlier studies have demonstrated a more severe clinical course of acute cholecystitis in diabetic patients as well as an increased risk of septic complications and death [42–44]. Diabetic patients treated surgically for acute cholecystitis have higher incidence rates of perioperative morbidity and mortality compared to non-diabetic patients [45]. As a result, diabetic patients with asymptomatic gallstones have been recommended prophylactic cholecystectomy.

However, others have shown similar rates of postoperative morbidity and mortality for biliary surgery in diabetic and non-diabetic patients [46–50]. Hickman et al. [45] demonstrated that infectious complications following acute cholecystitis in diabetics were three times that of non-diabetic patients and the mortality was entirely due to septic complications. The incidence of serious comorbidity, including cardiovascular and renal disease, was 35% in the diabetic patients compared with 15% in non-diabetics. This emphasizes the difficulty in attributing the increased morbidity and mortality to any single factor. Thus, as no prospective randomized controlled studies have been published, prophylactic cholecystectomy cannot be recommended for diabetic patients with asymptomatic gallstones. Cholecystectomy should only be performed in diabetic patients with symptomatic cholelithiasis [51]. Management of acute cholecystitis in patients with diabetes should be highly individualized due to the high incidence of coexisting medical diseases. As diabetic patients probably more frequently develop gangrenous cholecystitis and gallbladder perforation, early surgery should be recommended [49, 50]. The surgical approach – laparoscopic or open cholecystectomy – should depend on the cardiopulmonary status of the patient [52]. In medically severely compromised patients, other treatment modalities such as percutaneous cholecystostomy could be used [40, 53–55].

Acute Cholecystitis in High-Risk Patients

The morbidity and mortality following surgery for acute cholecystitis increases with age and concurrent medical diseases [56]. If the response to medical treatment is inadequate, emergency therapy is required to avoid progression of gallbladder inflammation to gangrene or perforation. If acute cholecystectomy is considered unacceptable, because of severe comorbid disease, open or laparoscopic cholecystostomy could be an alternative [56, 57]. Recently, less invasive methods used temporarily or definitively to treat the acute condition have emerged. These alternatives include percutaneous cholecystostomy, endoscopic retrograde cannulation of the gallbladder, and extracorporeal shock-wave lithotripsy. Ultrasonographic guided percutaneous drainage of the gallbladder can quickly reverse the local and systemic inflammatory process. Few technical complications are reported with transhepatic percutaneous cholecystostomy and success rates are reported in 73%–100% [53–55, 58, 59]. The patient should, if the general condition allows, undergo cholecystectomy after the inflammation has subsided [59]. In high-risk surgical patients, percutaneous cholecystolithotomy, stone dissolution with methyl *tert*-butyl ether, or endoscopic removal could be applied [53].

References

1. Mirizzi P (1937) Operative cholangiography. Surg Gynecol Obstet 65:702–710
2. Hunter J (1991) Avoidance of bile duct injury during laparoscopic cholecystectomy. Am J Surg 162:71–76
3. Savader SJ, Lillemoe KD, Prescott CA, Winick AB, Venbrux AC, Lund GB, et al. (1997) Laparoscopic cholecystectomy-related bile duct injuries: a health and financial disaster. Ann Surg 225(3):268–273
4. Deziel DJ, Millikan KW, Economou SG, Doolas A, Ko ST, Airan MC (1993) Complications of laparoscopic cholecystectomy: a national survey of 4,292 hospitals and an analysis of 77,604 cases. Am J Surg 165(1):9–14
5. Richardson MC, Bell G, Fullarton GM (1996) Incidence and nature of bile duct injuries following laparoscopic cholecystectomy: an audit of 5913 cases. West of Scotland Laparoscopic Cholecystectomy Audit Group (see comments). Br J Surg 83(10):1356–1360
6. Fletcher DR, Hobbs MS, Tan P, Valinsky LJ, Hockey RL, Pikora TJ, et al. (1999) Complications of cholecystectomy: risks of the laparoscopic approach and protective effects of operative cholangiography: a population-based study. Ann Surg 229(4):449–457
7. Andrén-Sandberg Å, Johansson S, Bengmark S (1985) Accidental lesions of the common bile duct at cholecystectomy. II. Results of treatment. Ann Surg 201:452–455
8. NIH (1992) Gallstones and laparoscopic cholecystectomy. NIH Consens Statement 10:1–20
9. Kullman E, Borch K, Lindström E, Svanvik J, Anderberg B (1996) Value of routine intraoperative cholangiography in detecting aberrant bile ducts and bile duct injuries during laparoscopic cholecystectomy. Br J Surg 83:171–175
10. Berggren U, Arvidsson D, Haglund U (1998) A survey of surgical treatment of gallstone disease and the diffusion of laparoscopic surgery in Sweden 1992–1993. Eur J Surg 164(4):287–295

11. Norrby S, Herlin P, Holmin T, Sjödahl R, Tagesson C (1983) Early or delayed cholecystectomy in acute cholecystitis? A clinical trial. Br J Surg 70:163–165
12. Elder S, Sabo E, Nash E, Abrahamson J (1997) Laparoscopic cholecystectomy for acute cholecystitis: prospective trial. World J Surg 21:540–545
13. Kiviluoto T, Siren J, Luukkonen P, Kivilaakso E (1998) Randomized trial of laparoscopic versus open cholecystectomy for acute and gangrenous cholecystitis. Lancet 351(9099):321–325
14. Lo C, Liu C, Lai E, Fan S, Wong J (1996) Early versus delayed laparoscopic cholecystectomy for treatment of acute cholecystitis. Ann Surg 223:37–42
15. Lai P, Kwong K, Leung K, Kwok S, Chan A, Chung S, et al. (1998) Randomized trial of early versus delayed laparoscopic cholecystectomy for acute cholecystitis. Br J Surg 85:764–767
16. Hill L, Johnson C, Lee R (1975) Cholecystectomy in pregnancy. Obstet Gynecol 46:291–293
17. Simon J (1983) Biliary tract disease and related surgical disorder during pregnancy. Clin Obstet Gynecol 26:810–821
18. Dixon N, Faddis D, Silberman H (1987) Aggressive management of cholecystitis during pregnancy. Am J Surg 154:292–294
19. Hiatt J, Hiatt J, Williams R, Klein S (1986) Biliary disease in pregnancy. Am J Surg 151:263–265
20. Printen K, Ott R (1978) Cholecystectomy during pregnancy. Am Surg 44:432–434
21. Hamlin E, Bartlett M, Smith J (1951) Acute surgical emergencies of the abdomen in pregnancy. N Engl J Med 244:128–131
22. Present D (1985) Disease of the biliary tract and pregnancy. In: Cherry S, Berkowitz R, Kase N (eds) Medical, surgical and gynecologic complications of pregnancy. Rovinsky and Gutmachers, Baltimore, pp 215–219
23. Shrinder S, Webster G (1965) Maternal and fetal hazards of surgery during pregnancy. Am J Obstet Gynecol 92:891–900
24. Green J, Roger A, Rubin L (1963) Fetal loss after cholecystectomy during pregnancy. Can Med Assoc J 88:576–577
25. Friley M, Douglas G (1972) Acute cholecystitis in pregnancy and the puerperium. Am Surg 38:314–317
26. Landers D, Carmona R, Cromblehome W, Lim R (1987) Acute cholecystitis in pregnancy. Obstet Gynecol 69:131–133
27. McKellar D, Anderson C, Boynton C, Peoples J (1992) Cholecystectomy during pregnancy without fetal loss. Surg Gynecol Obstet 174:465–468
28. Scott L (1992) Gallstone disease and pancreatitis in pregnancy. Gastroenterol Clin North Am 21:803–815
29. Talamini M (1993) Controversies in laparoscopic cholecystectomy: contraindications, pregnancy and avoidance of complications. Ballieres Clin Gastroenterol 7:881–896
30. Kammerer W (1979) Non obstetric surgery during pregnancy. Med Clin North Am 63:1157–1163
31. Lanzafame R (1995) Laparoscopic cholecystectomy. Surgery 118:627–631
32. Swisher S, Schmit P, Hunt K, Hiyama D, Bennion R (1994) Biliary disease during pregnancy. Am J Surg 168:576–581
33. Morrel D, Mullins J, PB H (1992) Laparoscopic cholecystectomy during pregnancy in symptomatic patients. Surgery 112:856–859
34. Eldring S (1993) Laparoscopic cholecystectomy during pregnancy. Am J Surg 165:625–627
35. Gadacz T, Talamini M, Lillemoe K, Yeo C (1990) Laparoscopic cholecystectomy. Surg Clin North Am 70:1249–1262
36. Ghumman E, Barry M, Grace P (1997) Management of gallstones in pregnancy. Br J Surg 84:1646–1650
37. Barone J, Bears S, Chen S, Tsai J, Russell J (1999) Outcome study of cholecystectomy during pregnancy. Am J Surg 177:232–236
38. Amos J, Schorr S, Norman P, Poole G, Thomae K, Mancino A, et al. (1996) Laparoscopic surgery during pregnancy. Am J Surg 171:435–437
39. Weber R, Smith R, Wright R (1993) Percutaneous cholecystostomy: a new treatment for acute cholecystitis in pregnancy. Contemp Surg Resident 1:21–23
40. Allmendinger N, Hallisey M, Ohki S, Straub J (1995) Percutaneous cholecystostomy: treatment for acute cholecystitis in pregnancy. Obstet Gynecol 86:653–654
41. Soper N (1993) Effect of nonbiliary problems on laparoscopic cholecystectomy. Am J Surg 165:522–526
42. Turner R, Becker W, Colleman W, Powell J (1969) Acute cholecystitis in the diabetic. South Med J 62:228–231
43. Mundth E (1962) Cholecystitis and diabetes mellitus. N Engl J Med 267:642–646

44. Goldstein M, Shein C (1963) The significance of biliary tract disease in the diabetics: its unique features. Am J Gastroenterol 39:630–634
45. Hickman M, Schwesinger W, Page C (1988) Acute cholecystitis in the diabetic. A case-control study of outcome. Arch Surg 123:409–411
46. Walsh D, Eckhauser F, Ramsburgh S, Burney R (1982) Risk associated with diabetes mellitus in patients undergoing gallbladder surgery. Surgery 91:254–257
47. Pickleman J, Gonzalez R (1986) The improving results of cholecystectomy. Arch Surg 121:930–934
48. Ransohoff D, Miller G, Forsythe S, Hermann R (1987) Outcome of acute cholecystitis in patients with diabetes mellitus. Ann Intern Med 106:829–832
49. Landau O, Deutsch A, Kott I, Rivlin E, Reiss R (1992) The risk of cholecystectomy for acute cholecystitis in diabetic patients. Hepatogastroenterology 39:437–438
50. Shpitz B, Sigal A, Kaufman Z, Dinbar A (1995) Acute cholecystitis in diabetic patients. Am Surg 61:964–967
51. Aucott JN, Cooper GS, Bloom AD, Aron DC (1993) Management of gallstones in diabetic patients. Arch Intern Med 153:1053–1058
52. Wittgen C, Andrus J, Andrus C, Kaminski D (1993) Cholecystectomy. Which procedure is best for the high-risk patient? Surg Endosc 7:395–399
53. Boland GW, Lee MJ, Mueller PR, Dawson SL, Gaa J, Lu DS, et al. (1994) Gallstones in critically ill patients with acute calculous cholecystitis treated by percutaneous cholecystostomy: nonsurgical therapeutic options. AJR Am J Roentgenol 162:1101–1103
54. Lo LD, Vogelzang RL, Braun MA, Nemcek AA Jr (1995) Percutaneous cholecystostomy for the diagnosis and treatment of acute calculous and acalculous cholecystitis. J Vasc Interv Radiol 6:629–634
55. Van Steenbergen W, Rigauts H, Ponette E, Peetermans W, Pelemans W, Fevery J (1993) Percutaneous transhepatic cholecystostomy for acute complicated calculous cholecystitis in elderly patients. J Am Geriatr Soc 41:157 162
56. Glenn F (1977) Cholecystostomy in the high risk patient with biliary tract disease. Ann Surg 185:185–191
57. Johnson AB, Fink AS (1998) Alternative methods for management of the complicated gallbladder. Semin Laparosc Surg 5(2):115–120
58. Patterson EJ, McLoughlin RF, Mathieson JR, Cooperberg PL, MacFarlane JK (1996) An alternative approach to acute cholecystitis. Percutaneous cholecystostomy and interval laparoscopic cholecystectomy. Surg Endosc 10(12):1185–1188
59. Davis CA, Landercasper J, Gundersen LH, Lambert PJ (1999) Effective use of percutaneous cholecystostomy in high-risk surgical patients: techniques, tube management, and results. Arch Surg 134(7):727–731, 731–732

Invited Comment

David Fromm

The impact of laparoscopic cholecystectomy has been extraordinary and has influenced the rates of cholecystectomy, technical issues and operative complications.

Indications for Cholecystectomy and Postoperative Symptoms

Since laparoscopy became the most commonly used approach to cholecystectomy in the early 1990s, the rates of cholecystectomy have increased by 20%–50% worldwide [1, 2]. Yet there are no reports of a concomitant increase of symptomatic cholelithiasis. We tend to lose sight of the fact that 13%–40% of patients undergoing cholecystectomy [3] have persisting abdominal pain after cholecystectomy. This may be due to preoperative selection or our inability to determine with greater precision symptoms due to cholelithiasis. Persisting symptom(s) without obvious cause after cholecystectomy, be it open or laparoscopic, are euphemistically referred to as the postcholecystectomy syndrome [4]. Although persisting symptoms occur more frequently than most of us would like to admit, the vast majority of patients are pleased with the outcome of their operative procedure. Much of this may be due to the variability in explaining the goals of the operation.

Open Surgery: Still a Viable Option

Laparoscopic cholecystectomy is the "procedure of choice" today because it is associated with almost less everything (except cost and biliary ductal injury) compared with open cholecystectomy. However, this precept is not supported by the much heralded prospective randomized study from Sheffield [5]. An open cholecystectomy through a minimal incision allowing safe operation may not, in fact, be much different from the laparoscopic approach. Nevertheless, the point may be moot because the public, physicians, media and instrument manufacturers believe in the more technologically "advanced" method. The Sheffield study indicates that one need not apologize for doing an open procedure for any reason, and, as virtually all agree, when safety is a concern the open approach is preferable. Even the open method can be precarious in certain circumstances. Haglund and Rasmussen remind us that cholecystostomy is a very defensible and safe procedure in difficult circumstances, including pregnancy.

Anatomic Considerations

Another impact of the laparoscopic approach is that there has been an almost complete reiteration in the literature of the anatomy and pitfalls of biliary surgery but with the implication that such features are unique to laparoscopy. However, anatomic considerations and the principles of cholecystectomy are no different whether the procedure is done through a large or small incision or through a laparoscope.

Cystic Duct Stump

In the heyday of open cholecystectomy, it was emphasized that one should not leave a long cystic duct stump because this could cause recurrent symptoms [6]. Laparoscopic cholecystectomy has shown that the length of the retained cystic duct is not critical. However, for cystic duct stump (irrespective of its length) to be asymptomatic, it must not be obstructed and must not conceal a stone.

Fundus-Down Approach

Most laparoscopic enthusiasts have neglected a principle that has withstood the test of time with the open approach [7]: safer exposure of the triangle of Calot can be achieved in difficult situations by a prograde dissection beginning with the fundus of the gallbladder, working toward the porta. This permits excellent exposure of the cystic-common duct junction and so-called accessory hepatic duct(s).

Cholangiography?

Laparoscopy has not solved the controversy about routine intraoperative cholangiography that exited during the open approach era. However, generically, we seem to be moving away from performing adjuvant procedures on a routine basis and focusing more on selective application. The data supporting routine cholangiography during laparoscopic cholecystectomy are not compelling, but a good rule is when there is question, do it! My bias is that much of the controversy surrounding the necessity of imaging studies pre-, intra- or postoperatively is overblown, and the decision depends on the clinical circumstances as well as the technical expertise (ERCP, intraoperative ultrasound, cholangiographic experience, etc.) available in a given institution.

Early Operation for Acute Cholecystitis

Controversy remains also about the timing of operation for acute cholecystitis. Many of us thought this issue was settled in the days of open cholecystectomy. Tissue planes are more easily discernible early in the course of disease than later. A laparoscopic approach does not make dissection of tissue planes easier, even though they may be more visible as the operative field is magnified on a screen. Several older randomized studies confirm the safety of early operation [8, 9].

Lost Stones

The issue of a lost stone(s) is new with laparoscopic cholecystectomy. During the open era, spilled stones were always removed as part of a prudent approach following the principle that it is undesirable to leave a foreign body floating in the peritoneal cavity. Thus, late "stone abscess" was almost unheard of until the advent of laparoscopic cholecystectomy. Most stones are lost during laparoscopy when a rent occurs in the gallbladder during dissection from its bed. Almost everyone makes an effort to remove lost stones but no one has precise data indicating how successful this is laparoscopically. The surgeon may not even be aware that a stone was "dropped" [10]. While complications relating to a spilled stone can be dramatic and may present more than 1 year after operation, the incidence is so low that there is little justification to routinely convert to an open approach to remove lost stones [11].

Carcinoma of the Gallbladder

Most agree with Eldar and Matter that in the presence of carcinoma, the laparoscopic approach should be converted to an open one in order to avoid contamination by tumor cells sloughing into the peritoneal cavity and subcutaneous tissues. What needs to be emphasized is that suspicion of extramural invasion in the gallbladder fossa is most often raised by a difficult tissue plane or one that, initially reasonable, becomes unreasonable. One study reports the incidence of port site metastases to be 9% for unsuspected carcinoma of the gallbladder laparoscopically removed without perforation, but the incidence increases to 40% if perforation occurs [12]. The appearance of port site metastases is independent of the port from which the gallbladder was extracted and may be a sign of disseminated disease. However, difficult extraction of an unprotected organ containing an unsuspected carcinoma penetrating the serosa or an unprotected gallbladder containing multiple small stones can result in frictional shedding of tumor cells or rupture leaving tumor cells or stones in the port site. There is good reason to enlarge the fascial opening to safely accommodate the gall bladder, since there are no substantive data suggesting that enlarging the port incision is associated with greater postoperative morbidity.

References

1. Steiner CA, Bass ER, Talamini MA, et al. (1994) Surgical rates and operative mortality for open and laparoscopic cholecystectomy in Maryland. N Engl J Med 330:403–408
2. Al-Mulhim AA, Al-Ali AA, Albar AA, et al. (1999) Increased rate of cholecystectomy after introduction of laparoscopic cholecystectomy in Saudi Arabia. World J Surg 23:458–462
3. O'Donnell LJD (1999) Post-cholecystectomy diarrhoea: a running commentary. Gut 45:796–797
4. Farthman EH, Radecke J (1993) Das Postcholecystektomie-Syndrom. Chirug 64:994–999
5. Majeed AW, Troy G, Nicholl JP, et al. (1996) Randomized, prospective, single-blind comparison of laparoscopic versus small-incision cholecystectomy. Lancet 347:989–994
6. Larmi TK, Mokka R, Kemppainen P, Seppala A (1975) A critical analysis of the cystic duct remnant. Surg Gynecol Obstet 141:48–52
7. Martin IG, Dexter SPL, Marton J, et al. (1995) Fundus-first laparoscopic cholecystectomy. Surg Endosc 9:203–206
8. McArthur P, Cushiere A, Sells RA, Shields A (1975) Controlled clinical trial comparing early with interval cholecystectomy for acute cholecystitis. Br J Surg 62:850–852
9. van der Linden W, Sunzel H (1970) Early versus delayed operation for acute cholecystitis: a controlled clinical trial. Am J Surg 120:7–13
10. Zamir G, Lyass S, Persemlidis D, Katz B (1999) The fate of dropped gallstones during laparoscopic cholecystectomy. Surg Endosc 13:68–70
11. Memon MA, Deeik RK, Maffi TR, Fitzgibbons RJ Jr (1999) The outcome of unretrieved gallstones in the peritoneal cavity during laparoscopic cholecystectomy. Surg Endosc 13:848–857
12. Z'graggen K, Birrer S, Maurer CA (1998) Incidence of port site recurrence after laparoscopic cholecystectomy for preoperatively unsuspected gallbladder carcinoma. Surgery 124:831–838

Editorial Comment

Drs. Eldar and Matter have provided us with an exhaustive outline of controversies associated with cholelithiasis. Professor Haglund and Dr. Rasmussen concentrated on controversies related to acute cholecystitis, and Dr. Fromm offered balancing comments.

Dr. Fromm's statement that "virtually all agree, when safety is a concern the open approach is preferable" represents words of wisdom floating in a sea of gimmicks. In addition to the "open" and percutaneous cholecystostomy mentioned by Haglund and Rasmussen, one should not forget the very important option of subtotal cholecystectomy. This method, which allows weathered surgeons to keep out of trouble in "difficult" open cholecystectomies [1] is also doable laparoscopically [2].

None of the discussants has emphasized enough the fact that the outcome of cholecystectomy for symptomatic cholelithiasis correlates with the symptoms of patients. The more "typical" are the symptoms (e.g., biliary colic) the better will be the results; removing the gallbladder for nontypical symptoms (e.g., dyspepsia) produces a greater number of dissatisfied patients [3].

The NIH Consensus Statement (1992) stated that "patients who are not good candidates for laparoscopic cholecystectomy include those with generalized peritonitis, septic shock from cholangitis, severe acute pancreatitis, end stage cirrhosis, and gallbladder cancer" [4]. Laparoscopic procedures are contraindicated in critically ill patients because the laparoscopic CO_2 pneumoperitoneum causes intra-abdominal hypertension. The latter, with its adverse cardiorespiratory and renal physiological effects, further compromises the condition of the already compromised patient [5]. Furthermore, experimental studies suggest that laparoscopic CO_2 pneumoperitoneum increases the infective-septic complications and mortality rate in "late peritonitis" [6]. As a general rule, during laparoscopic cholecystectomy the lowest possible intra-abdominal pressure should be used. This, together with gradual insufflation and limiting the head-up degree to minimum, avoids cardiovascular instability in high-risk patients [7].

And finally, are prophylactic antibiotics necessary and indicated in elective laparoscopic cholecystectomy? The verdict of level I evidence is no [8–10]; "small" wounds are associated with "little" infection - too "little" to allow antibiotic prophylaxis to be significantly beneficial.

References

1. Schein M (1991) Partial cholecystectomy in the emergency treatment of acute cholecystitis in the compromised patient. J Roy Coll Surg Edinb 36:295–297
2. Bornman PC, Terblanche J (1985) Subtotal cholecystectomy: for the difficult gallbladder in portal hypertension and cholecystitis. Surgery 98:1–6
3. Konsten J, Gouma DJ, von Meyenfeldt MF, Menheere P (1993) Long-term follow-up after open cholecystectomy. Br J Surg 80:100–102
4. NIH Consense Statement (1992) Sep 14–16; 10(3):1–28
5. Safran DB, Orlando R 3rd (1994) Physiologic effects of pneumoperitoneum. Am J Surg 167:281–286
6. Bloechle C, Emmermann A, Strate T, Scheurlen UJ, Schneider C, et al. (1998) Laparoscopic vs. open repair of gastric perforation and abdominal lavage of associated peritonitis in pigs. Surg Endosc 12:212–218
7. Dhoste K, Lacoste L, Karayan J, Lehuede MS, Thomas D, Fusciardi J (1996) Haemodynamic and ventilatory changes during laparoscopic cholecystectomy in elderly ASA III patients. Can J Anaesth 43:783–788
8. Tocchi A, Lepre L, Costa G, Liotta G, Mazzoni G, Maggiolini F (2000) The need for antibiotic prophylaxis in elective laparoscopic cholecystectomy: a prospective randomized study. Arch Surg 135:67–70
9. Illig KA, Schmidt E, Cavanaugh J, Krusch D, Sax HC (1997) Are prophylactic antibiotics required for elective laparoscopic cholecystectomy? Am Coll Surg 184:353–356
10. Higgins A, London J, Charland S, Ratzer E, Clark J, Haun W, Maher DP (1999) Prophylactic antibiotics for elective laparoscopic cholecystectomy: are they necessary? Arch Surg 134:611–613

CHAPTER 6

Non-Adenocarcinoma Pancreatic Tumors

Endocrine Tumors

Matthias Rothmund · D. Bartsch

Introduction

Diagnosis, localization and surgical as well as medical treatment of most endocrine pancreatic tumors is nowadays clearly established and not a matter of debate. This is especially true for sporadic benign insulinomas, gastrinomas or more rare tumors like VIPomas or glucagonomas. Controversies still exist in hereditary tumors, mainly in symptomatic gastrinomas and insulinomas, occurring within the syndrome of multiple endocrine neoplasia type I (MEN I). Since the recent description of the mutation in chromosome 11 associated with MEN I [1] the question of how we should deal with asymptomatic patients detected by genetic and/or biochemical screening also became controversial.

Nomenclature

In 1994, a group of noted European pathologists proposed a new classification of neuroendocrine tumors of the lung, pancreas and gut [2]. The classification is made according to the location of the tumors, their histopathological features and growth pattern. It should replace nonspecific terms like "carcinoid tumor" or "endocrine tumor" because it describes more clearly the degree of aggressiveness of these tumors and their expected outcome [3]. It certainly outdates older classifications such as the WHO classification of 1980. In the following chapters we will therefore use the term "neuroendocrine pancreatic" tumors (NPT).

Insulinoma

Sporadic Insulinomas

The insulinoma syndrome is diagnosed by history and a fasting test of up to 72 h duration, measuring glucose, insulin and C-peptide in serum. Before primary operations in sporadic insulinomas only cross-sectional imaging such as ultrasound is indicated to exclude a malignant metastasizing tumor, the localization of the mostly solitary and benign tumors being made during surgery by meticulous exploration and palpation of the pancreas, including intraoperative ultrasound (IOUS). Both palpation and IOUS have been shown to be more cost-effective than any other imaging procedure performed before surgery [4, 5]. Enucleation of the mostly small (0.5–2 cm) tumors from the head and body and distal resection for tumors in the tail are the preferred surgical procedures and are successful in more than 95% of patients [6].

More sophisticated localization procedures should only be utilized before re-operations. Endoscopic ultrasound and selective intra-arterial calcium injection are most efficient in this situation [7, 8]. Re-operations rather than medical treatment are preferred – the operation being performed in a specialized center [6].

MEN I Insulinoma

About 5% of all insulinomas are hereditary and occur as a part of the MEN I syndrome. MEN I insulinomas are rarely malignant and are localized within the pancreas without any preference to a certain region of the gland. They are almost always multiple and pathologists may describe adenomas, microadenomas and hyperplasia of β-cells within the same specimen together with other NPTs (e.g., PPomas). There is also nesidioblastosis in MEN I patients, mainly in children but a few authors have described this even in adults.

Since there is no good medical alternative for the treatment of hypoglycemia and hypoglycemic symptoms caused by MEN I insulinoma, surgery is indicated in these patients as soon as the diagnosis is made. There is some controversy concerning the type of procedure that should be used. Should one only excise tumors demonstrated by preoperative imaging or those which are palpated or demonstrated by IOUS during operation, or is there a standard procedure that can be used in all of these patients? Data published in the last 10 years show that distal pancreatic resection preserving the spleen, combined with enucleation of tumors in the head, can be considered as a standard procedure [9–11]. This makes the routine use of preoperative imaging tests questionable even in MEN I insulinomas.

Gastrinoma

Gastrinomas cause symptoms related to the hypersecretion of gastric acid stimulated by hypergastrinemia, mainly peptic ulcer disease and diarrhea, known as Zollinger-Ellison syndrome (ZES). The patient's life is threatened by both the complications of peptic ulcer disease and the progressive growth of the tumors themselves. Most gastrinomas are sporadic, while 20%–30% occur within the MEN I syndrome; 60%–90% of them are malignant, i.e., lymph node metastases and/or liver metastases are found during first exploration; 30% of patients with MEN I gastrinomas will have liver metastases at the time of diagnosis.

The main location of gastrinomas was in the last decade found to be the duodenum, either as solitary (sporadic) or as multiple (MEN I) tumors with diameters between 1 and 10 mm (microgastrinomas). The pancreas is the second most encountered location of gastrinomas. These tumors are mostly larger (1–4 cm in diameter) than duodenal gastrinomas. Other more rare locations in the gastrinoma triangle are the hepatoduodenal ligament, the liver or lymph nodes around the head of the pancreas [12–14].

Somatostatin receptor scintigraphy (SRS) has evolved as the most efficient procedure for staging of these tumors. After the diagnosis of a gastrinoma is made by acid secretory tests and serum gastrin measurement including secretin stimulation test SRS should be performed together with a cross-sectional study of the upper abdomen to localize the primary tumor and define the extent of disease [14–16].

Sporadic Gastrinoma

Though proton pump inhibitors are able to control acid secretion in ZES, surgery is the best initial treatment in patients with sporadic disease to prevent both complications from hypersecretion and tumor progression. If no diffuse liver metastases are present, 10-year cure and survival rates of 35% and 100%, respectively, can be reached by surgery [14, 17–19]. The operation of choice includes the resection of the primary tumor in the duodenum or pancreas and systematic sampling of lymph nodes around the head of the gland, the celiac axis and in the hepatoduodenal ligament. IOUS of the pancreas as well as the liver is an integral part of the procedure.

MEN I Gastrinoma

While the above mentioned approach to sporadic tumors is not questioned by most experts, surgical treatment of MEN I gastrinomas is considered as unnecessary or at least controversial by experienced gastroenterologists since the natural history of this disease is rather slow with median survival rates of 10–30 years. Besides the control of hypersecretion by proton-pump inhibitors, antiproliferative agents such as interferon and octreotide support a conservative approach. Recent data of the two institutions seeing the largest number of these patients (Hopital Bichat-Claude Bernard in Paris and the NIH, Bethesda, Md., USA) underline the dominant role of conservative treatment in these tumors [20–23].

Yu et al. showed that among 212 patients followed at the NIH, the mean disease duration was 30.8±0.6 years; 67 patients died, 34 of them from non-ZES-related causes but 33 from ZES-related disease, mostly from liver metastases and cachexia or liver and bone metastases or secondary endocrine disease such as hyperinsulinism or Cushing's syndrome. There was no difference in mortality whether these ZES patients had sporadic or MEN I gastrinomas [23]. It was also shown by this group that the occurrence of liver metastases was definitely related to the size of the gastrinomas [21]. Liver metastases were seen in tumors with a diameter up to 1 cm in 4% only, in patients with tumors between 1–3 cm in diameter in 28%, whereas in tumors above 3 cm in diameter metastases to the liver occurred in 61%. It was also shown that liver metastases at the time of diagnosis were the

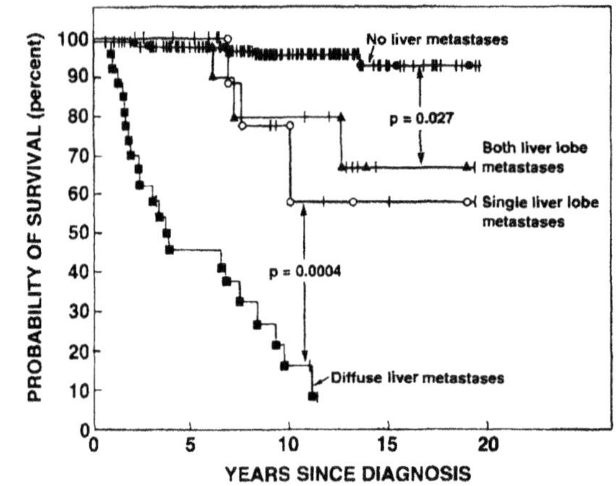

Fig. 1. Effect of the extent of liver metastases on survival. Survival rates were evaluated using death due to ZES-related causes as the outcome. Of 158 patients with no liver metastases, 6 died, of 14 patients with metastases in a single lobe of the liver, 3 died, of 13 patients with limited discrete lesions in both lobes, 3 died, and of 27 patients with diffuse metastases, 21 died. (From [23])

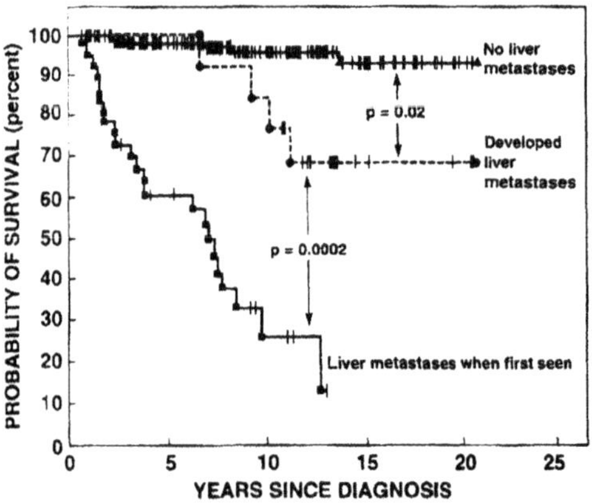

Fig. 2. Effect of the presence or absence of liver metastases or their development on survival. Survival rates were evaluated as described in Fig. 1. There were 158 patients with no liver metastases, 6 of whom died; 17 patients who did not initially have liver metastases developed liver metastases during follow-up period and 4 died; and of 37 patients with liver metastases present during an initial evaluation, 23 patients have died. (From [23])

main prognostic factor, patients without liver metastases showing a significantly longer survival. It is also important that patients who developed liver metastases during follow-up had a statistically significant worse survival than those who did not (Figs. 1, 2). Nevertheless, the authors recommend surgery only for patients with tumors of 3 cm in diameter or above [22, 23].

Early surgery would be justified if it could prevent the occurrence of liver metastases. Fraker et al. [24] showed that in 98 patients managed surgically, liver metastases occurred in 3 patients (3%) only, whereas in those managed medically they occurred in 6 of 26 patients (23%). In the same work it was shown that survival was different – in favor of those who had undergone surgery but the difference did not reach statistical significance.

As a "standard" procedure Thompson et al. [25] described an operation that encompasses distal pancreatectomy preserving the spleen, enucleation of tumors in the head, lymphadenectomy around the head of the pancreas, duodenotomy, sepa-

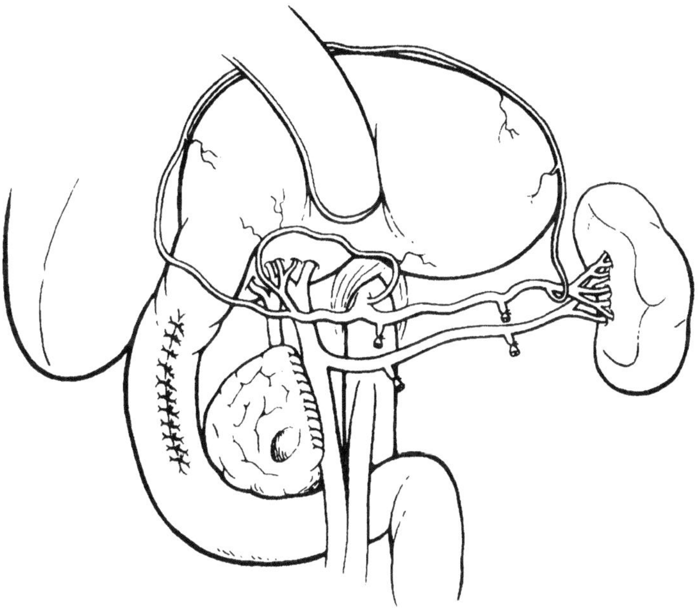

Fig. 3. The MEN I-ZES operation: (1) distal pancreatectomy (spleen saving), (2) enucleation of neuroendocrine tumors (head, uncinate), (3) duodenotomy, excision of neuroendocrine tumors, (4) regional lymph node dissection. (From [45])

rate palpation of the anterior and posterior wall of the duodenum for localization of microgastrinomas and excision of these tumors (Fig. 3). The procedure yielded excellent results in patients operated on for MEN I-ZES with 23 of 34 (68%) being normogastrinemic at follow-up; 9 of 27 (33%) had a negative secretin test [26].

There is limited experience with pancreatoduodenectomy for MEN I-ZES though it would make more sense compared to the procedure just mentioned, because also in the MEN I setting gastrinomas are almost always located in the gastrinoma triangle. On the other hand, pancreatoduodenectomy is a more demanding procedure and most likely accompanied by a higher morbidity than distal pancreatectomy. Data on pancreatoduodenectomy for MEN I-ZES show that patients at least for the years followed were biochemically cured with negative secretin stimulation tests [27, 28]. Our own experience includes another four patients with pancreatoduodenectomy for MEN I-ZES. Both have normal serum gastrin levels (basal and stimulated) 2 years after surgery.

In our view, there is a clear indication for surgery in MEN I gastrinoma patients if the tumors are 1 cm in diameter or more, since the risk for the development of liver metastases exceeds 4%. Local excision of duodenal gastrinomas and/or endocrine tumors within the pancreas is not successful. The operation described by Thompson et al. (Fig. 3) seems presently to be the most accepted procedure. Pancreatoduodenectomy is probably a better alternative to cure these patients.

Management of Neuroendocrine Pancreatic Tumors Detected by Genetic Screening

Since 1997, when the mutation associated with MEN I syndrome was described, almost all groups interested in these patients screened their families and have published data on the results of the screening. In our own material there were 15 unrelated kindred with MEN I. The mutations were first found in 12 of the 15 families [29] and later in the remaining three. Until recently, 35 unaffected members of the 15 families were screened. In eight of them a mutation was found, four of them had retrospectively symptoms of MEN I, mostly related to primary hyperparathyroidism and four patients were symptom-free. Among these symptom-free patients there was one with a positive secretin test for ZES. Microgastrinomas could be proven by duodenoscopy and biopsy. According to current recommendations this patient should be followed until the tumor diameter is 3 cm [22, 23].

There are data by Skogseid et al. [30, 31] showing that the disease of patients detected by biochemical or genetic screening, before symptoms develop, is more often limited than in symptomatic patients. The same is true for patients whose tumors are not yet demonstrable by imaging methods vs. those who are already visible. Though the number of patients observed is small and a good comparison cannot be made because of the retrospective design of the study, we believe that there is evidence that patients with NPTs detected by genetic and biochemical screening should undergo surgery before they develop symptoms and/or before their tumors are visible by imaging procedures.

Certainly this is a controversial issue since the natural history of MEN I NPTs is rather "benign." Also, since liver metastases are the main predictive factor and start to occur only after the tumors are bigger than 1 cm in size, one could wait for this stage of the disease. On the other hand, it is clear from data by Doherty et al. (1998) that patients may die from MEN I NPTs, showing that there is the same mortality in MEN I patients from MEN I-specific disease as well as from other reasons, but mortality from MEN I-specific disease occurs significantly earlier in life than from unrelated disease [32]. The question whether one should operate on these patients early or wait until the primary tumors are 3 cm in diameter can only be answered by a prospective controlled trial [33]. Such a trial seems to be warranted.

Malignant Neuroendocrine Pancreatic Tumors

The recognition of malignant neuroendocrine pancreatic tumors (NPTs) and their differentiation from exocrine malignancies is important in order to offer the patients an aggressive treatment even in an advanced stage of disease. One option to separate NPTs from exocrine tumors is, besides their appearance on CT scan or MRI, the use of somatostatin receptor scintigraphy. In contrast to exocrine tumors, NPTs express receptor subtype II that allows their imaging (Fig. 4).

About half of malignant NPTs are functioning (gastrinomas, insulinomas, glucagonomas etc.) and half are nonfunctioning [34]. Malignant NPTs threaten the patient's life by their growth (local invasion and/or metastases) and additionally – if present – by their excessive hormone production. To classify an NPT as malignant

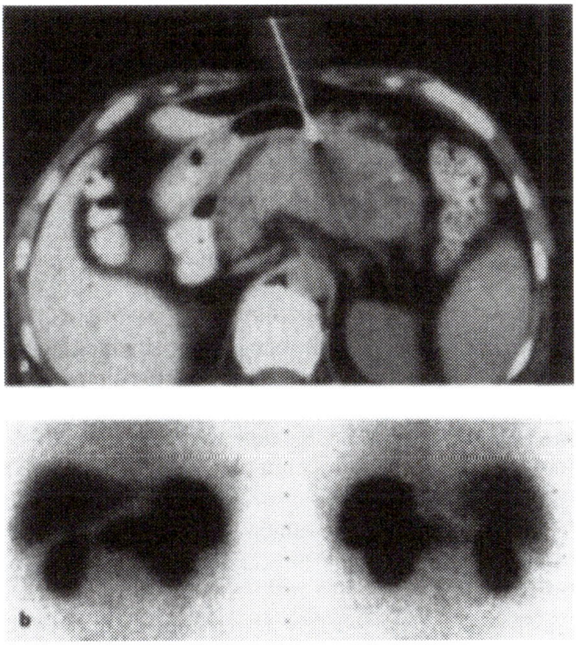

Fig. 4. a CT-guided needle aspiration from a huge pancreatic tumor, cytology showing evidence for adenocarcinoma. **b** The tumor is imaged by somatostatin receptor scintigraphy and was after resection diagnosed as a neuroendocrine tumor histologically (*left:* a–p projection, *right:* p–a projection)

usually requires the demonstration of distinct local invasion of surrounding soft tissue or vessels, or the presence of metastases, most commonly to the lymph nodes and liver.

Therapeutic options for a metastatic NPT include treatment with somatostatin alone or combined with interferon, chemotherapy, hepatic artery embolization and surgery. There are no prospective controlled trials for any of these modalities to prove their value. There is some evidence that surgery remains the most effective therapy for metastasizing NPTs, but aggressive resection of the primary and/or the metastases remains controversial. Also, only a minority of patients with metastasizing disease are suitable for potentially curative surgery [34, 35]. In a study from the Mayo Clinic encompassing 425 patients with neuroendocrine tumors of the intestine or pancreas, resection for liver metastases was performed only in 9% [36]. However, five of six potentially curative operated patients were alive and tumor-free at a mean follow-up of 20 months. Similar results were obtained by Frilling et al. [37] and Dousset et al. [38], who performed curative liver resections in 13% and 35% of their patients with NPT, respectively. In addition, Carty et al. [35] were able to show that patients with unresectable NPT had a 2-year survival of 60% and a 5-year survival of only 28%. The survival was 79% at 5 years when the hepatic metastases were completely removed. This is an impressive difference, although the patient groups were most likely not really comparable. Also, one has to keep in mind that recurrent disease is reported to be frequent [39].

The most controversial issue regarding metastatic NPTs is that of *orthotopic liver transplantation* (OLT). Whereas OLTs in patients with hepatic metastases of colorectal carcinoma, exocrine pancreatic carcinoma, or melanoma are very disappointing, highly selected patients with diffuse liver metastases from NPTs may benefit from this procedure. Pichlmayer et al. reported a 5-year survival rate of 81.8% after OLT for metastasized endocrine tumors [40]. Starzl's group had already documented five patients with metastases from NPT, including one gastrinoma and two glucagonomas, in whom OLT was performed [41]. Three patients were followed and were alive and tumor-free at 7, 16 and 34 months, respectively. On the other hand, Dousset et al. [38] reported early postoperative deaths due to surgical complications, graft rejection, or tumor recurrence in five of eight patients with OLT for liver metastases of NPT. The authors emphasized that technical difficulties of OLT in patients who had undergone either major surgery or chemoembolization should not be underestimated. Although their results were disappointing for patients with metastasized NPT, three patients grafted for metastasized neuroendocrine tumors of the gut ("carcinoid" tumors) survived tumor-free for a longer period of time. The seemingly better results of OLT for metastases from intestinal primaries were confirmed by the study of Le Treut et al. [42], who reported an actuarial 5-year survival rate of 78% for patients grafted because of intestinal neuroendocrine tumors, whereas patients grafted for NPT had a 2-year actuarial survival rate of 9% only. Thus, the benefit of OLT in patients with NPTs metastasizing to the liver will remain a matter of debate.

Multivisceral abdominal resections combined with cluster transplantations, as introduced by Starzl et al. in 1989 [43], offer a very radical but promising approach in highly selected patients with large neuroendocrine tumors of the pancreas or duodenum and nonresectable liver metastases. The actuarial 3-year survival rate for NPT was 64% with a postoperative mortality rate of 18%. However, in the Pittsburgh group's follow-up, the more aggressive procedure of abdominal exenteration with cluster transplantation has failed to reduce the rate of tumor recurrence when compared to standard OLT [44].

References

1. Chandrasekharappa SC, Guru SC, Manickam P, Olufemi S-E, Collins FS, Emmert-Buck MR, Debelenko LV, Zhuang Z, Lubensky IA, Liotta LA, Crabtree JS, Wang Y, Roe BA, Weisemann J, Boguski MS, Agarwal SK, Kester MB, Kim YS, Heppner C, Dongs Q, Spiegel AM, Burns AL, Marx SJ (1997) Positional cloning of the gene for multiple endocrine neoplasie-type 1. Science 276:404–406
2. Capella C, Heitz PU, Höfler H, Solcia E, Klöppel G (1994) Revised classification of neuroendocrine tumors of the lung, pancreas and gut. Digestion 55 [Suppl 3]:11–23
3. Klöppel G, Heitz PU, Capella C, Solcia E (1996) Pathology and nomenclature of human gastrointestinal neuroendocrine (carcinoid) tumors and related lesions. World J Surg 20:132–141
4. Van Heerden JA, Grant CS, Czako PF, Service J, Charboneau JW (1992) Occult functioning insulinomas: which localizing studies are indicated? Surgery 112:1010–1015
5. Rothmund M (1994) Localization of endocrine pancreatic tumours. Br J Surg 81:161–163
6. Rothmund M, Angelini L, Brunt M, Farndon JR, Geelhoed G, Grama D, Herfarth C, Kaplan E, Largiader F, Morino F, Peiper H-J, Proye C, Röher H-D, Rückert K, Kümmerle F, Thompson NW, van Heerden JA (1990) Surgery for benign insulinoma: an international review. World J Surg 14:393–399
7. Rösch R, Lightdale CJ, Botet JF, Boyce GA, Sivak MV, Yasuda K, Heyder N, Palazzo L, Dancygier H, Schusdziarra V, Classen M (1992) Localization of pancreatic endocrine tumors by endoscopic ultrasonography. N Engl J Med 326:1721–1726

8. Doppman JL, Miller DL, Chang R, Shawker TH, Gorden P, Norton JA (1991) Insulinomas: localization with selective intraarterial injection of calcium. Radiology 178:237–241
9. Demeure MJ, Klonoff CC, Karam JH, Duh Q-Y, D, Clark O (1991) Insulinomas associated with multiple endocrine neoplasia type I: the need for a different surgical approach. Surgery 110:998–1005
10. O'Riordain DS, O'Brien T, van Heerden JA, Service FJ, Grant CS (1994) Surgical management of insulinoma associated with multiple endocrine neoplasia type I. World J Surg 18:488–494
11. Thompson NW (1998) Current concepts in the surgical management of multiple endocrine neoplasia type 1 pancreatic-duodenal disease. Results in the treatment of 40 patients with Zollinger-Ellison-syndrome, hypoglycaemia or both. J Intern Med 243:495–500
12. Thompson NW, Vink AI, Eckhauser FE (1989) Microgastrinomas of the duodenum. A cause of failed operations for the Zollinger-Ellison syndrome. Ann Surg 9:396–404
13. Arnold WS, Fraker DL, Alexander HR, Weber HC, Norton JA, Jensen RT (1994) Apparent lymph node primary gastrinomal. Surgery 116:1123–1130
14. Norton JA, Fraker DL, Alexander HR, Venzon DJ, Doppman JL, Serrano J, Goebel SU, Peghini PL, Roy PK, Gibril F, Jensen RT (1999) Surgery to cure the Zollinger-Ellison syndrome. N Engl J Med 341:635–644
15. Gibril F, Reynolds JC, Doppman JL, Chen CC, Venzon DJ, Termanini B, Weber C, Stewart CA (1996) Somatostatin receptor scintigraphy: its sensitivity compared with that of other imaging methods in detecting primary and metastatic gastrinomas. Ann Intern Med 135:26–34
16. Kisker O, Bartsch D, Weinel RJ, Joseph K, Welcke UH, Zaraca F, Rothmund M (1997) The value of somatostatin-receptor scintigraphy in newly diagnosed endocrine gastroenteropancreatic tumors. J Am Coll Surg 184:487–492
17. Norton JA, Doppman JL, Jensen RT (1992) Curative resection in Zollinger-Ellison syndrome. Ann Surg 215:8–18
18. Kisker O, Bastian D, Bartsch D, Nies C, Rothmund M (1998) Localization, malignant potential, and surgical management of gastrinomas. World J Surg 22:651–658
19. Farley DR, van Heerden JA, Grant CS, Miller LJ, Ilstrup DM (1992) The Zollinger-Ellison syndrome. A collective surgical experience. Ann Surg 215:561–570
20. Mignon M, Ruszniewski P, Podevin P, Sabbagh L, Cadiot G, Rigaud D, Bonfils S (1993) Current approach to the management of gastrinoma and insulinoma in adults with multiple endocrine neoplasia type I. World J Surg 17:489–497
21. Weber C, Venzon DJ, Lin J-T, Fishbein VA, Orbuch M, Strader DB, Gibril F, Metz DC, Fraker DL, Norton JA, Jensen RT (1995) Determinants of metastatic rate and survival in patients with Zollinger-Ellison-syndrome: a prospective long-term study. Gastroenterology 108:1637–1649
22. Cadiot G, Vuagnat A, Doukhan I, Murat A, Bonnaud G, Delemer B, Thiéfin G, Beckers A, Veyrac M, Proye C, Ruszniewski P, Mignon M (1999) Prognostic factors in patients with Zollinger-Ellison-syndrome and multiple endocrine neoplasia type I. Gastroenterology 116:286–293
23. Yu F, Venzon DJ, Serrano J, Goebel SU, Doppman JL, Gibril F, Jensen T (1999) Prospective study of the clinical course, prognostic factors, causes of death, and survival in patients with long-standing Zollinger-Ellison-sydrome. J Clin Oncol 17:615–630
24. Fraker DL, Norton JA, Alexander R, Venzon DJ, Jensen RT (1994) Surgery for Zollinger-Ellison-syndrome alters the natural history of gastrinoma. Ann Surg 220:320–330
25. Thompson NW (1992) The surgical treatment of the endocrine pancreas and the Zollinger-Ellison syndrome in the MEN I syndrome. Henry Ford Hospital Med J 40:195–198
26. Thompson NW (1998) Current concepts in the surgical management of multiple endocrine neoplasia type I pancreatic-duodenal disease. Results in the treatment of 40 patients with Zollinger-Ellison-syndrome, hypoglycaemia or both. J Intern Med 243:495–500
27. Delcore R, Friesen SR (1992) Role of pancreatoduodenotomy in the management of primary duodenal wall gastrinomas in patients with Zollinger-Ellison-syndrome. Surgery 112:1016–1023
28. Stadil F, Bardram L, Gustafsen J, Efsen F (1993) Surgical treatment of the Zollinger-Ellison-syndrome. World J Surg 17:463–467
29. Bartsch D, Kopp I, Bergenfelz A, Rieder H, Münch K, Jäger K, Deiss Y, Schudy A, Barth P, Arnold R, Rothmund M, Simon B (1998) MEN1 gene mutations in 12 MEN1 families and their associated tumors. Eur J Endocrinol 139:416–420
30. Skogseid B, Öberg K, Eriksson B, Juhlin D, Granberg D, Akerström G, Rastad J (1996) Surgery for asymptomatic pancreatic lesion in multiple endocrine neoplasia type I. World J Surg 20:872–877
31. Skogseid B, Öberg K, Akerström G, Eriksson B, Westlin J-E, Janson ET, Eklöf H, Elvin A, Juhlin C, Rastad J (1998) Limited tumor involvement found at multiple endocrine neoplasia type I pancreatic exploration: can it be predicted by preoperative tumor localization? World J Surg 22:673–678

32. Doherty GM, Olson JA, Frisella MM, Lairmore TC, Wells SA, Norton JA (1998) Lethality of multiple endocrine neoplasia type I. World J Surg 22:581–587
33. Wells SA Jr (1999) Surgery for the Zollinger-Ellison syndrome. N Engl J Med 341:689–690
34. Lo CY, van Heerden JA, Thompson B, Grant CS, Söreide JA, Harmsen WS (1996) Islet cell carcinoma of the pancreas. World J Surg 20:878–884
35. Carty SE, Jensen RT, Norton JA (1992) Prospective study of aggressive resection of metastatic pancreatic endocrine tumors. Surgery 112:1024–1032
36. McEntee GP, Nagorney DM, Kvols LK, Moertel CG, Grant CSS (1990) Cytoreductive hepatic surgery for neuroendocrine tumors. Surgery 108:1091–1096
37. Frilling A, Rogiers X, Malago M, Liedke OM, Kaun M, Broelsch CE (1998) Treatment of liver metastases in patients with neuroendocrine tumors. Langenbecks Arch Surg 383:62–70
38. Dousset B, Saint-Marc O, Pitre J, Soubrane O (1996) Metastatic endocrine tumors: medical treatment, surgical resection, or liver transplantation. World J Surg 20:908–915
39. Norton JA (1994) Neuroendocrine tumors of the pancreas and duodenum. Curr Probl Surg 31:77–164
40. Pichlmayr R, Weimann A, Oldhafer KJ, Schlitt HJ, Klempnauer J, Bornscheuer A, Chavan A, Schmoll E, Lang H, Tusch G, Ringe B (1995) Role of liver transplantation in the treatment of unresectable liver cancer. World J Surg 19:807–813
41. Makowka L, Tzakis AG, Mazzaferro V, Teperman L, Demetris AJ, Iwatsuki S, Starzl TE (1989) Transplantation of the liver for metastatic endocrine tumors of the intestine and pancreas. Surg Gynecol Obstet 168:107–111
42. Le Treut YP, Delpero JR, Dousset B, Cherqui D, Segol P, Mantion G, Hannoun L, Benhamou G, Launois B, Boillot O, Domergue J, Bismuth H (1997) Results of liver transplantation in the treatment of metastatic neuroendocrine tumors. A 31 case French multicentric report. Ann Surg 225:355–364
43. Starzl TE, Todo S, Tzakis A, Podesta L, Mieles L, Demetris A, Teperman L, Selby R, Stevenson W, Stieber A, Gordon R, Iwatsuki S (1989) Abdominal organ cluster transplantation for the treatment of upper abdominal malignancies. Ann Surg 210:374–386
44. Alessiani M, Tzakis A, Todo S, Demetris AJ, Fung JJ, Starzl TE (1995) Assessment of 5-year experience with abdominal organ cluster transplantation. J Am Coll Surg 180:1–6

Cystic Tumors

Claudio Bassi · Massimo Falconi · Paolo Pederzoli

Introduction

Our knowledge of pancreatic cystic tumors (PCTs) dates back to 1830 [1]. Despite this, more than 150 years later, a report was published with the suggestive title "Spectrum of Cystic Tumors of the Pancreas" [2], bearing witness to the extent to which the identification, classification, natural history and therapeutic strategy of PCTs are still unresolved issues.

For many years, no more than a rough distinction was made between mucinous (macrocystic) and serous (microcystic) forms, but PCTs are now classified according to a system that defines each type on the basis of its epithelial lining (this latter element being the factor distinguishing PCTs from nonneoplastic cysts!) in conjunction with precise histological typing (Table 1) [3].

Mucinous PCTs are subdivided into two groups [4] with distinct anatomico-clinical characteristics, namely, *mucinous cystic tumors* (MCTs) and *intraductal papillary mucinous tumors* (IPMTs). The former, which occur exclusively in female subjects [5–8], are located mainly in the body tail and present one or more loculi

Table 1. Histological classification of pancreatic cystic tumors

a.	Microcystic/macrocystic serous tumor	**B**/M
b.	Mucinous cystic tumor	**B/UB**/M
c.	Intraductal papillary tumor with mucin hypersecretion	B/**UB**/M
d.	Solid (papillary) cystic tumor	**B**/M
e.	Mature cystic teratoma	**B**
f.	Acinar cystadenocarcinoma	**M**
g.	Endocrine cystic tumor	**B/UB**/M

B, benign; UB, uncertain biology; M, malignant. Boldface denotes the prevalent pattern.

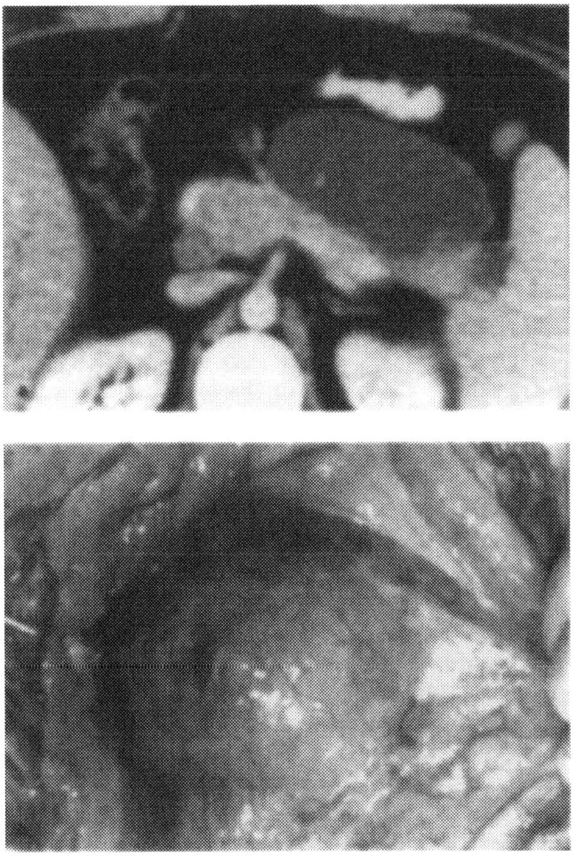

Fig. 5. a CT scan revealing encapsulated cystic mass of the body-tail of the pancreas suggestive of MCT. **b** Corresponding intraoperative appearance on opening the gastrocolic ligament. After splenopancreatectomy, histological examination confirmed the mucinous nature of the tumor with borderline aspects

unconnected to the ductal system (Fig. 5). The mucin-secreting epithelium is supported by ovarian-like stroma. Depending on the degree of epithelial dysplasia in these tumors, we can distinguish between *adenomas*, *borderline* forms and *adenocarcinomas*, the latter in turn being divided into *invasive* and *noninvasive* forms.

Histopathological examination by means of *multiple inclusions of the entire lesion* is mandatory for the correct classification of MCTs. This consideration in itself presents the surgeon with a clear-cut message: all MCTs are to be regarded as potentially malignant even if stromal invasion is the only useful parameter for identifying patients with a poor prognosis. None of our 49 cases with mild and borderline atypias presented recurrence or metastases after removal; in contrast, in the cystadenocarcinoma cases, the prognosis was strongly influenced by the type of intratumoral or capsular or extrapancreatic stromal invasiveness. The simultaneous presence of different degrees of dysplasia in the same tumor is suggestive of progression from adenoma to carcinoma [9–11].

In light of our most recent experience [8], we can conclude that the malignancy of MCTs correlates with multilocularity and presence of papillary projections or mural nodules, loss of ovarian-like stroma and p53 immunoreactivity. Moreover, the similarities between MCT and its ovarian, hepatobiliary and retroperitoneal counterparts suggest a common pathway for their development.

IPMT was long misdiagnosed, included among mucinous tumors in general and reported under various names [4, 11–13]. Its particular characteristics are prevalence in male subjects with a mean age of around 40 years, ERCP findings of dilation of the main and/or secondary ducts, dilation of the major and/or minor papilla with leakage of mucus, a clinical picture mimicking that of chronic obstructive pancreatitis, and intraductal growth.

In the case of these tumors, too, we distinguish between *adenomas, borderline* forms and *invasive* and *noninvasive adenocarcinomas.* In the early stage, the simple dilation of a secondary duct may point towards a misdiagnosis of MCT or pseudocyst in the course of chronic pancreatitis [11–16], but this aspect will be addressed later.

Serous cystic tumors (SCTs) consist of multiple cysts lined with epithelium characterizd by the absence of dysplasia. The clinical course is generally "silent" [17]. Only three malignant cases, all microcystic, have been reported in the literature [18–20]. Macroscopically, we distinguish between two variants, namely, microcystic and macrocystic SCTs. The former (52% of our 58 surgical observations) present a central scar and small cysts with a honey-comb appearance which often make radiological identification impossible (Fig. 6). Macrocystic SCTs are characterized by one or more cysts of various sizes with a serous content, no central scar and poorly demarcated growth. These features make it hard to differentiate preoperatively between these tumors and both pseudocysts and MCT [21, 22].

Despite their comparative rarity, we should also consider solid (papillary) cystic tumors (SPCT), which generally occur in young women. Although cases presenting malignant characteristics have been described, only one death due to metastasis has been reported to date; the finding of progesterone receptors suggests that the hormone may play a pathogenetic role in these tumors [23–27].

Natural History of PCT

Can the natural history of PCT be reliably outlined? In an attempt to answer this question, we feel that a number of important aspects should be addressed:

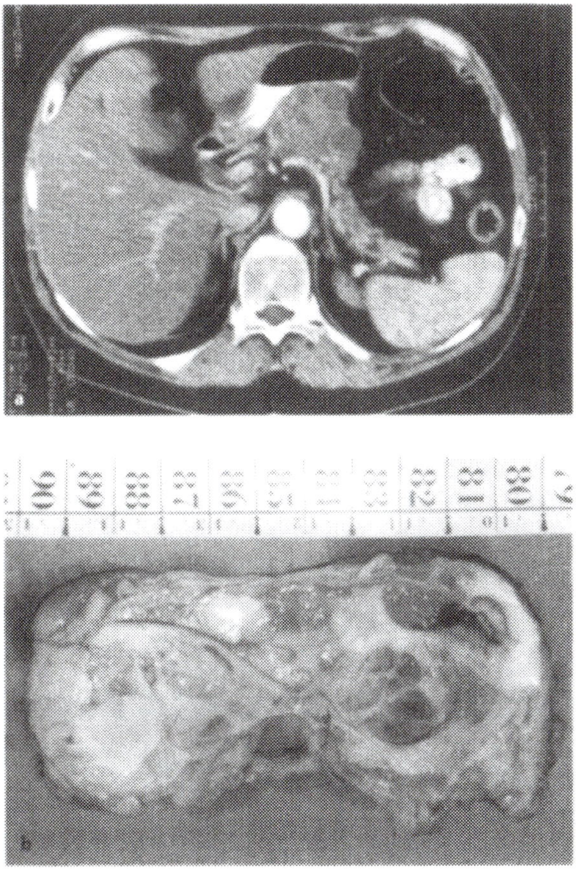

Fig. 6. a CT scan of "typical" serous tumor with multilocular-polycystic appearance and central scar. **b** Corresponding surgical specimen after intermediate resection of the pancreas

- These are lesions which should no longer be regarded as extremely rare, but rather as fairly frequent, as demonstrated by the progressive increase in reported cases of PCT as a result of the systematic use of US in the diagnosis of abdominal conditions. Since 1985 we ourselves have observed 209 cases, with an exponential increase in the number of cases over the three 5-year periods since that date. Also particularly noteworthy in this connection are the results of the autopsy study conducted by Kimura et al. [5], who report a 24% incidence of small PCTs (73/300 autopsy cases). The lesions detected are below the resolution capacity of the imaging techniques. This finding prompts one to postulate suggestive theories that may correlate well with the natural history of PCT: both the frequency and the tendency towards degeneration are high in such small lesions and are proportional to the age of the subjects.
- The possible malignant course even of serous forms is documented today not only in autopsy studies, but also in clinical studies [18, 20].
- The progression of MCTs to carcinoma is confirmed by the fact that patients treated initially with incomplete resection or erroneously by anastomosis subse-

quently presented malignant transformation [7, 17]. Our own experience in this connection is a good example [28]: seven patients with mucinous forms were treated by anastomosis and one by repeated external drainage. Possible progression to malignancy can also be deduced from the fact that the mean age of patients suffering from malignant forms is 10–12 years higher than that of patients with benign tumors.

- In the same tumor, the epithelium may vary from structurally benign to frankly malignant (how can we place any reliance on negative aspirate findings?!), passing through intermediate forms of atypicity defined as borderline. Furthermore, the extent of stromal invasion, meaning the progressive involvement of the intratumoral papillary stroma and of the capsula at peritumoral and extrapancreatic levels, provides evidence of the invasiveness or otherwise of a cystadenocarcinoma [4].

It would therefore appear both rational and prudent to consider PCTs as potentially malignant lesions and as almost certainly destined to develop into malignancies, if such development has not already occurred, when they contain mucin. We feel we should stress that, in the presence of mucin-secreting cystic tumors, thorough clinical observation and close monitoring cannot be a substitute for a *complete histological assessment* of their epithelium.

Role of Imaging: Pros and Cons

In cases of PCT, studied using US and/or CT scans, five distinct types of diagnostic situations may arise:

- A *firm diagnosis* can be formulated in no more than 15%–20% of cases and only in cases of serous cystadenoma presenting a "classic" appearance.
- A *highly probable diagnosis* can be formulated in 20%–25% of cases for cystic tumors belonging to the SPCT and IPMT categories. In the past, these tumors were mistaken for chronic obstructive pancreatitis. IPMTs of the secondary ducts are almost entirely tumors of the uncinate process, where they manifest themselves with a honey-comb appearance, in the context of which echogenic inclusions are detectable at traditional and/or endoscopic US or with solid density at CT. There is often involvement of the cephalic tract of Wirsung's duct with dilation upstream of it; in almost all such cases, dilation of the papilla protruding into the duodenal lumen is found. When an IPMT is suspected, the use of traditional ERCP or of MRI-ERCP is mandatory (Fig. 7), which in tumors of the secondary ducts shows the cystic mass in the uncinate process communicating with Wirsung's duct, while, in the case of tumors of the main duct, segmental or diffuse ductal ectasia is detected. Another characteristic element is the finding of amorphous defects in the context of the ducts, due to mucin or to actual papillary proliferations.
- A *probable diagnosis* can be formulated in 25%–30% of cases and refers to MCTs when manifesting as roundish masses, clearly demarcated with a distinct outline, and with macroscopic central cavities divided by sparse septations. Cal-

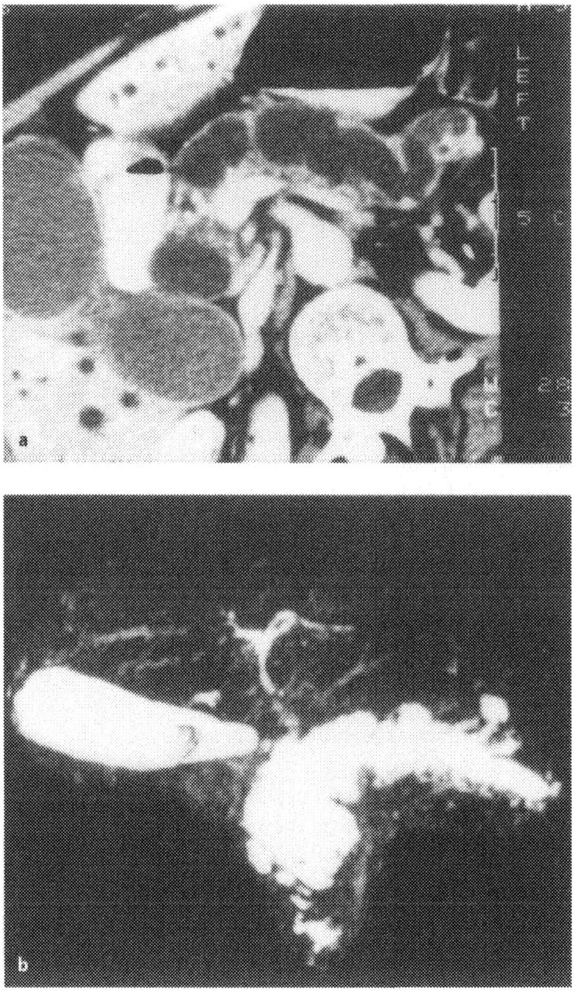

Fig. 7. CT scan (**a**) and MRI-ERCP (**b**) of diffuse IPMT affecting the entire pancreas and involving the main and secondary ducts. The patient was submitted to total pancreatectomy which revealed several degenerative areas along Wirsung's duct without either stromal or capsular infiltration

cifications are frequent. In no case is it possible to diagnose a malignancy on the basis of the morphological characteristics, except where remote metastases are detectable. The macrocystic appearance of MCTs cannot be regarded as pathognomonic, since, like pseudocysts, all PCTs can present themselves in this form. Hence the advisability, in the presence of a macrocystic lesion, of performing a needle aspiration, bearing in mind, however, the potential risk of dissemination of "malignant" mucus.

- A *nonspecific diagnosis* is inevitable in 15%–20% of cases, in the presence of a unilocular cystic mass. This aspect, which is more frequent in pseudocysts, can, in fact, be detected in all PCTs, particularly mucinous ones. In this case, preoperative characterization of the lesion can be achieved only by needle aspiration.

- *Misdiagnosis*, which occurs in approximately 20% of cases, is due to the abnormal appearance of the lesion, which makes it indistinguishable from other pancreatic diseases.

In conclusion, then, imaging techniques make a decisive contribution towards identifying PCTs and are important for their typing. Despite this, there are still situations in which the aspecificity of the findings or particular morphological and structural aspects do not allow a firm diagnosis to be achieved [29, 31].

Diagnostic Value of Cytology and Analysis of Cystic Content: Pros and Cons

Transcutaneous cytology can provide invaluable information such as findings of malignant cells. It is important to stress that information defined as "invaluable" is only such in the case of *clear-cut positivity* of the cytological examination (18 cases out of 59 in our experience). In actual fact, a negative cytological result does not necessarily mean the absence of malignant disease and invariably requires further diagnostic investigation. False-negatives amounted to 6.8% in our series.

Unfortunately, serum markers lack diagnostic reliability. CA 19-9 and CEA in the intracystic fluid do not in themselves help to distinguish between the various types of neoplasms [32–34].

One element which is only apparently banal is the visual evaluation of cystic aspirate. The appearance of the aspirate – fluid and transparent, on the one hand, and dense, streaky and/or hemorrhagic, on the other – clearly distinguishes between serous and mucinous forms. In the latter, high CA 19-9 and CEA protein concentrations are indicative of possible degeneration.

We can conclude that the combination of viscosity, CA 19-9, CEA and CA 125 levels, and cytology may afford a reasonable chance of distinguishing between malignant or potentially malignant PCTs and benign PCTs. The isoamylase content is fundamental (generally speaking, along with the clinical history!) in the differential diagnosis vs. pseudocysts. Table 2 gives the main differences in intracystic fluid characteristics that can be used in making the differential diagnosis [32, 34].

Lastly, we feel we should stress that, despite the importance attributed to evaluating the cystic content, we do not regard an exploratory puncture as necessary, reserving its use only for those patients in whom the diagnostic work-up fails to provide a clear indication for surgical exploration.

Table 2. Characteristics of intracystic fluid in pancreatic cystic tumors and pseudocysts

Type	Viscosity	CA 19-9	CEA	CA 125	Enzymes
Pseudocyst	Low	Variable	Low	Low	High
SCT	Low	Variable	Low	Variable	Variable
MCT	High	Elevated	High	Variable	Variable
CAK	High	Elevated	High	Variable	Variable

SCT, serous cystic tumor; MCT, mucinous cystic tumor; CAK, cystadenocarcinoma.

Therapy

The therapy of PCTs is generally surgical. Clinical, laboratory and radiological examinations are capable of yielding a correct diagnosis in no more than 80% of cases. In view of the degenerative potential of these tumors, surgery sometimes proves mandatory not only in therapeutic terms but also in order to define the tumors histologically.

The choice of type and extent of resection will depend upon the histotype since, if the lesion is malignant, the resection will have to be as radical as possible. Depending also on the site of the cystic tumor, conservative operations may be indicated in order to preserve parenchyma (duodeno-preserving resections of the head, spleen-preserving intermediate resections or resections of the tail) when the histotype appears to be reassuring with regard to present or future malignancy. In symptomatic cystic tumors of the head of the pancreas which cannot be treated by pancreatoduodenectomy, even an anastomosis may be an acceptable "conscious" option.

Lastly, a wait-and-see policy is a feasible proposition only if the preoperative characteristics are unquestionably typical of the serous forms, but if the tumor produces symptoms, the only acceptable solution once again is surgery.

With the sole exception, then, of the serous microcystic variant, all PCTs are potential candidates for surgical treatment. The absolute need for the pathologist to have the entire surgical specimen is another of the elements which make surgery mandatory in patients with "macrocystic" tumors or tumors belonging to the macrocystic SCT variant category.

Figures 8 and 9, in fact, are an attempt to summarize the diagnostic algorithm and the decision-making process in PCT. Recently, Le Borgne [35] has claimed that the discovery of a PCT should be followed by three steps: (1) confirmation of the intrapancreatic origin of the tumor; (2) investigation to rule out the diagnosis of a pseudocyst; and (3) identification of those PCTs which need resection owing to actual or potential malignancy. Substantially, we agree with this approach,

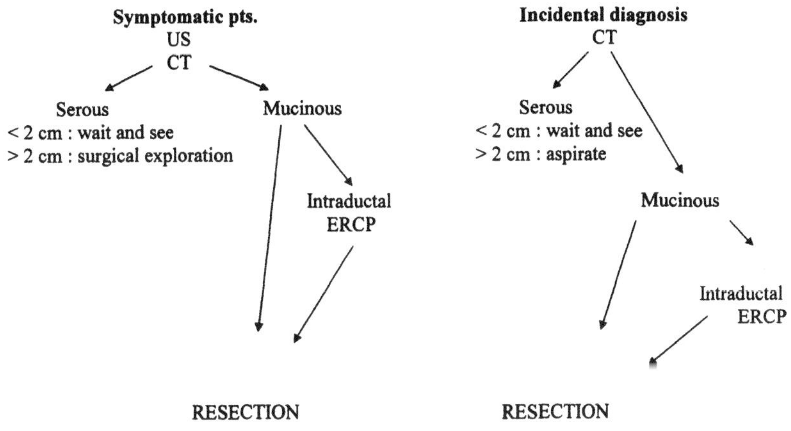

Fig. 8. Diagnostic algorithm in pancreatic cystic tumors

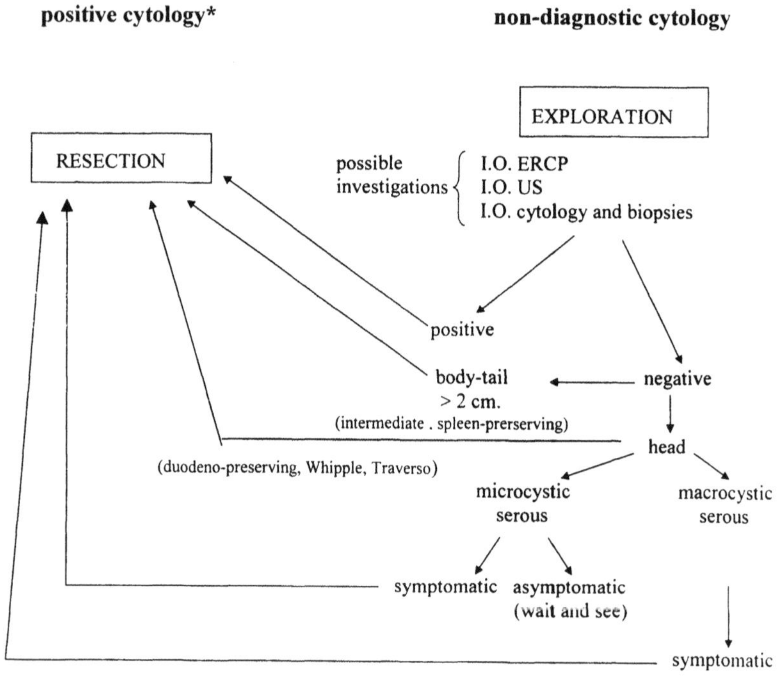

Fig. 9. Surgical decision-making in pancreatic cystic tumors* (*positive*-presence of malignant cells and/or mucin, *negative*-absence of malignant cells and/or mucin with presence of serous content)

though we would modify the emphasis and wording of step 3 so that it reads "identification of those (few) PCTs which can be left alone"!

References

1. Becourt PJ, Becourt G (1830) Recherches sur le pancréas: ses fonctions et ses alterations organiques. Levrautl, Strasbourg
2. Talamini MA, Pitt HA, Hruban RH, Boitnott JK, Coleman J, Cameron JL (1992) Spectrum of cystic tumors of the pancreas. Am J Surg 163:117–123
3. Klöppel G, Solcia E, Longnecker DS, et al. (1996) Histological typing of tumors of the exocrine pancreas, 2nd edn. Springer, Berlin Heidelberg New York
4. Yang EYT, Joehl RJ, Talamonti MS (1994) Cystic neoplasms of the pancreas. J Am Coll Surg 179:747–757
5. Kimura W, Nagai H, Kuroda A, Muto T, Esaki Y (1995) Analysis of small cystic lesions of the pancreas. Int J Pancreatol 18:197–206
6. Zamboni G, Scarpa A, Bogina G, et al. (1994) Cystic tumors of the pancreas. In: Pederzoli P, Cavallini G, Bassi C (eds) Facing the pancreatic dilemma. Springer, Berlin Heidelberg New York, pp 368–397
7. Compagno J, Oertel JE (1978) Mucinous cystic neoplasms of the pancreas with overt and latent malignancy (cystadenocarcinoma and cystadenoma). A clinicopathologic study of 41 cases. Am J Clin Pathol 69:573–580
8. Zamboni G, Scarpa A, Bogina G, et al. (1999) Mucinous cystic tumors of the pancreas: clinicopathological features, prognosis, and relationship with other mucinous cystic tumors. Am J Surg Pathol 23:410–422

9. Yamada M, Kozuka S, Yamano K, et al. (1991) Mucin-producing tumor of the pancreas. Cancer 68:159–168
10. Hodgkinson DJ, ReMine WH, Weiland LH (1978) A clinicopathologic study of 21 cases of pancreatic cystadenocarcinoma. Ann Surg 188:679–684
11. Obara T, Maguchi H, Saitoh Y, et al. (1991) Mucin-producing tumor of the pancreas: a unique clinical entity. Am J Gastroenterol 86:1619–1625
12. Rickaert F, Cremer M, Devière J, et al. (1991) Intraductal mucin-hypersecreting neoplasms of the pancreas. A clinicopathologic study of eight patients. Gastroenterology 101:512–519
13. Itai Y, Ohhashi K, Nagai H, et al. (1986) "Ductectatic" mucinous cystadenoma and cystadenocarcinoma of the pancreas. Radiology 161:697–700
14. Bastid C, Bernard JP, Sarles H, Payan MJ, Sahel J (1991) Mucinous ductal ectasia of the pancreas: a premalignant disease and a cause of obstructive pancreatitis. Pancreas 6:15–22
15. Sessa F, Solcia E, Capella C, et al. (1994) Intraductal papillary-mucinous pancreatic tumors represent a distinct group of pancreatic neoplasms: an investigation of tumor cell differentiation and K-ras, p53 and c-erbB-2 abnormalities in 26 patients. Virchows Arch 425:357–367
16. Nagai E, Ueki T, Ohijiiwa K, Tanaka M, Tsuneyashi M (1995) Intraductal papillary mucinous neoplasms of the pancreas associated with so-called "mucinous ductal ectasia". Am J Surg Pathol 19:576–589
17. Compagno J, Oertel JE (1978) Microcystic adenomas of the pancreas (glycogen-rich cystadenomas): a clinicopathologic study of 34 cases. Am J Clin Pathol 69:289–298
18. George DH, Murphy F, Michalski R, Ulmer BJ (1989) Serous cystadenocarcinoma of the pancreas: a new entity? Am J Surg Pathol 13:61–66
19. Kamei T, Funabiki M, Ochiai M, et al. (1992) Some considerations on the biology of pancreatic serous cystadenoma. Int J Pancreatol 11:97–104
20. Yoshimi N, Sugie S, Tanaka T, et al. (1992) A rare case of serous cystadenocarcinoma of the pancreas. Cancer 69:2449–2453
21. Lewandrowski K, Warshaw A, Compton C, et al. (1992) Macrocystic serous cystadenoma of the pancreas: a morphologic variant differing from microcystic adenoma. Hum Pathol 23:871–875
22. Egawa N, Maillet B, Schröder S, Mukai K, Klöppel G (1994) Serous oligocystic and ill-demarcated adenoma of the pancreas: a variant of serous cystic adenoma. Virchows Arch 424:13–17
23. Klöppel G, Maurer R, Hofmann E, et al. (1991) Solid-cystic (papillary-cystic) tumours within and outside the pancreas in men: report of two patients. Virchows Arch 418:179–183
24. Nishihara K, Nagoshi M, Tsuneyoshi M, Yamaguchi K, Hayashi I (1993) Papillary cystic tumors of the pancreas. Assessment of their malignant potential. Cancer 71:82–92
25. Compagno J, Oertel JE, Kremzar M (1979) Solid and papillary epithelial neoplasms of the pancreas, probably of small duct origin: a clinopathologic study of 52 cases. Lab Invest 40:248–249
26. Matsunou H, Konishi F, Yamamichi N, Takayanagi N, Mukai M (1990) Solid, infiltrating variety of papillary cystic neoplasm of the pancreas. Cancer 65:2747–2757
27. Zamboni G, Bonetti F, Scarpa A, et al. (1993) Expression of progesterone receptors in solid-cystic tumours of the pancreas: a clinicopathological and immunohistochemical study of ten cases. Virchows Arch 423:425–431
28. Pederzoli P, Bassi C, Falconi M, et al. (1996) I tumori cistici del pancreas. Atti Congresso Società Italiana di Chirurgia 1:96–113
29. Grieshop NA, Wiebke EA, Kratzer SS, Madura JA (1994) Cystic neoplasms of the pancreas. Am Surg 60:509–515
30. Procacci C (1994) Cystic tumours of the pancreas: possibilities of radiologic characterization. In: Pederzoli P, Cavallini G, Bassi C (eds) Facing the pancreatic dilemma. Springer, Berlin Heidelberg New York, pp 349–367
31. Procacci C, Graziani R, Bicego E, et al. (1996) Intraductal mucin-producing tumors of the pancreas: imaging findings. Radiology 198:249–257
32. Lewandrowski K, Lee J, Southern J, Centeno B, Warshaw A (1995) Cyst fluid analysis in the differential diagnosis of pancreatic cysts: a new approach to the preoperative assessment of pancreatic cystic lesions. Am J Roentgenol 164:815–819
33. Gupta RK, al-Ansari A (1994) Needle aspiration cytology in the diagnosis of mucinous cystadenocarcinoma of the pancreas. A study of five cases with an emphasis on utility and differential diagnosis. Int J Pancreatol 15:149–153
34. Lewandrowski KB, Southern JF, Pins MR, Compton CC, Warshaw AL (1993) Cyst fluid analysis in the differential diagnosis of pancreatic cysts. A comparison of pseudocysts, serous cystadenomas, mucinous cystic neoplasms, and mucinous cystadenocarcinoma. Ann Surg 217:41–47
35. Le Borgne J (1998) Cystic tumors of the pancreas. Br J Surg 85:577–578

Invited Comment

Richard A. Prinz · Constantine V. Godellas

The preceding sections outline some of the controversies facing physicians in the management of endocrine and cystic tumors of the pancreas. Some of these issues have been present for many years and others are the result of technologic advances that have increased our knowledge of these unusual lesions. Since these are two varied topics, they will be addressed separately.

Endocrine Tumors

Most surgeons in the United States still refer to endocrine tumors of the pancreas by the primary hormone which they secrete and not by the broad term of neuroendocrine pancreatic tumors. Most of the available data for endocrine tumors of the pancreas are obtained from tertiary centers where a relatively large number of these patients are seen. This is especially true for patients with multiple endocrine neoplasia type I (MEN I) associated pancreatic endocrine tumors. While some would recommend that all patients with these tumors be referred to specialized centers, the fact is that many patients will be initially worked-up and even treated at nonspecialized centers. We believe that the best method of localizing endocrine tumors of the pancreas is intraoperative exploration. Nevertheless preoperative imaging can be helpful to the surgeon and a cost-effective approach should be utilized in evaluating patients with insulinoma and gastrinoma. For both, we would start with CT scan. Although this study identifies the primary lesion in less than 20% of patients, it does image the liver and peripancreatic area and can identify metastatic disease. For insulinoma, our next preoperative study would be an endoscopic ultrasound. This can identify greater than 80% of these lesions. For gastrinomas, our second study would be an octreotide scan because of the high likelihood of positive somatostatin receptors on gastrinomas. This study can also identify extra pancreatic or metastatic disease. Arteriography with selective arterial calcium or secretin injection and venous sampling are only used in exceptional circumstances such as re-operations. Thorough intraoperative exploration by an experienced endocrine surgeon will find most insulinomas and gastrinomas. We consider intraoperative ultrasound as an essential part of the exploration procedure for these tumors. We do not advocate blind distal pancreatectomy for the patient with biochemical evidence of an insulinoma in whom no tumor has been found intraoperatively. A small biopsy should be obtained from the tail to rule out islet cell hyperplasia. This patient should then undergo further work-up to confirm the diagnosis and invasive localization procedures such as selective intra-arterial calcium injection.

The surgical management of patients with MEN I syndrome is much more controversial. The recent identification of the genetic abnormality of this syndrome has only added to this controversy. Currently there is no clinical utility for genetic screening of patients at risk for MEN I syndrome for possible pancreatic tumor.

The risk of pancreatic surgery is too great for patients to undergo prophylactic procedures. Likewise, the natural history of patients with MEN I disease has been rather indolent. We do not advocate genetic screening for pancreatic endocrine tumors in MEN I patients except under research protocols.

We would agree that symptomatic MEN I patients with insulinomas and gastrinomas should undergo surgery. Although there is controversy about what procedure should be utilized, we would perform distal pancreatectomy with enucleation of tumors in the head of the gland. For gastrinomas, the duodenum should be thoroughly evaluated because of the high likelihood of lesions being located there. Usually this requires opening the duodenum for complete bimanual palpation. We would also advocate surgical exploration in MEN I patients for lesions that are increasing in size, or that are greater than 2–3 cm in diameter.

We believe that an aggressive approach is warranted for malignant neuroendocrine tumors of the pancreas. Long survival is possible with these tumors so pancreatectomy and resection of metastatic disease can offer substantial palliation. Multivisceral transplantation for pancreatic endocrine tumors should be viewed as an experimental procedure and done under research protocol.

Cystic Tumors

Cystic tumors of the pancreas present no less controversy than endocrine tumors. It is critically important not to mistake a cystic tumor of the pancreas for a pseudocyst. This distinction can be made on clinical grounds. Pseudocysts will have a history of pancreatitis and a high likelihood of an elevated amylase. Cystic neoplasms will usually not have either of these. At operation, the remaining pancreas will be indurated with evidence of prior pancreatitis with a pseudocyst, but will be normal with a cystic neoplasm. Cystic neoplasms should be considered malignant or premalignant. The one exception might be serous tumors, but there have been rare reports of even these being malignant. Because of their malignant potential we believe that cystic tumors should be removed whenever this can be safely accomplished. In patients who are poor risks for surgery we would consider percutaneous aspiration of cyst fluid using a combination of measuring viscosity, CA 19-9, and CEA and evaluating cytology to distinguish between benign and potentially malignant cystic tumors. The benign lesions would then be followed with serial CT scans and the malignant lesions resected. Aspiration and cyst fluid evaluation is only used in patients in whom we are trying to avoid operation.

Complete surgical excision with formal pancreatectomy has been the approach for most mucinous tumors of the pancreas. This has been recommended because of the difficulty in distinguishing between benign and malignant disease. Even biopsy of the wall of the tumor has its shortcomings since the malignant growth may not be seen in all areas. Recent studies have reported enucleating small mucinous cystadenomas of the pancreas [1]. We believe this is a reasonable approach in patients with tumors less than 3–4 cm in diameter. Care must be taken not to injure the pancreatic duct when utilizing this approach or a high likelihood of pancreatic fistula and peripancreatic fluid collection problems will be encountered.

Intraductal papillary mucinous tumors have been reported with increasing frequency in the last decade. Our knowledge about their natural history remains incomplete. Nevertheless, this lesion should be kept in mind and not be mistaken for the ductal changes of chronic pancreatitis. The finding of mucus exuding from the ampulla of Vater is diagnostic. Complete excision of all the ductal mucosa containing this lesion is important to prevent recurrence and possible progression to frank malignancy. Nevertheless caution should be utilized in performing total pancreatectomy for this lesion. We currently perform pancreaticoduodenectomy or distal pancreatectomy depending on the disease location and utilize intraoperative frozen section to be certain that all of the diseased tissue has been cleared. Unfortunately there are shortcomings with this approach. We utilize MRCP to follow the ductal changes in the pancreatic remnant. Further follow-up studies will be helpful to identify the proper clinical approach to IPMT. In summary, cystic tumors of the pancreas pose problems in diagnosis. These lesions can be confused with benign lesions such as pseudocysts or chronic pancreatitis. If kept in mind they can be easily diagnosed and appropriately treated. This is extremely important because these patients usually have a very good prognosis when properly managed.

Reference

1. Talamini MA, Moesinger R, Yeo CJ, et al. (1998) Cystadenomas of the pancreas; is enucleation an adequate operation? Ann Surg 227:896–903

Editorial Comment

The average general surgeon is only seldom exposed to *endocrine pancreatic tumors*. Thus, we depend on experts such as Professor Rothmund and Dr. Bartsch who guide us in formulating diagnostic and therapeutic approaches to these rare conditions. In the second part of this chapter, Drs. Bassi, Falconi and Pederzoli share with us their experience with the multifaceted aspects of *cystic pancreatic tumors*, which although not commonplace, are diagnosed with an increasing frequency and are more amenable to curative surgery than their adenocarcinoma counterparts. And finally, Drs. Prinz and Godellas offer a balancing comment, emphasizing that the more common pancreatic pseudocysts have to be differentiated from cystic tumors and that intraductal papillary mucinous tumors should not be confused with chronic pancreatitis. If the readers would take notice of these two messages only, this section has achieved its purpose.

CHAPTER 7

Appendicitis

Acute Appendicitis

Shawn J. Pelletier · Timothy L. Pruett

Introduction

Acute appendicitis, with a 7% lifetime risk [1], remains the most common indication for emergency abdominal surgery. Considerable morbidity and mortality continue to be associated with appendicitis despite what is currently considered to be appropriate antibiotic and surgical care. Although the overall mortality rate is less than 1% in many series, the mortality associated with appendicitis in elderly patients ranges between 5% and 15% [2, 3]. The incidence of perforation commonly ranges from 17% to 40% [4, 5], is increased at both spectrums of age [2, 3, 6–12], and is well known to be associated with significant morbidity. Surgical doctrine suggests that a percentage of negative laparotomies are necessary and acceptable to limit the rate of perforation. Current studies demonstrate the negative laparotomy rate to range from 15% to 35% and to be associated with significant morbidity [4, 5, 13–15]. Because lower abdominal pain may be due to pelvic inflammatory disease or other obstetrical or gynecologic etiologies [4, 5, 16, 17], up to 45% of women of childbearing age are found to have normal appendices at exploration. Many controversies exist regarding the best method to improve accurate diagnosis, limit the number of negative laparotomies without increasing perforation rates, and the appropriate management of the complications of appendicitis to decrease morbidity and mortality.

Best Method to Obtain an Accurate Diagnosis

Attempts have been made to reduce the morbidity and mortality due to perforation or removal of normal appendices by improving the accuracy and decreasing the time for diagnosis. These attempts have included algorithm or computer-based diagnostic schemes [18–26], laboratory tests, or the utilization of imaging techniques such as ultrasound and CT scanning. Although varying degrees of success have been achieved, a balance of reasonable cost, timely diagnosis, and distribution of resources must be maintained.

History and Physical Examination

Although single evaluation of any one clinical variable alone has limited predictive value [27], a careful history and physical examination may remain the most effective and practical diagnostic modality [28, 29]. History and physical examination are increasingly underutilized and are being replaced with expensive technology. Although clinicians often do not collect sufficient data to make an accurate diagnosis [30, 31], careful clinical evaluation has been associated with a decrease in previously high rates of negative laparotomies.

Wagner et al. analyzed the results from 11 different publications evaluating different aspects of the history and physical examination for lower abdominal pain [32]. The authors calculated the sensitivity and specificity, respectively, of 13 characteristics of the history and physical examination including right lower quadrant pain (0.81/0.53), the presence of rigidity (0.27/0.83), migration of periumbilical pain to the right lower quadrant (0.64/0.82), the occurrence of pain before vomiting (1.00/0.64), the presence of the psoas sign (0.16/0.95), fever (0.67/0.79), rebound tenderness (0.63/0.69), guarding (0.74/0.57), absence of similar pain previously (0.81/0.41), rectal tenderness (0.41/0.77), anorexia (0.68/0.36), nausea (0.58/0.37), and vomiting (0.51/0.45). The three findings consistently found within these 11 studies to be most useful when present for identifying acute appendicitis included right lower quadrant pain, rigidity, and migration of initial periumbilical pain to the right lower quadrant. Another study demonstrated rebound tenderness, guarding, and gender to be independent predictors of appendicitis, while anorexia, nausea, and right-sided rectal tenderness had no diagnostic value [27].

An extended period of observation in patients with equivocal findings may be helpful [12, 18, 19]. Although a delay in patient presentation to the hospital is associated with an increased rate of perforation, admission and observation to clarify an uncertain diagnosis does not appear to increase findings consistent with late appendicitis in those patients requiring surgery [33]. The use of CT scanning early after presentation may be able to exclude appendicitis and has been advocated by some to allow early discharge and thus be cost effective. However, a proportion of patients will present with equivocal findings along with nausea, vomiting, and the inability to tolerate oral intake. This may represent a patient population that requires admission regardless of the need for surgery and may best be managed by observation and intravenous fluid replacement. The effectiveness of an observation period is dependent on the clinical skills of the caring physician.

Laboratory Evaluation

Although studies have evaluated many different laboratory tests to diagnose appendicitis, none have been completely reliable. An elevated white blood cell count with a predominance of polymorphonuclear cells ("left shift") remains the most commonly used and readily available. However, the white blood cell count has been demonstrated to only have a sensitivity and specificity of 81% and 36%, respectively [34]. Although currently having a limited role for diagnosis of appendicitis, investigators have evaluated the utility of other laboratory tests including acute phase reactants such as C-reactive peptide [35–38], proinflammatory cytokines such as interleukin-6 [39], and elastases [34].

Clearly history, physical examination, and basic laboratory evaluation including a white blood cell count with differential can accurately diagnose appendicitis in many patients. History and examination alone have an accuracy of 84% while addition of laboratory data including the white blood cell count with differential and C-reactive protein concentration improve the accuracy significantly to 92% [40]. Patients presenting with a clear clinical diagnosis of appendicitis should receive fluid resuscitation, antibiotics, and can be brought to the operating room without further investigation with a low rate of histologically normal appendices. Only those patients presenting with equivocal findings should be evaluated with imaging modalities.

Radiological Evaluation

The utility of radiographic diagnosis has been an area of recent attention. Previous studies evaluating plain abdominal radiographic imaging and barium enemas have demonstrated these modalities to be neither specific nor sensitive [41]. Although considerable effort has been directed toward studying the utility of ultrasound for the evaluation of acute appendicitis, its role will likely be limited. Abdominal ultrasound is more effective to detect distention of the appendix rather than perforation [9, 41–49]. Studies have not demonstrated ultrasound to be clearly superior to history and physical examination. Implementing the use of ultrasound may also not be widely applicable outside of research protocols because of high operator variability associated with this modality.

Compared to ultrasound, CT has been demonstrated to be superior in both adult and pediatric populations [50, 51]. CT scan of the appendix has been demonstrated to have a sensitivity ranging from 96% to 100%, a specificity of 89–97%, a positive-predictive value of 92–97%, and a negative predictive value of 95–100% [50, 52–54]. The utilization of appendiceal CT has been associated with a decrease in the negative appendectomy rate by 13% [55–57], a reduction in the perforation rate by 8% [55], and a lowering of total costs by decreasing the average length of stay for observation by allowing the diagnosis of an abnormal appendix or an alternative diagnosis to be made sooner [56, 57]. Similar results have been reproduced in a community hospital setting [58]. In addition, CT can also be beneficial for evaluating patients with suspected recurrent or chronic appendicitis [59]. However, conflicting results exist suggesting that radiological misdiagnosis of diverticulitis and appendicitis leads to unnecessary hospitalization, medical treatment, and overuse of hospital resources [60].

Imaging modalities have a clear benefit for clarifying the diagnosis in patients with lower abdominal pain but perhaps should be restricted to those with an uncertain diagnosis. High positive and negative predictive values have been demonstrated for abdominal CT scanning, allowing the ability to include or exclude the diagnosis of appendicitis. Ultrasound is not as accurate for detecting ruptured appendices and is limited for ruling out appendicitis but may have a role for evaluation of pelvic organs in women of childbearing age.

Nonoperative Versus Surgical Management

Appendiceal Abscess

Although removal of the appendix in almost any patient is probably safe with antibiotic coverage, a nonoperative approach, including intravenous fluid replacement and antibiotics, has been previously advocated for the treatment of a nontoxic patient with a clear diagnosis of appendiceal abscess. Patients not responding within 24–48 h as assessed by clinical parameters are then usually treated with operative management. With antibiotic therapy, periappendiceal abscesses usually resolve in 10–14 days without surgical or percutaneous drainage. Although CT-guided drainage is now possible with the advantage of faster resolution of the periappendiceal abscess, drainage is frequently not required. Although the standard transabdominal approach using CT or sonographic guidance is preferred, a variety of approaches, including transgastric, transrectal, transvaginal and transgluteal, may be used [61]. Limitations include difficulty draining multiloculated abscesses, inaccessible locations or the need for general anesthesia in the pediatric population. Conservative therapy was typically followed by an interval appendectomy at 6 weeks to 3 months after nonoperative treatment and has been associated with low morbidity without prolonged hospitalization [62, 63].

Controversy exists regarding the necessity of interval appendectomy following conservative treatment for periappendiceal abscess. When interval appendectomy was not performed, the rate of recurrent appendicitis requiring surgical intervention was approximately 10% in the adult and pediatric population [64, 65]. Others argue that although initial drainage of periappendiceal abscess is effective, the possibility of recurrence suggests that interval appendectomy should be a critical component of management [66].

Perforated Appendicitis

Bufo and colleagues demonstrated that nonoperative treatment of perforated appendicitis with IV fluid administration and antibiotic therapy in pediatric patients followed by interval appendectomy was a safe alternative. When successful, length of hospitalization, overall costs, and morbidity were less [67]. Others have treated perforated appendicitis in children with immediate appendectomy, intra-abdominal antibiotic irrigation, transperitoneal drainage through the wound, and 10-day treatment with triple-therapy intravenous antibiotics with a major complication rate of 6.4% [68].

Acute Appendicitis

A prospective controlled study demonstrated that 2 days of antibiotics intravenously followed by oral treatment for 8 days was as effective as surgery for acute appendicitis. Patients treated conservatively had short hospital stays, less pain and required less analgesia but the recurrence rate of appendicitis requiring surgical intervention within 1 year was 35% [69]. Although ultrasound examination can be used in the evaluation for failure of treatment [70], the high rate of recurrence without surgery and the minimal morbidity and mortality associated with surgical therapy suggests that operative intervention should be the preferred method of treatment.

Laparoscopic Versus Open Appendectomy

Although numerous studies have been performed comparing open to laparoscopic appendectomy, most randomized studies have only enrolled approximately 100 patients and inconsistent results have been demonstrated. Theoretically, laparoscopy offers the advantage of allowing a more complete examination of the abdomen, avoids the misplacement of a small incision, and may be useful when appendiceal pathology is not encountered. Debate exists regarding whether the laparoscopic technique should be routinely used for all appendectomies.

When compared to open appendectomy, laparoscopic appendectomy has not been consistently shown to be advantageous. A meta-analysis of ten studies demonstrated an increased risk for surgical site infection for open appendectomy [71]. Minimal or no difference has been demonstrated with respect to hospital stay, cost, and time until returning to work or usual activity. Laparoscopic appendectomy was consistently associated with a longer operative time ranging from a mean of 5–29 min [71, 72]. Cost analysis studies also have had varying results.

The routine use of laparoscopic appendectomy may be indicated in some subgroups of patients. Because the typical presentation of appendicitis could be due to a number of pathological processes in young women, up to 45% of lower abdominal pain in this population may be misdiagnosed. Laparoscopy can be used as a potential diagnostic and therapeutic tool.

Patients with AIDS presenting with lower abdominal pain have been shown to have HIV-related processes as well as appendicitis. However, those with appendicitis presented with a considerably increased rate of rupture and had a significantly increased morbidity [73, 74]. For patients with AIDS, consideration should be given to evaluation with CT scanning and intervention with laparoscopy.

Morbidly obese patients often require an extended right lower quadrant incision for adequate exposure during an open appendectomy. In addition, physical examination is often difficult due to body habitus. The morbidly obese patient may represent a population that may benefit from preoperative CT scanning when diagnosis is equivocal and laparoscopic appendectomy to avoid difficult exposure and an extended incision.

Some investigators have evaluated the potential of microlaparoscopes (2 mm) used with local anesthesia to assess the abdomen in patients with right lower quadrant pain [75]. Although some have claimed that microlaparoscopy should be more widely utilized [76], the quality of the image using the microlaparoscope is, at present, limited and does not allow adequate exclusion of acute appendicitis.

Barrat et al. attempted to reduce the number of normal appendices removed by not removing macroscopically normal appendices at laparoscopy. The rate of removal of normal appendices was 25% in the control group, which underwent open appendectomy, compared to 8% in the laparoscopic group [77]. However, the false-negative rate was approximately 10%, limiting the utility of this approach. To decrease the possibility of future diagnostic dilemmas and because of a considerable false-negative rate on inspection, appendectomy should still be performed with the finding of a normal appendix on exploration without any other explanation for symptoms [78, 79].

Prevention of Postoperative Infectious Complications

Intraoperative Peritoneal Culture

Altemeier previously demonstrated that polymicrobial flora could be isolated from the peritoneum of patients with perforated appendicitis [80] and has led to routine intraperitoneal culturing during appendectomy at some centers. However, one study has demonstrated similar infectious complication rates whether intra-abdominal culture was obtained or not [81]. This may be due to the fact that cultures in the majority of cases have little variation and include aerobic and anaerobic colonic flora [82–84]. In addition, the considerable time, cost and difficulty in culturing anaerobic organisms likely leads to incomplete isolation of all pathogens [81, 85]. Bilik et al. demonstrated that the return of cultures 2–3 days after appendectomy did not lead to a change in the empiric antibiotic regimen in the vast majority of cases [81] and other studies have demonstrated that changing of empiric therapy based on culture results did not decrease morbidity [83, 85]. Furthermore, management of postoperative infectious complications was not guided by prior intraoperative cultures [81]. Similar results have been demonstrated in the pediatric population [86, 87]. These data indicate that surgeons select antibiotic therapy for perforated appendicitis based on assumptions of which organisms are likely to be present and not on culture data. Obtaining cultures from patients with appendicitis contributes little to the initial management of the patient or to later management of infectious complications.

Prophylactic Antibiotic Therapy

The most commonly used prophylactic antibiotics for acute appendicitis are designed to cover aerobic and anaerobic colonic flora as well as gram-positive skin flora. Unfortunately, a "gold standard" regimen of antibiotic prophylaxis has not been clearly defined. Regimens including metronidazole for anaerobic coverage have been shown to effectively decrease postoperative infections [88–91]. Interestingly, no difference was noted between prophylaxis for appendicitis when antibiotics were started before or during the operation [92].

For perforated appendicitis, an optimal antibiotic regimen also has not been defined, although triple therapy, including ampicillin, gentamicin and metronidazole, is commonly used to include both aerobic and anaerobic coverage. A number of studies have demonstrated the efficacy and safety of varying combination or monotherapies, including ticarcillin/clavulanate, imipenem/cilistatin, piperacillin, meropenum, tobramycin and clindamycin, and cefotetan [93–97]. Hopkins et al. demonstrated that monotherapy with a second-generation cephalosporin was an economical and efficacious adjunct for complicated appendicitis treated surgically [96].

Wound Closure for Perforated Appendicitis

Primary wound closure is universally accepted in cases of nonperforated appendicitis; however, delayed primary or secondary closure are often routine in cases of ruptured appendicitis. Recently, primary closure of cases with ruptured appendicitis has been advocated in an attempt to decrease morbidity. A cost-utility analysis demonstrated primary closure to be advantageous compared with delayed primary closure and secondary closure for contaminated right lower quadrant incisions [98]. Serour et al. demonstrated a wound infection rate of 6% among children with perforated appendicitis who underwent appendectomy with primary wound closure with interrupted absorbable subcuticular sutures and 7–10 days of triple antibiotic therapy [99]. Primary closure offers significant advantages in the pediatric population and appears to be a safe method for closure in this population. In contrast, another study demonstrated increased readmission rates, wound infections, and length of hospital stays with primary closure for appendicitis [100]. Because of similar cosmetic results as the primary closure and a lower surgical site infection rate, delayed primary closure may be the best option for the adult population.

Conclusion

Many controversies for the diagnosis and management of appendicitis persist or have recently developed with advances in technology. Notwithstanding the advances in technology, the mainstay for diagnosis of appendicitis should remain a careful history and physical examination supplemented with basic laboratory evaluation. Imaging modalities should be reserved for patients presenting with an unclear diagnosis. Although laparoscopy has clear advantages in some patient populations, the associated increase in costs and operative time may not justify the routine use of this technique in all patients. Despite recent advances for diagnosis and treatment, considerable morbidity and mortality continue to be associated with acute appendicitis.

References

1. Irvin TT (1989) Abdominal pain: a surgical audit of 1190 emergency admissions. Br J Surg 76:1121–1125
2. Balsano N, Cayten CG (1990) Surgical emergencies of the abdomen. Emerg Med Clin North Am 8:399–410
3. Fenyo G (1974) Diagnostic problems of acute abdominal diseases in the aged. Acta Chir Scand 140:396–405
4. Lewis F, Holcroft J, Boey J, Dunphy E (1975) Appendicitis: a critical review of diagnosis and treatment in 1000 cases. Arch Surg 110:677–684

5. Addiss DG, Shaffer N, Fowler BS, Tauxe RV (1990) The epidemiology of appendicitis and appendectomy in the United States. Am J Epidemiol 132:910–925
6. Jess P, Bjerregaard B, Brynitz S, Holst-Christensen J, Kalaja E, Lund-Kristensen J (1981) Acute appendicitis. Prospective trial concerning diagnostic accuracy and complications. Am J Surg 141:232–234
7. Mittelpunkt A, Nora PF (1966) Current features in the treatment of acute appendicitis: an analysis of 1,000 consecutive cases. Surgery 60:971–975
8. Franz MG, Norman J, Fabri PJ (1995) Increased morbidity of appendicitis with advancing age. Am Surg 61:40–44
9. Wade DS, Marrow SE, Balsara ZN, Burkhard TK, Goff WB (1993) Accuracy of ultrasound in the diagnosis of acute appendicitis compared with the surgeon's clinical impression. Arch Surg 128:1039–1044, 1044–1046
10. Bugliosi TF, Meloy TD, Vukov LF (1990) Acute abdominal pain in the elderly. Ann Emerg Med 19:1383–1386
11. Owens BJ, Hamit HF (1978) Appendicitis in the elderly. Ann Surg 187:392–396
12. White J, Santillana M, Haller J (1975) Intensive in-hospital observation: a safe way to decrease unnecessary appendectomy. Am Surg 41:793–798
13. Jerman RP (1969) Removal of the normal appendix: the cause of serious complications. Br J Clin Pract 23:466–467
14. Chang FC, Hogle HH, Welling DR (1973) The fate of the negative appendix. Am J Surg 126:752–754
15. Howie JG (1966) Death from appendicitis and appendicectomy. An epidemiological survey. Lancet 2:1334–1337
16. Bongard F, Landers DV, Lewis F (1985) Differential diagnosis of appendicitis and pelvic inflammatory disease. A prospective analysis. Am J Surg 150:90–96
17. Berry J Jr, Malt RA (1984) Appendicitis near its centenary. Ann Surg 200:567–575
18. Jones PF (1990) Practicalities in the management of the acute abdomen. Br J Surg 77:365–367
19. Schwartz SI (1987) Tempering the technological diagnosis of appendicitis. N Engl J Med 317:703–704
20. Neutra RR (1978) Appendicitis: decreasing normal removals without increasing perforations. Med Care 16:956–961
21. Adams ID, Chan M, Clifford PC, et al. (1986) Computer aided diagnosis of acute abdominal pain: a multicentre study. Br Med J (Clin Res Ed) 293:800–804
22. De Dombal FT, Leaper DJ, Horrocks JC, Staniland JR, McCann AP (1974) Human and computer-aided diagnosis of abdominal pain: further report with emphasis on performance of clinicians. Br Med J 1:376–380
23. de Dombal FT (1993) Educational assessment of clinical diagnostic skills: studies across Europe on acute abdominal pain. Postgrad Med J 69:S94–S96
24. Alvarado A (1986) A practical score for the early diagnosis of acute appendicitis. Ann Emerg Med 15:557–564
25. Bond GR, Tully SB, Chan LS, Bradley RL (1990) Use of the MANTRELS score in childhood appendicitis: a prospective study of 187 children with abdominal pain. Ann Emerg Med 19:1014–1018
26. Fenyo G, Lindberg G, Blind P, Enochsson L, Oberg A (1997) Diagnostic decision support in suspected acute appendicitis: validation of a simplified scoring system. Eur J Surg 163:831–838
27. Andersson RE, Hugander AP, Ghazi SH, et al. (1999) Diagnostic value of disease history, clinical presentation, and inflammatory parameters of appendicitis. World J Surg 23:133–140
28. Peterson MC, Holbrook JH, Von Hales D, Smith NL, Staker LV (1992) Contributions of the history, physical examination, and laboratory investigation in making medical diagnoses. West J Med 156:163–165
29. Hampton JR, Harrison MJ, Mitchell JR, Prichard JS, Seymour C (1975) Relative contributions of history-taking, physical examination, and laboratory investigation to diagnosis and management of medical outpatients. Br Med J 2:486–489
30. Lavelle SM, Kanagaratnam B (1990) The information value of clinical data. Int J Biomed Comput 26:203–209
31. Todd BS, Stamper R (1993) Limits to diagnostic accuracy. Med Inform (Lond) 18:255–270
32. Wagner JM, McKinney WP, Carpenter JL (1996) Does this patient have appendicitis? JAMA 276:1589–1594
33. Eldar S, Nash E, Sabo E, et al. (1997) Delay of surgery in acute appendicitis. Am J Surg 173:194–198
34. Eriksson S, Granstrom L, Olander B, Pira U (1995) Leucocyte elastase as a marker in the diagnosis of acute appendicitis. Eur J Surg 161:901–905

35. Gronroos JM, Gronroos P (1999) Leucocyte count and C-reactive protein in the diagnosis of acute appendicitis. Br J Surg 86:501–504
36. Albu E, Miller BM, Choi Y, Lakhanpal S, Murthy RN, Gerst PH (1994) Diagnostic value of C-reactive protein in acute appendicitis. Dis Colon Rectum 37:49–51
37. Hallan S, Asberg A (1997) The accuracy of C-reactive protein in diagnosing acute appendicitis – a meta-analysis. Scand J Clin Lab Invest 57:373–380
38. Gronroos JM, Forsstrom JJ, Irjala K, Nevalainen TJ (1994) Phospholipase A2, C-reactive protein, and white blood cell count in the diagnosis of acute appendicitis. Clin Chem 40:1757–1760
39. Eriksson S, Granstrom L, Olander B, Wretlind B (1995) Sensitivity of interleukin-6 and C-reactive protein concentrations in the diagnosis of acute appendicitis. Eur J Surg 161:41–45
40. Hallan S, Asberg A, Edna TH (1997) Additional value of biochemical tests in suspected acute appendicitis. Eur J Surg 163:533–538
41. Brazaitis MP, Dachman AH (1993) The radiologic evaluation of acute abdominal pain of intestinal origin. A clinical approach. Med Clin North Am 77:939–961
42. Lim HK, Bae SH, Seo GS (1992) Diagnosis of acute appendicitis in pregnant women: value of sonography. AJR Am J Roentgenol 159:539–542
43. Taourel P, Baron MP, Pradel J, Fabre JM, Seneterre E, Bruel JM (1992) Acute abdomen of unknown origin: impact of CT on diagnosis and management. Gastrointest Radiol 17:287–291
44. Kang WM, Lee CH, Chou YH, et al. (1989) A clinical evaluation of ultrasonography in the diagnosis of acute appendicitis. Surgery 105:154–159
45. Anteby SO, Schenker JG, Polishuk WZ (1975) The value of laparoscopy in acute pelvic pain. Ann Surg 181:484–486
46. Davies AH, Mastorakou I, Cobb R, Rogers C, Lindsell D, Mortensen NJ (1991) Ultrasonography in the acute abdomen. Br J Surg 78:1178–1180
47. John H, Neff U, Kelemen M (1993) Appendicitis diagnosis today: clinical and ultrasonic deductions. World J Surg 17:243–249
48. Puylaert JB, Rutgers PH, Lalisang RI, et al. (1987) A prospective study of ultrasonography in the diagnosis of appendicitis. N Engl J Med 317:666–669
49. Gamal R, Moore TC (1990) Appendicitis in children aged 13 years and younger. Am J Surg 159:589–592
50. Balthazar EJ, Birnbaum BA, Yee J, Megibow AJ, Roshkow J, Gray C (1994) Acute appendicitis: CT and US correlation in 100 patients. Radiology 190:31–35
51. Jabra AA, Shalaby-Rana EI, Fishman EK (1997) CT of appendicitis in children. J Comput Assist Tomogr 21:661–666
52. Schuler JG, Shortsleeve MJ, Goldenson RS, Perez-Rossello JM, Perlmutter RA, Thorsen A (1998) Is there a role for abdominal computed tomographic scans in appendicitis? Arch Surg 133:373–376, 377
53. Rao PM, Feltmate CM, Rhea JT, Schulick AH, Novelline RA (1999) Helical computed tomography in differentiating appendicitis and acute gynecologic conditions. Obstet Gynecol 93:417–421
54. Rao PM, Rhea JT, Novelline RA, et al. (1997) Helical CT technique for the diagnosis of appendicitis: prospective evaluation of a focused appendix CT examination. Radiology 202:139–144
55. Rao PM, Rhea JT, Rattner DW, Venus LG, Novelline RA (1999) Introduction of appendiceal CT: impact on negative appendectomy and appendiceal perforation rates. Ann Surg 229:344–349
56. Rhea JT, Rao PM, Novelline RA, McCabe CJ (1997) A focused appendiceal CT technique to reduce the cost of caring for patients with clinically suspected appendicitis. AJR Am J Roentgenol 169:113–118
57. Rao PM, Rhea JT, Novelline RA, Mostafavi AA, McCabe CJ (1998) Effect of computed tomography of the appendix on treatment of patients and use of hospital resources. N Engl J Med 338:141–146
58. Funaki B, Grosskreutz SR, Funaki CN (1998) Using unenhanced helical CT with enteric contrast material for suspected appendicitis in patients treated at a community hospital. AJR Am J Roentgenol 171:997–1001
59. Rao PM, Rhea JT, Novelline RA, McCabe CJ (1998) The computed tomography appearance of recurrent and chronic appendicitis. Am J Emerg Med 16:26–33
60. Rao PM, Rhea JT, Wittenberg J, Warshaw AL (1998) Misdiagnosis of primary epiploic appendagitis. Am J Surg 176:81–85
61. Fulcher AS, Turner MA (1996) Percutaneous drainage of enteric-related abscesses. Gastroenterologist 4:276–285
62. Yamini D, Vargas H, Bongard F, Klein S, Stamos MJ (1998) Perforated appendicitis: is it truly a surgical urgency? Am Surg 64:970–975

63. Mazziotti MV, Marley EF, Winthrop AL, Fitzgerald PG, Walton M, Langer JC (1997) Histopathologic analysis of interval appendectomy specimens: support for the role of interval appendectomy. J Pediatr Surg 32:806–809
64. Ein SH, Shandling B (1996) Is interval appendectomy necessary after rupture of an appendiceal mass? J Pediatr Surg 31:849–850
65. Jamieson DH, Chait PG, Filler R (1997) Interventional drainage of appendiceal abscesses in children. AJR Am J Roentgenol 169:1619–1622
66. Price MR, Haase GM, Sartorelli KH, Meagher DP Jr (1996) Recurrent appendicitis after initial conservative management of appendiceal abscess. J Pediatr Surg 31:291–294
67. Bufo AJ, Shah RS, Li MH, et al. (1998) Interval appendectomy for perforated appendicitis in children. J Laparoendosc Adv Surg Tech A 8:209–214
68. Lund DP, Murphy EU (1994) Management of perforated appendicitis in children: a decade of aggressive treatment. J Pediatr Surg 29:1130–1133, 1133–1134
69. Eriksson S, Granstrom L (1995) Randomized controlled trial of appendicectomy versus antibiotic therapy for acute appendicitis. Br J Surg 82:166–169
70. Eriksson S, Tisell A, Granstrom L (1995) Ultrasonographic findings after conservative treatment of acute appendicitis and open appendicectomy. Acta Radiol 36:173–177
71. Fingerhut A, Millat B, Borrie F (1999) Laparoscopic versus open appendectomy: time to decide. World J Surg 23:835–845
72. Lujan Mompean JA, Robles Campos R, Parrilla Paricio P, Soria Aledo V, Garcia Ayllon J (1994) Laparoscopic versus open appendicectomy: a prospective assessment. Br J Surg 81:133–135
73. Savioz D, Lironi A, Zurbuchen P, Leissing C, Kaiser L, Morel P (1996) Acute right iliac fossa pain in acquired immunodeficiency: a comparison between patients with and without acquired immune deficiency syndrome. Br J Surg 83:644–646
74. Flum DR, Steinberg SD, Sarkis AY, Wallack MK (1997) Appendicitis in patients with acquired immunodeficiency syndrome. J Am Coll Surg 184:481–486
75. Mutter D, Navez B, Gury JF, et al. (1998) Value of microlaparoscopy in the diagnosis of right iliac fossa pain. Am J Surg 176:370–372
76. Palter SF, Olive DL, Rosser JC (1995) Diagnosis of acute appendicitis by microlaparoscopy under local anesthesia. J Am Assoc Gynecol Laparosc 2:S40
77. Barrat C, Catheline JM, Rizk N, Champault GG (1999) Does laparoscopy reduce the incidence of unnecessary appendicectomies? Surg Laparosc Endosc 9:27–31
78. Deutsch AA, Zelikovsky A, Reiss R (1982) Laparoscopy in the prevention of unnecessary appendicectomies: a prospective study. Br J Surg 69:336–337
79. Olsen JB, Myren CJ, Haahr PE (1993) Randomized study of the value of laparoscopy before appendicectomy. Br J Surg 80:922–923
80. Altemeier W (1938) The bacterial flora of acute perforated appendicitis with peritonitis. Ann Surg 107:517–528
81. Bilik R, Burnweit C, Shandling B (1998) Is abdominal cavity culture of any value in appendicitis? Am J Surg 175:267–270
82. Brook I (1980) Bacterial studies of peritoneal cavity and postoperative surgical wound drainage following perforated appendix in children. Ann Surg 192:208–212
83. Mosdell DM, Morris DM, Voltura A, et al. (1991) Antibiotic treatment for surgical peritonitis. Ann Surg 214:543–549
84. David IB, Buck JR, Filler RM (1982) Rational use of antibiotics for perforated appendicitis in childhood. J Pediatr Surg 17:494–500
85. McNamara MJ, Pasquale MD, Evans SR (1993) Acute appendicitis and the use of intraperitoneal cultures. Surg Gynecol Obstet 177:393–397
86. Kokoska ER, Silen ML, Tracy TF Jr, et al. (1999) The impact of intraoperative culture on treatment and outcome in children with perforated appendicitis. J Pediatr Surg 34:749–753
87. Mosdell DM, Morris DM, Fry DE (1994) Peritoneal cultures and antibiotic therapy in pediatric perforated appendicitis. Am J Surg 167:313–316
88. Banani SA, Talei A (1999) Can oral metronidazole substitute parenteral drug therapy in acute appendicitis? A new policy in the management of simple or complicated appendicitis with localized peritonitis: a randomized controlled clinical trial. Am Surg 65:411–416
89. Shubing W, Litian Z (1997) Preventing infection of the incision after appendectomy by using metronidazole preoperatively to infiltrate tissues at the incision. Am J Surg 174:422–424
90. Kumarakrishnan S, Srinivasan K, Sahai A, Kate V, Ananthakrishnan N (1997) A trial of various regimens of antibiotics in acute appendicitis. Trop Gastroenterol 18:177–179
91. Soderquist-Elinder C, Hirsch K, Bergdahl S, Rutqvist J, Frenckner B (1995) Prophylactic antibiotics in uncomplicated appendicitis during childhood – a prospective randomised study. Eur J Pediatr Surg 5:282–285

92. Almqvist P, Leandoer L, Tornqvist A (1995) Timing of antibiotic treatment in non-perforated gangrenous appendicitis. Eur J Surg 161:431–433
93. Ciftci AO, Tanyel FC, Buyukpamukcu N, Hicsonmez A (1997) Comparative trial of four antibiotic combinations for perforated appendicitis in children. Eur J Surg 163:591–596
94. Allo MD, Bennion RS, Kathir K, et al. (1999) Ticarcillin/clavulanate versus imipenem/cilistatin for the treatment of infections associated with gangrenous and perforated appendicitis. Am Surg 65:99–104
95. Berne TV, Yellin AE, Appleman MD, Heseltine PN, Gill MA (1996) Meropenem versus tobramycin with clindamycin in the antibiotic management of patients with advanced appendicitis. J Am Coll Surg 182:403–407
96. Hopkins JA, Wilson SE, Bobey DG (1994) Adjunctive antimicrobial therapy for complicated appendicitis: bacterial overkill by combination therapy. World J Surg 18:933–938
97. Salam IM, Abu Galala KH, el Ashaal YI, Chandran VP, Asham NN, Sim AJ (1994) A randomized prospective study of cefoxitin versus piperacillin in appendicectomy. J Hosp Infect 26:133–136
98. Brasel KJ, Borgstrom DC, Weigelt JA (1997) Cost-utility analysis of contaminated appendectomy wounds. J Am Coll Surg 184:23–30
99. Serour F, Efrati Y, Klin B, Barr J, Gorenstein A, Vinograd I (1996) Subcuticular skin closure as a standard approach to emergency appendectomy in children: prospective clinical trial. World J Surg 20:38–42
100. Lemieur TP, Rodriguez JL, Jacobs DM, Bennett ME, West MA (1999) Wound management in perforated appendicitis. Am Surg 65:439–443

Appendiceal Mass and Abscess

Roger Saadia · Jeremy Lipschitz

Introduction

Semantic confusion persists about this inflammatory complication of acute appendicitis [1]. A mass is a palpable conglomerate, consisting of the inflamed (usually perforated) appendix, adjacent viscera and the greater omentum. When pus formation occurs within this mass, it is referred to as "abscess." In the absence of pus, the generic description of "mass" is commonly retained ("phlegmon" being rarely used nowadays).

There are differences in opinion amongst practicing general surgeons about the treatment of this condition, a fact surprisingly belied by the dearth of recent published literature. As astonishing is the uneven coverage of the subject by modern surgical textbooks. For example, Hamilton Bailey's book [2] provides a reasoned, in-depth account, while Sabiston's [3] dismissively devotes a mere six lines to a dogmatic approach that fails to differentiate between mass and abscess.

The contemporary controversies relate to:

- The differential diagnosis of mass or abscess
- The initial management of the appendiceal mass
- The initial management of the appendiceal abscess
- The role of laparoscopy
- The need for interval appendicectomy

Mass or Abscess?

In the classical textbook description [4], an appendix mass forms around the third day after an acute attack and sometimes develops into an abscess around the fifth to tenth day. The recommendation used to be made that pyrexia, the aggravation of the local signs and a rising leukocyte count are strong indicators of pus formation. In practice, however, it was noted long ago that it is usually very difficult to differentiate clinically between mass and abscess [5]. Since the mid-1980s, imaging (in the form of ultrasonography or CT) has become a routine component in the assessment of these patients. While some investigators report good results with ultrasonography [6, 7], others prefer CT imaging [8–10]. Which imaging technique is superior is more a matter of individual preference and expertise than a major controversy. The important point is the necessity to involve the radiologist if one is to offer rational, individualized treatment.

Appendiceal Mass: Immediate Surgery Versus Conservative Treatment

Management needs to be considered in three different clinical settings. In the first one, a palpable mass is first discovered on palpation of the right iliac fossa in an anesthetized patient about to undergo an appendicectomy. There is little discussion about how to proceed, provided the symptoms have been present for a few days only. Appendicectomy must be performed as scheduled. The findings rarely correspond to the definition given above of an appendiceal perforation walled-off by thickened neighboring bowel loops and omentum. More commonly, it is an appendix enlarged by the inflammatory process that happens to be palpable through a lean, relaxed abdominal wall. Occasionally, the greater omentum is found loosely wrapped around the appendix. There is no evidence that appendicectomy is attended by a higher complication rate. In the second scenario, in the course of an operation for presumed acute appendicitis, the appendix is found to be engulfed in a mass of uncertain etiology. The safe approach is a segmental intestinal resection with primary ileocolonic anastomosis. Whether a limited ileocaecal resection through the same incision is preferred to a formal right hemicolectomy depends on the likelihood of malignancy [11].

It is a different matter with the patient presenting late after an acute attack with a mass already palpable on admission to hospital. The management controversy relates to the need for immediate surgery vs. an initial trial of nonoperative treatment consisting mainly of antibiotics (usually intravenously) with variable measures to rest the bowel if necessary. The classical treatment used to be conservative (the so-called Ochsner-Sherren regimen). It was based mainly on the fear of disturbing the natural barriers erected in order to localize the peritoneal inflammation. Having satisfied themselves with appropriate imaging that no pus is present, the modern advocates of nonoperative treatment present three additional arguments. Firstly, immediate appendicectomy is technically more difficult, with a greater risk of postoperative fecal fistula. Secondly, operation can always be resorted to, should the initial conservative trial fail. And thirdly, the legendary pudding is here for all to taste: this approach works in over 80% of cases [1, 12].

Nevertheless, there are still those who favor immediate operation. Before the advent of radiological imaging, when masses and abscesses were by necessity lumped together, the case for immediate operation could be argued as some studies found less complications with this approach. Today, the proponents of surgery for the phlegmonous mass concede a somewhat more difficult operation but are able to present evidence supporting the safety of the approach. Shorter hospital stays are also claimed, especially if interval appendicectomy requiring a second hospitalization is considered a compulsory component of the conservative option. *We believe that if two treatment options are equally safe, the preferred one should be the least invasive.* And, for most patients, a slightly longer absence from home is acceptable if the alternative is an operation. There is little to support the claim that "the trend is in favor of immediate appendectomy, since it is more expeditious and appears to be just as safe" [13]. Hospital costs considerations may factor into the decision for a more aggressive early surgical approach, but should not prevail to the detriment of the patient.

Appendiceal Abscess: Drainage, Antibiotics Alone, Expectant Treatment?

The standard traditional treatment of an appendiceal abscess is drainage. This used to require an operation in all cases, but with the advent of interventional radiology, it is now best achieved percutaneously (or transrectally) under ultrasound or CT guidance. Open operation, usually via an extraperitoneal approach, is reserved for complex multilocular collections or after failure of percutaneous drainage. When operative drainage used to be the norm, classical teaching dictated no prolonged attempt to perform an appendicectomy unless the appendix is found free in the abscess cavity [14], "begging to be resected." In most cases, an immediate appendicectomy was not performed as the appendix used to be found incorporated in the abscess walls. However, some modern authors favor early operative abscess drainage and report an easy immediate appendicectomy in most cases [15].

Whatever the method of drainage and whether or not an immediate appendicectomy is performed, until recently, most authors recommended drainage as soon as the diagnosis of abscess was established either on clinical grounds, or by imaging, when this became available. This approach was underpinned by the surgical dogma that whenever pus is present it must be drained. Furthermore, in the case of appendiceal abscesses, it was held in the old days that there are hazards attached to prolonged antibiotic therapy. Antibiotics were said to sterilize an abscess which then behaves as an irritant, causing "obscure subacute intestinal obstruction." They were also claimed to promote the formation of granulation tissue "leading to a frozen pelvis with consequent stricture of the rectum" [14]. This warning is repeated in a recent edition [4] of the same textbook. Similar warnings about the formation of an "antibioticoma" [16] persist to this day, but without well-documented evidence.

Nowadays, even the necessity to drain pus in all cases is being challenged. Small, recently formed abscesses may regress with antibiotic therapy alone. Indeed, conservative treatment of intra-abdominal septic collections following appendicectomy in the child seems highly successful [17]. A CT classification of appendiceal masses was recently proposed [8]. Group I comprises phlegmons and abscesses with a maximum diameter smaller than 3 cm; group II larger but well-localized abscesses; and group III includes extensive periappendicular abscesses involving multiple intra- or extraperitoneal compartments. Complete resolution was obtained with antibiotics alone in 88% of group I patients, while the treatment of choice for group II and group III was percutaneous catheter drainage and surgical drainage, respectively.

An even more conservative management policy of appendiceal abscesses - termed "ultra-conservative" - has met with a significant measure of success [18]. Hospital observation alone, without enforced bed rest, special diet or antibiotics, resulted in complete resolution in all 28 patients selected for this treatment. There was only one patient with recurrent acute appendicitis and another with a recurrent abscess. Admittedly, some of these patients may have had phlegmonous masses despite their clinical presentation suggestive of an abscess, but at least eight abscesses were diagnosed ultrasonographically. The authors explain their success by contending that the withholding of antibiotics encourages spontaneous drainage of the septic collections into the bowel. The only reported disadvantage of this management policy was prolonged hospitalization, since 14% of the patients had to remain in hospital for 3 weeks or longer.

Surgical Approach: Open Versus Laparoscopic

Diagnostic laparoscopy is currently accepted in the diagnosis of patients with right iliac fossa pain [19], and may have its greatest role in females during their child-bearing years [20]. Laparoscopic appendicectomy is equivalent to the open procedure in treating acute appendicitis, and may be beneficial in reducing post-operative pain, returning patients to work, and reducing wound infections [21-23]. Appendiceal abscess is considered a relative contraindication to laparoscopy [24, 25], although the presumed reasons, such as spread of sepsis by the pneumoperitoneum, may be mitigated by the ability to irrigate the peritoneal cavity under laparoscopic guidance. The risk of injury to the bowel and its mesentery is a major concern with laparoscopy [19], and periappendiceal adhesions account for the majority of conversions to the open procedure. In addition, the length of hospitalization for appendicitis relates to the degree of sepsis present rather than the method of appendicectomy [26]. It is our opinion that there is little justification for approaching an inflammatory right iliac fossa mass (presumed appendiceal in origin) laparoscopically.

Interval Appendicectomy: Always, Never, Sometimes?

Interval appendicectomy used to be the unavoidable complement to conservative treatment of the phlegmonous mass. And classical teaching required a 3-month waiting period, which is nowadays shortened to the time required for complete resolution of the mass [4]. An elective appendicectomy after the drainage of an abscess was also the norm, although it was conceded that, by the time this was performed, in many cases the appendix would have shriveled to a fibrotic cord, unlikely to cause further problems. There are still modern advocates for this approach [2, 27]. The justification for interval appendicectomy rests on the possibility of a recurring acute attack and on the fear of an erroneous initial diagnosis of appendicitis in the context of a caecal or appendiceal malignancy.

But many have questioned the practice of interval appendicectomy [6, 12, 28–30], since the recurrence rate of acute appendicitis is low (3%–15%) over a long follow-up period. And it could be argued, therefore, that routine interval appendicectomy is unnecessary in the majority of patients. As for the minority presenting with recurrent acute (or chronic) appendicitis, emergency appendicectomy is nowadays a safe operation. An argument can be made in favor of interval appendicectomy in patients who, in the future, may not have easy access to modern surgical facilities [31]. The issue of misdiagnosing a malignancy is a real one. It is recommended that patients over the age of 40 undergo a barium enema examination or a colonoscopy after successful conservative treatment of an appendiceal mass [1]. Concern about a tumor undetected by conventional means or occurring in younger patients may persist, but it is unclear how many of these extremely rare tumors would be detected in the course of interval appendicectomy if they arise in the cecum.

Conclusion

No management recommendations are presently evidence-based. The following is our preferred management policy:

- Modern imaging is essential in distinguishing an appendiceal mass from abscess.
- A phlegmonous mass should be treated nonoperatively, at least initially.
- Small abscesses can be given a trial of nonoperative treatment with appropriate antibiotics. Drainage should be performed if there is persistence of local pain or systemic symptoms beyond 36–48 h of treatment, or unresolving intestinal obstruction.
- Larger abscesses should be drained. The drainage modality should depend on the characteristics of the abscess and the expertise available.
- There is no role for laparoscopy in the management of the appendiceal mass or abscess.
- After successful nonoperative treatment of a mass or drainage of an abscess, interval appendicectomy is not routinely performed. Adult patients must be suitably investigated to exclude a malignancy.

References

1. Nitecki S, Assalia A, Schein M (1993) Contemporary management of the appendiceal mass. Br J Surg 80:18–20
2. Ellis BW, Paterson-Brown S (eds) (1995) Hamilton Bailey's emergency surgery, 12th edn. Butterworth Heinemann, Oxford

3. Sabiston DC, Lyerly HK (eds) (1997) Sabiston's textbook of surgery: the biological basis of modern surgical practice, 15th edn. Saunders, Philadelphia
4. Mann CV, Russell RCG (eds) (1991) Bailey and Love's short practice of surgery, 21st edn. Chapman and Hall, London
5. Jordan JS, Kovalcic PJ, Schwab CW (1981) Appendicitis with a palpable mass. Ann Surg 193:227–229
6. Bagi P, Dueholm S (1987) Nonoperative management of the ultrasonically evaluated appendiceal mass. Surgery 101:602–605
7. Bagi P, Dueholm S, Karstrup S (1987) Percutaneous drainage of appendiceal abscess. Dis Colon Rectum 30:532–535
8. Jeffrey RB (1989) Management of the periappendiceal inflammatory mass. Semin Ultrasound CT MR 10:341–347
9. Van Sonnenberg E, Wittich GR, Casola G, et al. (1987) Periappendiceal abcesses: percutaneous drainage. Radiology 163:23–26
10. Nunez D, Yrizarry JM, Casillas VJ, Becerra J, Russell E (1989) Percutaneous management of appendiceal abscesses. Semin Ultrasound CT MR 10:384–391
11. Poon RT, Chu KW (1999) Inflammatory cecal masses in patients presenting with appendicitis. World J Surg 23:713–716
12. Hoffmann J, Lindhard A, Jensen H-E (1984) Appendix mass: conservative management without interval appendectomy. Am J Surg 148:379–382
13. Way LL (ed) (1994) Current surgical diagnosis and treatment, 10th edn. Appleton and Lange, Norwalk
14. Rains AJH, Capper WM (eds) (1971) Bailey and Love's short practice of surgery, 15th edn. Lewis, London
15. Ridings P (1993) Contemporary management of the appendiceal mass. Br J Surg 80:810
16. Monson J, Duthie G, O'Malley K (eds) (1999) Surgical emergencies. Blackwell Science, Oxford
17. Okoye BO, Rampersad B, Marantos A, Abernethy LJ, Losty PD, Lloyd DA (1998) Abscess after appendicectomy in children: the role of conservative management. Br J Surg 85:1111–1113
18. Hoffmann J, Rolff M, Lomborg V, Franzmann M (1991) Ultraconservative management of appendiceal abscess. J R Coll Surg Edinb 36:18–20
19. Memon MA, Fitzgibbons RJ (1997) The role of minimal access surgery in the acute abdomen. Surg Clin North Am 77:1333–1353
20. Laine S, Rautala A, Gullichsen R, et al. (1997) Laparoscopic appendectomy – is it worthwhile? A prospective, randomised study in young women. Surg Endosc 11:95–97
21. Hansen JB, Smithers BM, Schache D, et al. (1996) Laparoscopic vs. open appendectomy: a prospective randomised trial. World J Surg 20:17–20
22. Ortega AE, Hunter JG, Peters JH, et al. (1995) A prospective randomised trial of laparoscopic appendectomy with open appendectomy. Am J Surg 169:208–212
23. Kazemer G, de Zeeuw GR, Lange JF, et al. (1997) Laparoscopic vs. open appendectomy. Surg Endosc 11:336–340
24. Freezee RC, Bohannon WF (1996) Laparoscopic appendectomy for complicated appendicitis. Arch Surg 131:509–511
25. Negebauer E, Troidl H, Kum CK, et al. (1995) The European Association for Endoscopic Surgery consensus development conferences on laparoscopic cholecystectomy, appendectomy and hernia repair. Consensus statements (September 1994). Surg Endosc 9:550–563
26. Cuschieri A (1997) Appendectomy – laparoscopic or open? Surg Endosc 11:319–320
27. Jarvinen HJ (1998) Invited commentary. Eur J Surg 164:775
28. Lewin J, Fenyo G, Engstrom L (1988) Treatment of appendiceal abscess. Acta Chir Scand 154:123–125
29. Ranson JHC (1987) Nonoperative treatment of the appendiceal mass: progress or regression? Gastroenterology 93:1439–1445
30. Eriksson S, Styrud J (1998) Interval appendicectomy: a retrospective study. Eur J Surg 164:771–774
31. Sargeant ID, Mason PF (1993) Contemporary management of the appendiceal mass. Br J Surg 80:810

Invited Comment

Zygmunt H. Krukowski

Introduction

When considering controversies in managing appendicitis it is timely to consider why we treat the condition operatively with the risks of surgical misadventure, complications and hazards of general anesthesia. It is difficult for any physician with a conventional education to reflect on something so fundamental. The perceived wisdom of generations is that the clinical suspicion of acute appendicitis requires an urgent operation. This approach harks back to the nineteenth century and the introduction of the relative safety of surgery under general anesthesia.

In the "old days" appendicitis was treated nonoperatively in the expectation of resolution or progression to peritonitis or localization into an abscess. An abscess was then incised and drained. Peritonitis either as a result of rapid progression or rupture of an abscess was usually fatal. The relative safety of removing the appendix before progression transformed management into the familiar pattern essentially pursued today. The risk of removing a large number of normal or nonperforated appendices was outweighed by the reduction in mortality resulting from severe septic complications. In the risk/benefit analysis of the day the complications of the operation were perceived to be less than the risk of nonoperative management. Would this risk assessment be the same today?

Antibiotics

The introduction of antibiotics 50 years ago did not affect the management of appendicitis until the plethora of studies during the 1970s and 1980s. These antibiotic trials were directed at preventing the complications of the surgery rather than the consequences of the disease. Indeed, most trials specifically excluded perforated appendicitis. The morbidity of the treatment was greater than that of the disease for the majority of patients with nonperforated disease. The alternative of medical management of acute appendicitis with antibiotics has been the subject of speculation but only limited study in both perforated [1] and nonperforated disease [2] with interesting results. The majority of patients settled uneventfully with only a minority requiring surgery for recurrence.

Contemporary Risks of Appendicitis

Serious complications of acute appendicitis are rare and there is a paucity of unbiased reporting of large unselected series. The Scottish Audit of Surgical Mortality (SASM) is a national confidential peer review study in which every surgical death in Scotland (population 5,100,000) is subject to independent scrutiny. An average of 3,500 appendectomies are performed annually and in the 5 years between 1994 and 1998 there were 41 deaths in patients with a presenting diagnosis of acute appendicitis. This translates into a contemporary mortality of 0.2%.

Diagnosis

Despite some evidence of efficacy for medical treatment for appendicitis contemporary practice equates a diagnosis of appendicitis with an operation. Early diagnosis by imaging or laparoscopy may have the merit of expediency and appeal to the surgical psyche with connotations of immediacy, but is this in the best interest of the patient? An abdominal CT scan carries the risk of ionizing radiation and *diagnostic laparoscopy the risk of penetrating abdominal trauma.* If every patient who might have appendicitis were exposed to this level of radiation or invasive investigation, there must be a cumulative risk. *Lack of published evidence of harm is not equivalent to proof of safety.*

Although the pressure on hospital resources varies remarkably between countries, there are always cost considerations. The extra cost of an immediate CT scan has been compared favorably with a period of inpatient observation [3]. However, as Pelletier and Pruet rightly indicate, this will not prevent the admission of patients with a negative scan who require admission for management of symptoms which may well prove self-limiting.

Clinical Investigation

The objective in managing appendicitis should be to make appropriate management decisions with the minimum use of resource. Pelletier and Pruett make a cogent case for a continuing key role for clinical evaluation. This may be underused in favor of more esoteric investigations. No investigation is perfectly reliable and it is important not *to substitute clinical uncertainty for radiological ambivalence.* Reports of highly accurate, sensitive and specific investigations are biased by the inclusion of patients in whom clinical evaluation was already clear.

There is ample evidence that a management scheme based on careful clinical assessment is both safe and effective with a low negative appendectomy rate of only 4%–8% [4]. This requires continuity of the observer and constant practice with regular review of the normal appendectomy rate.

Laboratory Investigation

There have been many analyses of the utility of a variety of assays and none is foolproof. The confounding effect of the timing of the investigation in relation to the onset of symptoms is important. Repeating the test can be helpful but the results must always be interpreted in the context of the clinical picture.

Imaging

A good review [5] of the place of ultrasound concluded that this was of benefit in patients with continuing and indeterminate symptoms but there is no indication for the routine use of ultrasound. Furthermore in 10% of patients with a negative scan, exploration on clinical grounds reveals an inflamed appendix [6]. The utility of helical CT [3] must be tempered with the risk of inducing cancer quoted at 1:2000 for conventional CT. Whilst this may be less with a targeted scan, the radiation exposure resulting from widespread adoption of such a policy in a young population seems entirely unjustified.

Laparoscopic/Open Approach

This is an argument which looks set to run for some considerable time. In a slim patient the appendix can be removed through a 3-cm incision and the benefit of a laparoscopic approach then becomes inconsequential. Whilst a laparoscopic approach in women of child-bearing age is regularly promoted because of the increased diagnostic yield, it is surprising that the benefits of a laparoscopic approach in men are not more strongly canvassed. The most difficult open appendectomies in both sexes can be in the obese and heavily muscled where larger, often extended, incisions and excessive retraction may be required. The advantages of the laparoscopic approach are greatest in these circumstances and to be preferred in my view.

Prevention of Complications

The argument against routine culture of the peritoneum is persuasive. The bacteriology of peritoneal and parietal contamination in appendicitis is established and by the time the bacteriology report is to hand the patient has been long discharged. The choice of prophylactic and therapeutic antibiotics is straightforward and nowadays normally a matter for a decision of the antibiotic policy committee rather than a belated report on an individual patient. I would dispute the guarded approval for delayed primary closure in adults with perforated appendicitis. Delayed wound closure is not an option which we use after the first operation for abdominal sepsis. Prospective audit of wound sepsis, including late follow-up, in our unit since 1977 confirms that primary closure in perforated and gangrenous appendicitis is associated with a wound sepsis rate of less than 5%. In the last 147 such cases between 1990 and 1999, there were one in-hospital and five late wound infections (including one at 6 months): a rate of 4.1%. Furthermore, we do not give therapeutic antibiotics for more than 3 days for peritonitis.

Appendix Mass/Abscess

Saadia and Lipschitz give a good overview of the subject of the appendicular mass and abscess and correctly identify that the management of the appendicular mass is greatly influenced by the timing of the observation of the mass. None would abandon appendicectomy upon palpating a mass in the right lower quadrant of an anesthetized patient and few would not image a mass palpable in the same area on presentation.

Treatment

The efficacy of a conservative approach to the appendix mass [7] has been established and the question needs to be asked "why operate"? Operation depends on the interpretation of the evolution of the inflammatory process and other factors including socio-economic pressures and coincidental pathology. If return to work, particularly in an isolated situation, is critical and a phlegmonous mass without suppuration is demonstrated, then appendectomy may be the more attractive option. Equally, knowledge that the great majority of appendiceal masses will resolve without surgery can avoid a difficult and bloody operation in the established acute situation of several days duration. This may be particularly advantageous in the presence of serious cardiorespiratory disease. Operation can then be offered to those who either wish interval appendectomy or the minority (14%) who experience recurrent symptoms during the first year.

It appears logical to use antibiotics in the conservative management of a mass or abscess but even this has been questioned [8]. Whilst this study confirmed the feasibility of this approach, there seems little doubt that resolution is expedited by antibiotics. The need to drain abscesses demonstrated on CT is debatable. Simply identifying a collection is no indication to drain and a trial of conservative therapy should precede intervention.

Conclusion

In truth there are not as many controversies in appendicitis as alternatives. There is too small an evidence base to resolve many of the issues addressed in these two papers and accordingly the potential for the exercise of clinical judgment remains. However, a wholesale move to the routine use of spiral CT for the diagnosis of appendicitis will emasculate the clinical skills of the next generation of surgeons. The cynic might argue that it will generate income for radiologists and open a new area of legal activity when anyone who had a CT to diagnose appendicitis develops cancer in the years ahead. There is every reason for acute appendicitis to retain its primacy as the proving ground of the novice surgeon and the rock against which the reputation of the established surgeon is constantly tested.

References

1. Bufo AJ, Shah RS, Li MH, et al. (1998) Interval appendicectomy for perforated appendicitis in children. J Laparoendosc Adv Surg Tech A 8:209–214
2. Ericksson S, Ranstom L (1995) Randomized controlled trial of appendicectomy versus antibiotic therapy for acute appendicitis. Br J Surg 82:166–169
3. Rao PM, Rhea JT, Novelline RA, et al. (1998) Effect of computed tomography of the appendix on treatment of patients and use of hospital resources. N Engl J Med 338:141–146
4. Jones PF, Bagley FH (1998) Acute appendicitis. In: Jones PF, Krukowski ZH, Youngson GG (eds) Emergency abdominal surgery, 3rd edn. Chapman and Hall, London
5. Orr RK, Porter D, Hartmann D (1995) Ultrasonography to evaluate adults for appendicitis. Acad Emerg Med 2:644–650
6. Ramachandra R, Sivit CJ, Newman KD, et al. (1996) Ultrasonography as an adjunct in the diagnosis of acute appendicitis: a 4 year experience. J Pediatr Surg 31:164–169
7. Nitecki S, Assalia A, Schein M (1993) Contemporary management of the appendiceal mass. Br J Surg 80:18–20
8. Hoffman J, Rolff M, Lomborg V, Franzmann M (1991) Ultraconservative management of appendiceal abscess. J R Coll Surg Edinb 36:18–20

Editorial Comment

In this chapter, Drs. Pelletier and Pruett emphasize that history and physical examination are still the gold standard in the diagnosis of acute appendicitis. Drs. Saadia and Lipschitz lay down a reasonable case for the nonoperative management of appendiceal mass and abscess, and Professor Krukowski shares with us his enlightened vision – decorated with exquisite pearls.

A few points to supplement the above discussion:

- Pelletier and Pruett mention, en passant, recurrent and chronic appendicitis. Do these conditions exist? There are those who report large series of patients allegedly suffering from such entities [1]. This most probably represents a liberal policy of appendectomies in patients with nonspecific abdominal pain, combined with pathologists reporting appendiceal "inflammation" or "scarring" – the true significance of which is unknown. That most patients "feel better" after such an operation may be explained by a placebo effect, the unpredictable natural history of nonspecific abdominal pain, and probably by the removal of a true pathological appendix in a few patients. It appears that the science behind liberal usage of appendectomies for subacute or chronic appendicitis is as flimsy as that behind lysis of multiple adhesions for abdominal pain. Most authors, however, agree that *very rarely* acute appendicitis can resolve spontaneously and recur repeatedly in the same individual and that a history of prior similar episodes of pain should not dissuade one from considering the diagnosis of acute, subacute or chronic appendicitis [2]. Contemporary American series report only a small number of such patients [3–5], which are very scarcely seen – if ever – in our daily practice. Interestingly, acute appendicitis has been described in patients who had a prior appendectomy – which left them with an excessively long appendicular stump; this is supposedly becoming more common after laparoscopic appendectomy (stump appendicitis) [6].

- All our discussants support selective imaging in suspected appendicitis. We agree: we have to be careful before adopting an investigation claimed to be "effective" by others. You read, for example, that in a Boston ivory tower routine CT of the abdomen has been proven cost-effective in the diagnosis of acute appendicitis [7]. Prior to succumbing to the temptation to order a CT for any suspected acute appendicitis check out whether the methods used in the original study can be duplicated in your own environment. Do you have senior radiologists to read the CT at 3 a.m. - or would the CT be reported on only in the morning - after the appendix is, or should be, in the formalin jar?
- Pelletier and Pruett quote a study which advocates the use of (transincisional) drains. As they did not condemn such practice, we will have to do so. That transincisional drains are obsolete and promoting wound complications, has not been controversial for a long time. But what is the role of peritoneal drainage after appendectomy - if any? Although drains were found beneficial in some retrospective studies [8], there is no good evidence to suggest that they are advantageous or necessary at all. The only prospective study - from India [9] - that examines the value of peritoneal drainage in perforated appendicitis shows a higher rate of complications associated with the use of drains. What is true for diffuse peritonitis in general may also be true for acute appendicitis - drains are useless and not indicated except when there is a well-formed abscess cavity that does not collapse or disappear after drainage.
- We agree with Professor Krukowski who disputes the "guarded approval" by Drs. Pelletier and Pruett for delayed primary closure of wounds in adults with perforated appendicitis. A recent meta-analysis supports the notion that the majority of such wounds should be primarily closed [10].
- Drs. Pelletrier and Pruett discuss antibiotic therapy in acute appendicitis but - in common with the literature - ignore the issue of *duration* of administration. Professor Krukowski, however, points out that he does not "give therapeutic antibiotics for more than 3 days in peritonitis" - achieving a wound infection rate of 4.1%. This mimics the experience with "minimal antibiotic" therapy [11, 12], also discussed in a previous volume of *Crucial Controversies in Surgery* [13].
- As all our contributors mention, the majority of patients with acute appendicitis would respond to nonoperative therapy - if so managed; in this respect acute appendicitis may behave as acute diverticulitis. Moreover, after successful nonoperative therapy the majority of patients do not need an "interval" appendectomy or sigmoidectomy, respectively. That this is so is only logical since both conditions represent a minute perforation of a hollow viscus containing the same type of bacteria. So why do we usually manage appendicitis with an operation and diverticulitis with antibiotics? The different approach is based on dogma and tradition, which derive from the fact that the operative management of acute appendicitis was and is associated with a lesser morbidity and mortality than that of diverticulitis.

References

1. Croce E, Olmi S, Azzola M, Russo R (1999) Laparoscopic appendectomy and minilaparoscopic approach: a retrospective review after 8-years' experience. J Surg Laparosc Surg 3:285–292
2. Mattei P, Sola JE, Yeo CJ (1994) Chronic and recurrent appendicitis are uncommon entities often misdiagnosed. J Am Coll Surg 178:385–389
3. Crabbe MM, Norwood SH, Robertson HD, Silva JS (1986) Recurrent and chronic appendicitis. Surg Gynecol Obstet 163:11–13
4. Savrin RA, Clausen K, Martin EW Jr, Cooperman M (1979) Chronic and recurrent appendicitis. Am J Surg 137:355–357
5. Hawes AS, Whalen GF (1994) Recurrent and chronic appendicitis: the other inflammatory conditions of the appendix. Am Surg 60:217–219
6. Walsh DC, Roediger WE (1997) Stump appendicitis – a potential problem after laparoscopic appendicectomy. Surg Laparosc Endosc 7:357–358
7. Rao PM, Rhea JT, Novelline RA, Mostafavi AA, McCabe CJ (1998) Effect of computed tomography of the appendix on treatment of patients and use of hospital resources. N Engl J Med 15;338:141–146
8. Kokoska ER, Silen ML, Tracy TF Jr, Dillon PA, Cradock TV, Weber TR (1998) Perforated appendicitis in children: risk factors for the development of complications. Surgery 124:619–625, 625–626
9. Dandapat MC, Panda C (1992) A perforated appendix: should we drain? J Indian Med Assoc 90:147–148
10. Rucinski J, Fabian T, Panagopoulos G, Schein M, Wise L (2000) Gangrenous and perforated appendicitis: a meta-analytic study of 2532 patients indicates that the incision should be closed primarily. Surgery 127:136–141
11. Schein M, Assalia A, Bachus H (1994) Minimal antibiotic therapy after emergency abdominal surgery: a prospective study. Br J Surg 81:989–991
12. Wittmann DH, Schein M (1996) Let us shorten antibiotic prophylaxis and therapy in surgery. Am J Surg 172(6A):26S–32S
13. Schein M, Wise L (1977) Editorial comment. Peritonitis. In: Schein M, Wise L (eds) Crucial controversies in Surgery. Karger Landes Systems, pp 253–256

CHAPTER 8

Mesenteric Ischemia

Acute Mesenteric Arterial Ischemia

Jon S. Thompson · Thomas G. Lynch

Controversies

- Role of arteriography in diagnosis and management
- Determination of intraoperative viability
- Should massive resection be performed?
- Role of second-look procedures

Role of Arteriography in Diagnosis and Management

The diagnosis of acute arterial mesenteric ischemia remains challenging, but of critical importance, since early exploration can lead to the reversal of ischemia in many cases and prompt resection of gangrenous bowel can improve outcome. Timely diagnosis requires a high index of suspicion, and the prompt recognition of suggestive signs of ischemia. While characteristic laboratory findings (leukocytosis, lactic acidosis) and radiologic abnormalities (bowel wall thickening, pneumatosis, portal venous air) have been described, the accuracy of clinical diagnosis continues to be notoriously poor [1].

The value of imaging studies in the diagnosis and management of acute mesenteric ischemia has been the subject of continuing debate. Plain films of the abdomen have a low diagnostic accuracy. The value of duplex ultrasonography is often limited by the presence of abdominal distention and small bowel gas, both of which are typical of mesenteric ischemia. CT imaging has proved useful in the diagnosis of mesenteric venous thrombosis [2–4]. Recent reports have begun to assess its value in acute arterial mesenteric ischemia [5–7]. Klein et al. [6] reported that arteriography and CT imaging had a comparable sensitivity to mesenteric infarction, 87.5% and 82%, respectively. Magnetic resonance imaging of the mesenteric circulation has also been evaluated in normal volunteers [8–10] and in experimentally induced mesenteric ischemia [11].

Currently, however, arteriography is the only imaging technique with diagnostic and therapeutic potential. Arterial mesenteric ischemia may be secondary to embolic occlusion, thrombosis or nonocclusive mesenteric ischemia (NOMI). Some feel that arteriography in patients with acute embolic or thrombotic occlusive disease will only unnecessarily delay surgery and is of no value in patients with a classic presentation. Other authors [12-15] have suggested that arteriography may further define the extent of disease and permit the use of adjunctive pharmacologic therapy in patients without peritoneal signs. Recent reports have described the successful use of adjunctive lytic therapy [16-19]. Simo et al. [19] reported on the use of urokinase in ten patients with mesenteric emboli and the absence of peritoneal signs. Successful lysis was achieved in nine and clinical success, defined as the resolution of abdominal pain, in seven. Three patients subsequently underwent laparotomy.

Boley [20] has suggested that the aggressive use of arteriography may increase the frequency with which mesenteric ischemia, and NOMI in particular, is diagnosed. NOMI accounts for 20%-30% of episodes of acute mesenteric ischemia and can be secondary to vasoactive medications, decreased cardiac output with associated hypotension, dysrhythmias, myocardial injury or hypovolemia. A high index of suspicion, and early arteriography, in this group of patients may result in diagnosis prior to intestinal infarction and a reduction in operative mortality.

In addition, Boley [20] and others [13-15] have advocated the adjunctive use of papaverine in the patients with NOMI. Boley has proposed selective superior mesenteric artery infusion of papaverine (30-60 mg/h). The infusion is continued during and following surgical exploration in patients with persistent peritoneal signs. For those without peritoneal signs the infusion is continued for 24 h, after which arteriography is repeated. Other authors have reported the use of phenoxybenzamine, and have provided experimental evidence for the use of glucagon and prostaglandin I_2 [21, 22].

In summary, arteriography is certainly indicated in patients presenting with a stable hemodynamic profile and absence of peritoneal signs. If arteriography can be performed promptly prior to planned exploration and during the process of resuscitation in patients with early peritoneal signs, catheters may also be of value in the interoperative and perioperative period for the adjunctive infusion of vasodilatory or thrombolytic agents. Arteriography should be performed in all patients at risk for NOMI who have symptoms of prolonged ileus, abdominal distention or tenderness.

Determination of Intraoperative Viability

There is a significant body of literature describing the methods used to determine the viability of ischemic and acutely reperfused bowel at the time of initial surgical exploration. The use of technetium-labeled microspheres [23, 24], electromyography [25], Doppler ultrasound [26, 27], fluorescein fluorescence pattern recognition [28, 29], fluorescein time-distribution curves [30, 31], He-Ne laser Doppler [32] and photoplethysmography [33] have been evaluated by various authors. The majority of these techniques, however, require specialized equipment that limits routine applicability. As a result, Doppler ultrasound and fluorescein fluorescence pattern recognition continue to be commonly employed because of the simplicity of the techniques.

Wright and Hobson [26] first reported on the use of Doppler ultrasound in the assessment of bowel viability. Doppler flow was evaluated at three locations: the mesenteric vascular pedicle, the mesenteric border of the bowel and the anti-mesenteric surface of the bowel. The authors reported that all segments with Doppler flow present in each of the three zones were viable at 24 h. Bulkley et al. [28] subsequently compared Doppler ultrasound and fluorescein fluorescence patterns seen using a long wave ultrasound ("Woods") light, following the intravenous administration of sodium fluorescein. In a feline model, they reported only a 33% sensitivity with Doppler ultrasound and a 100% sensitivity with fluorescence pattern recognition. In a subsequent clinical trial [29], the authors reported a 100% sensitivity using fluorescence pattern recognition, a 78% sensitivity with clinical judgment alone and a 63% sensitivity with Doppler ultrasound. In comparison to quantitative fluorometric assessment of fluorescein distribution, however, Silverman et al. [8] found the pattern recognition method had a sensitivity of only 40%. In a canine model of mesenteric ischemia, a comparison of Doppler ultrasound, laser Doppler flow velocimetry and quantitative fluorometry demonstrated sensitivities of 86%, 85% and 95%, respectively.

Clinical practice would suggest that physical findings are useful in the determination of intestinal viability and their accuracy has ranged between 75% and 80% [29]. The appearance of the ischemic intestine will depend on the duration of the ischemia as well as its cause [34]. Early arterial obstruction may produce little change in the external appearance of the bowel. Reliance on physical findings alone, however, can lead to inaccurate conclusions regarding intestinal viability and more quantitative methods are desirable. It would appear that Doppler ultrasound and fluorescence pattern recognition provide a viable alternative. More quantitative techniques, while demonstrating increased accuracy, require expensive equipment and have not enjoyed wide clinical acceptance.

Should Massive Resection Be Performed?

The appropriateness of massive resection remains controversial when irreversible intestinal ischemia is extensive. Death is inevitable if all nonviable bowel is not resected, but massive resection may merely result in less timely demise [35, 36]. Furthermore, there are concerns about the quality of life in the survivors who may require long-term parenteral nutrition (PN) and have an ostomy. These are important issues, since many patients with mesenteric ischemia are elderly patients with co-morbid conditions.

Rates of resection usually reflect the surgeon's bias since a preoperative discussion of these issues with the patient and family is not often feasible. Resection for massive infarction was undertaken in 53%–92% of patients in reported series (Table 1) [35–41]. Of course, in some cases the diagnosis is suspected and no operation is performed.

Clearly the morbidity and mortality of massive resection for mesenteric ischemia are significant. Massive resection for infarction has a mortality rate of 31%–

Table 1. Resection for massive infarction

Author	No. of patients explored	No. of massive infarctions	No. (%) resected
Sitges-Serra [35]	105	83	44 (53%)
Ottinger [36]	103	61	28 (46%)
Sachs [37]	30	24	22 (92%)
Pierce [38]	56	30	20 (67%)
Singh [39]	18	12	10 (83%)
Krausz [40]	26	16	14 (88%)
Levy [41]	77	32	17 (53%)
Total	415	258	155 (60%)

65% [35, 37, 42]. Complications occur in as many as 80% of patients [42]. Early reoperation is required in one-fourth of patients and survivors have a mean hospital stay of approximately 2 months. However, approximately one-half of patients will survive massive resection and its associated complications.

Enterostomy is performed in 11%–67% of patients at the time of massive resection [35, 42]. This is prudent when bowel viability is questionable and the operation needs to be completed expeditiously. The anticipated functional outcome is another important issue, as diarrhea and perianal complications are frequent if remnants of less than 90 cm of small bowel are anastomosed to the left colon. An enterostomy performed at the time of resection is often permanent in these patients because further operations are avoided. However, elderly patients usually tolerate ostomies quite well.

Approximately 20% of patients require home PN after massive resection for ischemia [35]. The need for permanent PN is usually predictable since it is based on the site and extent of resection [43, 44]. Patients with >180 cm small intestine will generally not require parenteral nutrition (PN). Patients with <60 cm small intestine are likely to require long-term PN. Patients with remnant lengths in between will require PN for a period of months but are likely to eventually discontinue PN. Compared to an end jejunostomy a jejunoileal anastomosis is equivalent to adding 80 cm of small bowel and a jejunocolic anastomosis is the equivalent to adding 26 cm of small bowel in terms of improved absorptive function [44]. Unfortunately, an end jejunostomy is frequently the result of massive resection for acute mesenteric arterial ischemia.

While long-term survival in these patients is reduced with advanced age, overall 5-year survival is approximately 60% in patients with mesenteric infarction requiring PN [45]. Rehabilitation to normal age-related activity is possible in the majority of these patients [46]. While long-term PN results in some physical distress and psychological limitations, quality of life is quite acceptable in most patients [47].

Massive resection should always be given consideration in patients with mesenteric infarction due to mesenteric ischemia. Approximately 50% of patients will survive massive resection. Following the initial hospitalization these patients have a reasonable quality of life. Most patients will not require permanent PN. The main contraindication to massive resection should be preexisting quality of life and co-morbid conditions.

Second-Look Procedures

A second-look procedure is an option when viability of extensive segments is unclear and resection would result in the short bowel syndrome. With this approach, clearly necrotic bowel is resected and re-anastomosis performed only in viable-appearing bowel. Potentially salvageable bowel is retained and reevaluated at a planned second look carried out in approximately 24 h irrespective of the patient's subsequent clinical course. Depending on the patient's overall condition and situation, reexploration may reveal extensive ischemic bowel that will not have to be resected, ischemic bowel that will have to be resected but perhaps less extensively than predicted at the initial procedure, or no evidence of ischemic bowel. The merit of the second-look procedure should be determined based on the frequency of these findings.

The diagnosis of ongoing intestinal ischemia is difficult. Clinical assessment is notoriously inaccurate. While creation of a stoma is another way to assess viability of the remnant postoperatively, it may not permit adequate visualization of the entire remnant [48]. Thus, the use of second-look procedures should result in more timely diagnosis and management. The outcome of second-look procedures may be influenced by how selectively they are applied (Table 2). The frequency of second-look procedures ranges from 13% to 100% in various reports [36, 37, 41, 49, 50]. When performed more selectively, the diagnosis of ongoing ischemia may be delayed. Wilson et al. [50] only performed second-look procedures in 13% of patients but had another 17% patients undergo clinical deterioration due to recurrent ischemia. Ottinger [36] found that three (18%) of 17 revascularized patients not undergoing a second look would have benefited from reexploration. He also reported that 20% of patients died before a planned second-look procedure could be carried out.

Ischemic bowel is found at planned reexploration in 50% to 75% of cases. Overall, 80% of these patients will undergo further resection. The important issue is whether or not this approach leads to lesser resection. Sachs et al. [36] performed second-look procedures in 12 revascularized patients. Nine had ischemic bowel and seven underwent resection but only one underwent a lesser resection. Levy et al. [37] reported that all ten patients with intestinal ischemia had further resection at the second look and that three patients underwent lesser resection using this approach. Thus second-look procedures reduce the extent of resection in a number of patients.

Table 2. Outcome of second-look procedures for acute arterial ischemia

Author	No. of patients	No. (%) 2nd look	No. (%) positive	No. (%) resected	No. (%) lesser resection
Ottinger [36]	103	15 (15%)	10 (67%)	8 (53%)	-
Sachs [37]	30	12 (40%)	9 (75%)	7 (58%)	1 (8%)
Ballard [19]	16	16 (100%)	10 (63%)	6 (38%)	
Levy [41]	45	18 (40%)	10 (56%)	10 (56%)	3 (17%)
Wilson [50]	30	4 (13%)	2 (50%)	2 (50%)	-
Total	224	65 (29%)	41 (63%)	33 (80%)	-

Whether or not revascularization was performed at the initial procedure also influences outcome. Levy et al. [37] found that all of their patients not undergoing initial resection or revascularization required subsequent resection. However, only one (16%) of six patients undergoing revascularization had subsequent resection, suggesting that the second-look procedure may have prevented unnecessary resection in these patients.

Second-look procedures have a role in selected patients with acute mesenteric arterial ischemia. The primary role is in patients with questionable bowel viability in whom massive resection would lead to the need for permanent PN. This approach may be especially useful after revascularization. Compiled reports suggest that second-look procedures will lead to less extensive resection and more timely diagnosis of ongoing ischemia.

References

1. Sarr MG, Bulkley GB, Zurdema GD (1983) Preoperative recognition of intestinal strangulation obstruction. Am J Surg 145:176–182
2. Franquet T, Bescos JM, Reparaz B (1989) Noninvasive methods in the diagnosis of isolated superior mesenteric vein thrombosis: US and CT. Gastrointest Radiol 14:321–325
3. Rosen A, Korobkin M, Silverman P, et al. (1984) Mesenteric vein thrombosis; CT identification. AJR 143:83–86
4. Clemett AK, Chang J (1975) The radiological diagnosis of spontaneous mesenteric venous thrombosis. Am J Gastroenterol 63:209–215
5. Catalano O (1995) Computed tomography in the diagnostic approach to acute mesenteric ischemia. Radiol-Med-Torino 89:440–446
6. Klein HM, Lensing R, Klosterhalfen B, Tons C, Gunther RW (1995) Diagnostic imaging of mesenteric infarction. Radiology 197:79–82
7. Suzuki T (1996) CT diagnosis of acute occlusion of the superior mesenteric artery. Nippon-Igaku-Hoshasen-Gakkai-Zasshi 56:83–88
8. Shirkhoda A, Konez O, Shetty AN, Bis KG, Ellwood RA, Kirsch MJ (1997) Mesenteric circulation: three-dimensional MR angiography with a gadolinium-enhanced multiecho gradient-echo technique. Radiology 202:257–261
9. Heiss SG, Li KC (1998) Magnetic resonance angiography of mesenteric arteries. A review. Invest Radiol 33:670–681
10. Shirkhoda A, Konez O, Shetty AN, Bis KG, Ellwood RA, Kirsch MJ (1998) Contrast-enhanced MR angiography of the mesenteric circulation: a pictorial essay. Radiographics 18:851–861
11. Klein HM, Klosterhalfen B, Kinzel S, Jansen A, Seggewiss C, Weghaus P, Kamp M, Tons C, Gunther RW (1996) CT and MRI of experimentally induced mesenteric ischemia in a porcine model. J Comput Assist Tomogr 20:254–261
12 Geelkerken RH, van Bockel JH (1995) Mesenteric vascular disease: a review of diagnostic methods and therapies. Cardiovasc Surg 3:247–260
13. Bassiouny HS (1997) Nonocclusive mesenteric ischemia. Surg Clin North Am 77:319–326
14. McKinsey JF, Gewertz BL (1997) Acute mesenteric ischemia. Surg Clin North Am 77:307–318
15. Mansour MA (1999) Management of acute mesenteric ischemia. Arch Surg 134:328–331
16. Boyer L, Delorme JM, Alexandre M, Boissier A, Gimbergues P, Glanddier G, Viallet JF (1994) Local fibrinolysis for superior mesenteric artery thromboembolism. Cardiovasc Intervent Radiol 17:214–216
17. Kwauk ST, Bartlett JH, Hayes P, Chow KC (1996) Intra-arterial fibrinolytic treatment for mesenteric arterial embolus: a case report. Can J Surg 39:163–166
18. Badioloa CM, Scoppetta DJ (1997) Rapid revascularization of an embolic superior mesenteric artery occlusion using pulse-spray pharmacomechanical thrombolysis with urokinase. Am J Roentgenol 169:55–57
19. Simo G, Echenagusia AJ, Camunez F, Turegano F, Cabrera A, Urbano J (1997) Superior mesenteric arterial embolism: local fibrinolytic treatment with urokinase. Radiology 204:775–779
20. Kaleya RN, Sammartano RJ, Boley SJ (1992) Aggressive approach to acute mesenteric ischemia. Surg Clin North Am 72:157–182

21. Athanasoulis CA, Wittenberg J, Bernstein R, Williams LF (1975) Vasodilatory drugs in the management of nonocclusive bowel ischemia. Gastroenterology 68:146–150
22. Kazmers A, Zwolak R, Appelman HD, Whitehouse WM, Wu SCH, Zelenock GB, Cronenwett JL, Lindenauer SM, Stanley JC (1984) Pharmacologic interventions in acute mesenteric ischemia: improved survival with intravenous glucagon, methylprednisolone, and prostacyclin. J Vasc Surg 1:472–481
23. Moosa AF, Skinner DB, Stark U, Hoffer P (1974) Assessment of bowel viability using 99 m technetium tagged albumin microspheres. J Surg Res 16:466–472
24. Zarins CK, Skinner DB, Rhodes BA, James AE (1974) Predictions of the viability of revascularized intestine with radioactive microspheres. Surg Gynecol Obstet 138:576–580
25. Katz S, Wahab A, Murray W, William LF (1974) New parameters of viability in ischemic bowel disease. Am J Surg 127:136–141
26. Wright CB, Hobson RW (1975) Prediction of intestinal viability using Doppler ultrasound technics. Am J Surg 129:642–645
27. Cooperman M, Pace WG, Martin EW Jr, Pflug B, Keith LM Jr, Evan WE, Carey LC (1978) Determination of viability of ischemic intestine by Doppler ultrasound. Surgery 83:705–710
28. Bulkley GB, Wheaton LG, Strandberg JD, Zuidema GD (1979) Assessment of small intestinal recovery from ischemic injury after segmental, arterial, venous, and arteriovenous occlusion. Surg Forum 30:210–213
29. Bulkley GB, Zuidema GD, Hamilton SR, O'Mara CS, Klacksman PG, Horn SD (1981) Intraoperative determination of small intestinal viability following ischemic surgery. Ann Surg 193:628–637
30. Silverman DG, Hurford WE, Cooper HS, Robinson M, Brousseau DA (1983) Quantification of fluorescein distribution to strangulated rat ileum. Surg Res 34:179–186
31. Carter MS, Fantini GA, Sammartano RJ, Mitsuda S, Silverman DG, Boley SJ (1984) Qualitative and quantitative fluorescein fluorescence in determining intestinal viability. Am J Surg 147:117–123
32. Rotering RH, Dixon JA, Holloway, GA Jr, McCloskey DW (1982) A comparison of the He Ne laser and ultrasound Doppler systems in the determination of viability of ischemic canine intestine. Ann Surg 196:705–708
33. Pearce WH, Jones ON, Warren GH, Bartle EJ, Whitehill TA, Rutherford RB (1987) The use of infrared photoplethysmography in identifying early intestinal ischemia. Arch Surg 122:308–310
34. Mitsudo S, Brandt LS (1992) Pathology of intestinal ischemia. Surg Clin North Am 72:43–63
35. Sitges-Serra A, Mas X, Roqueta F, Figueras J, Sanz F (1988) Mesenteric infarction: an analysis of 83 patients with prognostic studies in 44 patients undergoing a massive small bowel resection. Br J Surg 75:544–548
36. Ottinger LW (1978) The surgical management of acute occlusion of the superior mesenteric artery. Ann Surg 188:721–731
37. Sachs SM, Morton JH, Schwartz SI (1982) Acute mesenteric ischemia. Surgery 92:646–653
38. Pierce GE, Brockenbrough EC (1970) The spectrum of mesenteric infarction. Am J Surg 119:233–239
39. Singh RP, Shah RC, Lec ST (1975) Acute mesenteric vascular occlusion: a review of 32 patients. Surgery 78:613–617
40. Krausz MM, Manny J (1978) Acute superior mesenteric arterial occlusion: a plea for early diagnosis. Surgery 83:482–485
41. Levy PH, Krausz MM, Manny J (1990) Acute mesenteric ischemia: improved results – a retrospective analysis of 92 patients. Surgery 107:372–380
42. Nguyen BT, Blatchford GJ, Thompson JS, Bragg LE (1989) Should intestinal continuity be restored after massive intestinal resection. Am J Surg 158:577–580
43. Gouttebel MC, Saint-Aubert B, Astre C, Joyeux H (1986) Total parenteral nutrition needs in different types of short bowel syndrome. Dig Dis Sci 31:718–723
44. Carbonnel F, Cosnes J, Chevret S, Beaugerie L, Ngo Y, Malefusse M, Parc R, Quintrec YL, Gendre JP (1996) The role of anatomic factors in the nutritional autonomy after extensive small bowel resection. JPEN 20:275–280
45. Messing B, Lemann M, Landais P, et al. (1995) Prognosis of patients with nonmalignant chronic intestinal failure receiving long-term home parenteral nutrition. Gastroenterology 108:1005–1010
46. Howard L, Amentim Fleming CR, Shike M, Steiger E (1995) Current use and clinical outcome of home parenteral and enteral nutritional therapies in the United States. Gastroenterology 109:355–365
47. Ladefoged K (1981) Quality of life in patients on permanent home parenteral nutrition. JPEN 5:132–137

48. Snyder CL, Kaufman DB (1991) A simple technique for assessing the viability of stomas of intestines. Surg Gynecol Obstet 172:399–400
49. Ballard JL, Stone WM, Hallett JW, Pairolero PC, Cherry KJ (1993) A critical analysis of adjuvant techniques used to assess bowel viability in acute mesenteric ischemia. Am Surg 59:309–311
50. Wilson C, Gupta R, Gilmour DG, Imrie CW (1987) Acute superior mesenteric ischemia. Br J Surg 74:279–281

Acute Mesenteric Venous Ischemia

Hannes A. Rüdiger · Pierre-Alain Clavien

Introduction

Elliot [1] first reported mesenteric infarction due to vascular occlusion in 1895. Mesenteric venous thrombosis, a cause of 5%–15% of all mesenteric ischemias [2–5], was described as a clinical entity distinct from arterial occlusion in 1935 [6]. While the incidence of mesenteric ischemia has increased over the past two decades due to increased life expectancy [7], the diagnosis and treatment have remained challenging and controversial [2]. The mortality associated with venous mesenteric ischemia ranges between 13% and 50%, which is still better than that of other forms of acute mesenteric venous ischemia [4, 8–12].

The extent of thrombosis in small vessels is a major determinant for the severity of the disease since thrombosis solely localized in main venous channels in the mesentery is better tolerated due to extensive collateralization [13]. The most frequent cause of venous mesenteric ischemia is thrombosis of the superior mesenteric vein (SMV) typically causing ischemia in the mid jejunum and ileum [5]. Intestinal ischemia is exceptional in presence of portal vein thrombosis alone [14].

A variety of predisposing conditions have been incriminated in mesenteric ischemia due to mesenteric venous thrombosis [5]: the most important are previous abdominal surgery [4, 10], hypercoagulable states [4, 15, 16], malignancy [4, 10], cirrhosis [4], abdominal trauma [4, 17], irradiation [3, 4, 10, 17], and the use of oral contraceptives [4, 18, 19].

Diagnosis

Mesenteric venous infarction is rarely diagnosed preoperatively since it lacks a typical clinical presentation [9]. The diagnosis is usually only made during laparotomy or even autopsy. However, early diagnosis and rapid intervention are important to preserve small bowel function and to increase patient survival [20]. Patients with mesenteric venous ischemia usually present with symptoms consistent with acute bowel ischemia with abdominal pain as the main feature [4, 11, 21]. Abdominal pain is usually out of proportion to physical findings. A few signs may suggest a venous etiology rather than an arterial obstruction. Venous mesenteric ischemia is associated with a prolonged duration of pain prior to admission [9]. This prolonged clinical course may be related to the development of a large number of collaterals within the mesenteric venous system including the portal vein, the superior and inferior mesenteric veins and the splenic vein [22]. These collaterals may partially prevent a rapid progression of the ischemic event with subsequent development of transmural infarction.

Since laboratory tests are unspecific and do not allow to confirm or exclude a diagnosis [4], immediate radiologic evaluation should be performed. Roentgenographic and other imaging studies can definitively establish the diagnosis of mesenteric venous thrombosis before intestinal infarction occurs [11]. Ultrasonography, computed tomography (CT) and magnetic resonance imaging have been used to demonstrate venous thrombi before the bowel becomes necrotic [11].

Doppler Ultrasonography

Inderbitzi et al. [23] have shown that Doppler ultrasonography can be very sensitive in detecting portal and mesenteric vein thrombosis. However, in our experience, Doppler ultrasonography is rarely diagnostic and is often difficult to apply because of the overlying air due to concomitant ileus. Therefore we generally recommend performing a CT scan as first radiologic investigation.

Computed Tomography

While the literature concerning CT examination in mesenteric venous thrombosis is limited, it is widely used as a screening method in the evaluation of patients with an acute abdomen, particularly in the United States. It provides information about the intestinal wall, mesenteric circulation and peritoneal cavity [24]. Contrast-enhanced CT scan represents a useful alternative to arteriography. With optimal enhancement, mesenteric venous thrombosis is easily detectable even in peripheral branches [24]. The diagnostic triad of CT scan findings diagnostic for venous mesenteric ischemia include (1) a sharply defined enhancing venous wall with a central area of low density in the superior mesenteric vein (thrombosis) [24], (2) thickening of the intestinal wall and valvulae conniventes localized to a jejuno-ileal segment (ischemic bowel), and (3) peritoneal fluid usually in presence of transmural infarction [25]. When venous etiology is suspected, we recommend performing a CT scan as the sole diagnostic test [25].

Gadolinium-Enhanced Magnetic Resonance Venography

Few data are available regarding this novel modality in the setting of mesenteric venous thrombosis. However, recent reports suggest high sensitivity in detecting occlusions in the mesenteric venous system [26, 27]. Gadolinium-enhanced three-dimensional MR portal venography is an accurate, noninvasive method of imaging the mesenteric-portal vein that does not require the administration of either ionizing radiation or an iodine-based contrast reagent [26]. Magnetic resonance venography (MRV) might become the gold standard diagnostic test for venous mesenteric thrombosis.

Arteriography

Arteriography may provide important information regarding the anatomic extent of arterial obstruction and usually enables to differentiate proximal from distal arterial occlusion in the superior mesenteric artery. Proximal occlusion is due to thrombosis, while distal occlusions in the superior mesenteric artery are related to arterial emboli. Delayed imaging provides information about the mesenteric venous system. However, the extent of the thrombosis is better assessed by CT scan. An arteriography should be performed only if an arterial etiology is suspected. A possible advantage of arteriography is the possibility of using the catheter selectively placed in the superior mesenteric artery for continuous delivering of drugs such as vasodilatators [28]. However, if a venous etiology is suspected, a CT scan should be preferred since arteriography is invasive, time-consuming, and may lead to a further delay of life-saving laparotomy [25].

Treatment

The primary goal of treatment of mesenteric ischemia is the prevention of bowel gangrene [4] and resection of the infarcted bowel. It has been long accepted that suspicion of mesenteric venous ischemia should be immediately treated with laparotomy. In the 1960s, mortality without surgical treatment was reported to approach 100% [10]. Due to considerable improvement of diagnostic modalities over the past two decades, mesenteric venous ischemia can often be diagnosed before the presence of bowel infarction. At this stage, mesenteric venous ischemia can sometimes be successfully treated nonoperatively. If signs of peritonitis (rebound sign and tenderness) are present, immediate laparotomy should be performed without need for extensive diagnostics, and a CT scan should not be performed [5, 8]. In less urgent cases, we recommend performing a CT scan. The characteristic triad of CT scan findings including hypodensity in the trunk of the superior mesenteric vein, thickening of the intestinal wall and ascites [25] is in itself an absolute indication for immediate surgery. Normal laboratory values should not delay immediate laparotomy [4].

However, the radiographic findings of mesenteric venous thrombosis (MVT) alone do not necessarily mandate laparotomy [5]. In selected cases a conservative management may be superior to an operative approach. If the CT scan reveals hypodensity in the trunk of the superior mesenteric vein and thickening of the intestinal wall but no peritoneal fluid, conservative therapy seems reasonable using immediate anticoagulation with full-dose intravenous heparin [29]. Serial CT or ultrasonography should be performed to closely monitor the potential formation of peritoneal fluid. In cases of secondary accumulation of peritoneal fluid, surgery must be performed without delay [29].

Bowel Resection

Surgical intervention is warranted with the onset of peritoneal irritation [5, 8]. Two main strategies regarding the extent of the bowel resection were proposed, namely: (1) resection of the macroscopically nonviable bowel or (2) extended resection including 15 cm of macroscopically normal bowel. The approach with resection limited to nonviable bowel was proposed earlier by Russel [21]. However, in venous mesenteric infarction a recurrence rate of 50%–60% following resection of infarcted bowel was found at the site of anastomosis despite early anticoagulative prophylaxis [9]. The notoriously unreliable visual assessment of bowel viability together with damages due to reperfusion injury [30, 31] and persistent arterial spasms may contribute to the high incidence of recurrent thrombosis [9]. They usually involve the 10 cm adjacent to the end-to-end anastomosis [9]. To prevent recurrent or chronic mesenteric venous ischemia, several strategies had been described. We proposed in an earlier report extensive resection of 15 cm of macroscopically normal bowel proximal and distal to the demarcation lines [9]. This strategy might be contraindicated in presence of extensive infarction since wide resection may lead to short bowel syndrome [5] with subsequent dependence on long-term parenteral nutrition [7]. In this case, a more conservative resection might be performed including a second look after 24–48 h [5, 9].

Thrombectomy

Successful cases of thrombectomies have been reported during the 1970s [32, 33]. One author recently recommended thrombectomies in combination with resection of gangrenous bowel [22]. However, thrombectomy is only effective for thrombi localized in large venous trunks leaving behind obstruction in the small veins in the vicinity of the bowel, the main source of mesenteric ischemia [9]. Most patients with acute mesenteric vein thrombosis have a more diffuse pattern of venous obstruction, which makes a thrombectomy impossible [5]. In addition, Laufman et al. [34] showed in an animal model that a significant postoperative vasospasm occurs after removal of the venous occlusion. Therefore, we do not recommend thrombectomy for patients with acute mesenteric venous thrombosis.

Antegrade Thrombolysis

The antegrade arterial infusion of the thrombolytic drug urokinase has recently been described in a case report [13]. This might be a promising approach since it also addresses thrombosis in small veins of the mesentery [13]. However, further experience with this novel therapy is necessary since the possible high efficacy in lysing the thrombus might be outweighed by the increased risk of bleeding.

Anticoagulation

Immediate anticoagulative therapy is indicated once the diagnosis of mesenteric venous thrombosis is made [4], and an assessment regarding coagulopathies is mandatory in every case. The need for long-term postoperative anticoagulative therapy is widely accepted. As originally proposed by Boley et al. [4, 11], anticoagulative therapy should be initiated with a bolus dose of 5000 units heparin followed by intravenous infusion of 1000 units/h. A high incidence of recurrent thrombosis within the initial 6 weeks postoperative was reported, leading to the recommendation of anticoagulation well beyond this period. However, the exact duration of anticoagulation needed remains controversial. A subsequent conversion from heparin to dicoumarol or coumadin after 10 days is usually performed. These oral anticoagulatives are kept for 6 months [8, 10, 21] and might be considered as lifelong therapy [5], particularly in the presence of documented coagulopathies, such as activated protein C (APC) resistance, anti-thrombin III, protein C or S deficiencies [35].

Conclusions

Acute MVT has become more common with aging of the population. Contrast-enhanced CT scan is the most sensitive diagnostic modality. Immediate laparotomy is recommended if peritonitis is present or the characteristic triad of bowel wall thickening, hypodensity in the mesenteric vein and ascites is seen on CT scan. In the absence of peritonitis and ascites, an attempt at conservative treatment may be justified including full-dose intravenous heparin. In the presence of infarcted bowel, wide resection should be performed including 15 cm of viable bowel proximal and distal to the demarcation lines to prevent early and late recurrences. Anticoagulative therapy should be initiated at the time of diagnosis and maintained for at least 6 months.

References

1. Elliot J (1895) The operative relief of gangrene of intestine due to occlusion of the mesenteric vessels. Ann Surg 21:9–23
2. Clavien PA, Muller C, Harder F (1987) Treatment of mesenteric infarction. Br J Surg 74(6):500–503
3. Grendell JH, Ockner RK (1982) Mesenteric venous thrombosis. Gastroenterology 82(2):358–372
4. Rhee RY, Gloviczki P (1997) Mesenteric venous thrombosis. Surg Clin North Am 77(2):327–338
5. Rhee RY, Gloviczki P, Mendonca CT, et al. (1994) Mesenteric venous thrombosis: still a lethal disease in the 1990s. J Vasc Surg 20(5):688–697
6. Donaldson JK SB (1935) Mesenteric thrombosis. Arterial and venous types as separate clinical entities, a clinical and experimental study. Am J Surg 24(2):208–217
7. Horgan PG, Gorey TF (1992) Operative assessment of intestinal viability. Surg Clin North Am 72(1):143–155
8. Grieshop RJ, Dalsing MC, Cikrit DF, et al. (1991) Acute mesenteric venous thrombosis. Revisited in a time of diagnostic clarity. Am Surg 57(9):573–577, 578
9. Clavien PA, Durig M, Harder F (1988) Venous mesenteric infarction: a particular entity. Br J Surg 75(3):252–255

10. Naitove AWR (1964) Primary mesenteric venous thrombosis. Ann Surg 161(4):516–523
11. Boley SJ, Kaleya RN, Brandt LJ (1992) Mesenteric venous thrombosis. Surg Clin North Am 72(1):183–201
12. Wilson C, Walker ID, Davidson JF, Imrie CW (1987) Mesenteric venous thrombosis and antithrombin III deficiency. J Clin Pathol 40(8):906–908
13. Train JS, Ross H, Weiss JD, et al. (1998) Mesenteric venous thrombosis: successful treatment by intraarterial lytic therapy. J Vasc Intervent Radiol 9(3):461–464
14. Trinkle JK, Rush BF, Fuller MA, et al. (1969) The operative management of idiopathic mesenteric venous thrombosis with intestinal infarction. Am Surg 35(5):338–341
15. Gruenberg JC, Smallridge RC, Rosenberg RD (1975) Inherited antithrombin-III deficiency causing mesenteric venous infarction: a new clinical entity. Ann Surg 181(6):791–794
16. Peters TG, Lewis JD, Flip DJ, Morris L (1977) Antithrombin III deficiency causing postsplenectomy mesenteric venous thrombosis coincident with thrombocytopenia. Ann Surg 185(2):229–231
17. Moser G, Pouret JP (1977) [Mesenteric venous infarction. Report of twelve cases (author's translation)]. Ann Chir 31(2):157–161
18. Civetta JM, Kolodny M (1970) Mesenteric venous thrombosis associated with oral contraceptives. Gastroenterology 58(5):713–716
19. Miller DR (1971) Unusual focal mesenteric venous thrombosis associated with contraceptive medication: a case report. Ann Surg 173(1):135–138
20. Slutzker DM, Pigula F (1987) Small bowel infarction and death from primary mesenteric venous thrombosis. Am J Emerg Med 5(2):126–129
21. Russell JC, Bloom GP (1982) Mesenteric venous infarction: presenting as upper gastro-intestinal bleeding. Conn Med 46(10):563–565
22. Klempnauer J, Grothues F, Bektas H, Pichlmayr R (1997) Results of portal thrombectomy and splanchnic thrombolysis for the surgical management of acute mesentericoportal thrombosis. Br J Surg 84(1):129–132
23. Inderbitzi R, Wagner HE, Seiler C, et al. (1992) Acute mesenteric ischaemia. Eur J Surg 158(2):123–126
24. Kim JY, Ha HK, Byun JY, et al. (1993) Intestinal infarction secondary to mesenteric venous thrombosis: CT-pathologic correlation. J Comput Assist Tomogr 17(3):382–385
25. Clavien PA, Huber O, Mirescu D, Rohner A (1989) Contrast enhanced CT scan as a diagnostic procedure in mesenteric ischaemia due to mesenteric venous thrombosis. Br J Surg 76(1):93–94
26. Saddik D, Frazer C, Robins P, et al. (1999) Gadolinium-enhanced three-dimensional MR portal venography. AJR Am J Roentgenol 172(2):413–417
27. Wilson MW, Hamilton BH, Dong Q, et al. (1998) Gadolinium-enhanced magnetic resonance venography of the portal venous system prior to transjugular intrahepatic portosystemic shunts and liver transplantation. Original investigation. Invest Radiol 33(9):644–652
28. Boley SJ, Brandt LJ (1986) Selective mesenteric vasodilators. A future role in acute mesenteric ischemia? Gastroenterology 91(1):247–249
29. Clavien PA, Huber O, Rohner A (1989) Venous mesenteric ischaemia: conservative or surgical treatment? [letter]. Lancet 2(8653):48
30. Kuzu MA, Koksoy C, Kale IT, et al. (1998) Reperfusion injury delays healing of intestinal anastomosis in a rat. Am J Surg 176(4):348–351
31. Kong SE, Blennerhassett LR, Heel KA, et al. (1998) Ischaemia-reperfusion injury to the intestine. Aust NZ J Surg 68(8):554–561
32. Bergentz SE, Ericsson B, Hedner U, et al. (1974) Thrombosis in the superior mesenteric and portal veins: report of a case treated with thrombectomy. Surgery 76(2):286–290
33. Inahara T (1971) Acute superior mesenteric venous thrombosis: treatment by thrombectomy. Ann Surg 174(6):956–961
34. Laufman H, Martin W, Tuell S (1945) The pattern of vasospasm following acute arterial and venous occlusion. A micrometric study. Surg Gynecol Obstet 85:675–686
35. Wheeler HB (1998) Should surgical patients be screened for thrombophilia? Semin Thromb Hemost 24 [Suppl 1]:63–65

Chronic Visceral Ischemia

Darren B. Schneider · Louis M. Messina · Ronald J. Stoney

Supported in part by the Pacific Vascular Research Foundation.

Introduction

Atherosclerotic occlusive disease of the mesenteric arteries causes progressive impairment of blood flow to the abdominal viscera, eventually producing chronic visceral ischemia. Although occlusion of the visceral arteries was described well over a century ago [1], it was not until 1936 that Dunphy correctly established the relationship between chronic visceral artery occlusive disease, postprandial abdominal pain, and death from bowel infarction [2]. Classically, symptoms are precipitated by ingestion of food, causing postprandial abdominal pain ("intestinal angina"), food aversion, and progressive weight loss. While relatively uncommon, chronic visceral ischemia is a widely recognized entity and its incidence may be rising [3]. Establishing of the diagnosis, however, is frequently delayed and a percentage of patients will go on to develop fatal intestinal infarction if adequate visceral perfusion is not restored. Surgical visceral revascularization provides durable relief of visceral ischemia and, therefore, is the preferred treatment. Percutaneous visceral angioplasty with or without stenting may be effective in selected patients, but the durability of these catheter-based interventions is yet to be established. In this chapter we will focus on crucial issues regarding the diagnosis and management of chronic visceral ischemia, including: imaging techniques available to document impaired visceral blood flow, operative approaches for visceral artery revascularization, endovascular approaches for visceral revascularization, and the management of recurrent visceral ischemia.

Diagnostic Imaging Techniques

The diagnosis of chronic visceral ischemia is all too often delayed, due to the rarity of this syndrome and the reluctance on the part of referring physicians to obtain expensive or invasive imaging studies. On average, the delay from the onset of symptoms to the diagnosis of chronic visceral ischemia takes 1 year or more [4]. Because the classic symptoms (postprandial pain, food aversion, and weight loss) may be confused with symptoms of more common disorders, such as peptic ulcer disease, biliary colic, and gastrointestinal malignancies, chronic visceral ischemia is a diagnosis of exclusion. Endoscopic and imaging studies are appropriately performed to exclude these possibilities; however, when negative, a vascular etiology should be evaluated.

Traditionally, the diagnosis of chronic visceral ischemia is confirmed by anteroposterior and lateral aortography, which remains the gold standard and should be performed prior to undertaking operative or percutaneous revascularization procedures. Demonstration of significant stenosis or occlusion of at least two of the three mesenteric arteries (celiac artery, CA; superior mesenteric artery, SMA; or inferior mesenteric artery, IMA) is usually required to confirm the diagnosis due to the extensive collateral circulation between these vessels. Recent advances in imaging techniques, however, have led to the development of noninvasive imaging modalities capable of assessing the mesenteric blood flow. A high clinical index of suspicion and increased familiarity with noninvasive imaging techniques, such as mesenteric duplex ultrasonography or magnetic resonance angiography, is necessary to overcome unnecessary delays in diagnosis and treatment.

Duplex ultrasonography is a useful noninvasive means of identifying mesenteric artery stenoses in patients undergoing initial evaluation for chronic visceral ischemia. Using Doppler-derived blood flow velocities, Moneta et al. [5] have established criteria for detection of ≥70% stenosis of the CA or SMA, based upon measurement of peak systolic velocity (PSV). A 70% or greater CA stenosis could be predicted with a sensitivity of 87% and a specificity of 80% using a threshold PSV of ≥200 cm/s or no flow signal. A threshold PSV of ≥250 cm/s or no flow signal predicted a 70% or greater SMA stenosis with a sensitivity of 92% and a specificity of 96%. In contrast, Zwolak [6] and others [7, 8] have reported that end-diastolic velocity (EDV) thresholds are more accurate predictors of hemodynamically significant CA and SMA stenoses. A CA EDV ≥55 cm/s or detection of retrograde hepatic artery flow predicted >50% stenosis with a sensitivity of 93% and a specificity of 100%. Likewise, an SMA EDV ≥45 cm/s or no flow signal predicted a >50% stenosis with a sensitivity of 90% and a specificity or 91%. Comparison of pre- and postprandial velocity measurements may also be used to predict high-grade SMA stenoses, but offer limited benefit over fasting studies alone [9]. Although used as a screening test for chronic visceral ischemia, mesenteric duplex ultrasonography is technically difficult to perform and requires a well-trained, experienced vascular technician. Furthermore, overlying bowel gas, prior abdominal surgery, or obese body habitus can also interfere with duplex evaluation of the visceral arteries, and the CA may not be amenable to evaluation in up to 20% of patients [5].

Within the last decade magnetic resonance imaging (MRI) techniques have been developed and also provide a noninvasive means of evaluating the mesenteric circulation. The proximal CA and SMA are well visualized using gadolinium-enhanced magnetic resonance angiography (MRA) with 3-D reconstruction [10, 11]. While 3-D MRA provides detailed morphologic analysis, phase-contrast MRI (PC-MRI) techniques allow assessment of flow within the SMA and superior mesenteric vein (SMV). Increases in postprandial blood flow within the SMV out of proportion to SMA blood flow appear to be a sensitive marker of significant SMA stenosis [12]. In the presence of a hemodynamically significant SMA stenosis, the discrepancy in postprandial SMV and SMA blood flow reflects the recruitment of collateral blood flow.

Overall, mesenteric duplex ultrasonography, 3-D MRA, and PC-MRI are excellent noninvasive screening tests for patients with suspected chronic visceral ischemia. In addition, these imaging modalities may also be useful for postoperative surveillance of mesenteric revascularizations when baseline postoperative studies are compared with scans obtained at regular follow-up intervals [13, 14]. While duplex ultrasonography and MRA hold promise as diagnostic adjuncts, they cannot supplant arteriography at the present time. Before planning visceral revascularization, suspected hemodynamically significant visceral arterial disease detected by duplex or MRI techniques should be further defined by biplanar abdominal aortography.

Operative Revascularization Techniques

Surgical options for the treatment of chronic visceral ischemia include both transaortic endarterectomy and aortovisceral bypass grafting. Techniques for bypass can be further subdivided into retrograde grafts originating from the infrarenal aorta vs. antegrade grafts originating from the supraceliac aorta and they may be comprised of either prosthetic material or autogenous tissue. Reimplantation and transarterial endarterectomy techniques have been largely abandoned in favor of transaortic endarterectomy and aortovisceral bypass, which offer superior patency [15]. Both transaortic endarterectomy and aortovisceral bypass provide durable relief of visceral ischemic symptoms [16] with an operative mortality ranging from 5% to 12% in most series [13, 16–20].

Controversy exists regarding the number and priority of visceral arteries that should undergo revascularization. Hollier [17] found that the frequency of recurrent visceral ischemia was inversely related to the number of visceral vessels revascularized. When only a single vessel was revascularized the late recurrence rate was 50% compared to 11% when all three visceral arteries were revascularized. Based upon similar observations, others have also advocated revascularization of at least the CA and SMA in an effort to prevent recurrent visceral ischemia [19–22]. Revascularization of the IMA and the hypogastric arteries may also improve visceral perfusion. This approach, however, has been challenged by reports of relief of ischemic symptoms and low recurrence rates after isolated revascularization of the SMA [23, 24]. Nonetheless, our preferred approach is to revascularize at least the two main visceral arteries, the CA and the SMA, for several reasons. First, although revascularization of multiple vessels may slightly increase perioperative morbidity rates, the long-term symptom-free survival rate appears to be better [4, 20]. Second, revascularization of multiple vessels may prevent symptomatic recurrence due to reocclusion of a single graft or visceral artery [13]. Finally, complete visceral revascularization should also be performed in patients who lack intact visceral collaterals due to prior surgery [25].

Based upon over three decades of experience, antegrade aortovisceral bypass grafting and transaortic visceral endarterectomy are our preferred methods for operative visceral artery revascularization. These techniques have been described in detail, may be performed through an abdominal approach, and provide durable relief of visceral ischemic symptoms in over 90% of patients at 5 years [15, 16, 26]. Antegrade grafts originate from the supraceliac aorta, which is more likely to be disease-free than the infrarenal aorta. In contrast to retrograde grafts, the geometry of antegrade grafts allows for use of short lengths of conduit, which may have fewer propensities to kink or buckle. Moreover, antegrade bypass grafts with an end-to-end visceral anastomosis may have less turbulent flow than the end-to-side anastomoses of retrograde grafts. Autogenous saphenous vein does not appear to confer any benefit over prosthetic conduit and may actually be less durable than prosthetic visceral artery reconstructions [15].

The choice between antegrade prosthetic grafting and transaortic endarterectomy is governed by the overall medical condition of the patients and the experience of the surgeon. In good risk patients with concomitant renal artery or aortic disease, transaortic endarterectomy is our procedure of choice. In patients with transmural calcification or distal involvement of the visceral arteries by atheromatous disease antegrade bypass grafting may be more appropriate.

Percutaneous Visceral Angioplasty

Visceral angioplasty is not new [27] and the technique appears safe and effective in the short term [28–30]. However, most reports of visceral angioplasty are anecdotal and its role as a primary treatment for chronic visceral ischemia remains unsettled [29]. Early restenosis may occur, requiring repeat angioplasty, which can be performed with low complication rates [28, 30]. Stent placement as an adjunct to visceral angioplasty may reduce the incidence of restenosis and improve patency rates [31]. As experience accumulates with endovascular approaches angioplasty and stenting may become a reasonable option, especially for patients who are not surgical candidates or develop recurrent visceral ischemia.

Recurrent Chronic Visceral Ischemia

Despite the overall success of operative visceral revascularization late failures occur and patients may present with recurrent ischemic symptoms. In our own series of 109 visceral revascularizations recurrent visceral ischemia was documented in 19 patients (17%), and the outcome for these patients was determined by their clinical presentation. One-third of patients presented with acute visceral ischemia, which has a dismal prognosis, and 86% (six out of seven) died of bowel infarction. In contrast, two-thirds of the patients developed chronic recurrent visceral ischemia and most underwent successful reoperative visceral revascularization. A total of 30 reoperations for recurrent chronic visceral ischemia in 24 patients have been performed at UCSF with a 5-year survival rate of 75%. Moreover, the same techniques used for primary visceral revascularization (antegrade aortovisceral bypass grafting or transaortic endarterectomy) were performed in over 90% of the patients who underwent reoperation [4]. Mateo et al. [20] have reported similar results, confirming that operative reintervention may be successfully performed using established techniques when patients present with recurrent chronic visceral ischemia.

In some patients with recurrent chronic visceral ischemia diffuse reocclusion of previously repaired visceral arteries may occasionally preclude redo-revascularization of the CA or SMA. Under these unusual circumstances creative approaches are necessary to restore adequate visceral perfusion in order to prevent progression to fatal bowel infarction. Stenosis or occlusion of a prior graft may respond to angioplasty and stenting or thrombolysis. Isolated bypass to the hepatic artery

[32] or the IMA [25], which takes advantage of existing collateral pathways, has also been reported to restore adequate visceral perfusion when conventional revascularization techniques could not be applied.

Conclusions

Operative revascularization of both the CA and SMA remains the cornerstone of treatment for chronic visceral ischemia, achieving durable relief of ischemic symptoms with acceptable rates of morbidity and mortality. Endovascular treatment of mesenteric occlusive disease also appears to be technically feasible and clinically effective. Although durability is uncertain at the present time, percutaneous angioplasty and stenting may eventually become an option in the primary treatment of chronic visceral ischemia, especially in patients who are poor surgical candidates. Noninvasive imaging techniques may facilitate earlier identification of patients with impaired visceral blood flow, which should then be confirmed by biplanar aortography prior to revascularization. After revascularization, surveillance using duplex ultrasonography or MRA may allow identification of revascularization failures prior to the development of recurrent symptoms. In patients with recurrent chronic visceral ischemia, reintervention provides durable relief of symptoms with life expectancy rates comparable to primary visceral revascularization.

References

1. Chiene J (1869) Complete obliteration of celiac and mesenteric arteries: viscera receiving their blood supply through extra-peritoneal system vessels. J Anat Physiol 3:63–72
2. Dunphy JE (1936) Abdominal pain of vascular origin. Am J Med Sci 192:109–113
3. Hallett JW Jr, James ME, Ahlquist DA, et al. (1990) Recent trends in the diagnosis and management of chronic intestinal ischemia. Ann Vasc Surg 4:126–132
4. Schneider DB, Schneider PA, Reilly LM, et al. (1998) Reoperation for recurrent chronic visceral ischemia. J Vasc Surg 27:276–284
5. Moneta GL, Lee RW, Yeager RA, et al. (1993) Mesenteric duplex scanning: a blinded prospective study. J Vasc Surg 17:79–84
6. Zwolak RM, Fillinger MF, Walsh DB, et al. (1998) Mesenteric and celiac duplex scanning: a validation study. J Vasc Surg 27:1078–1087, 1088
7. Bowersox JC, Zwolak RM, Walsh DB, et al. (1991) Duplex ultrasonography in the diagnosis of celiac and mesenteric artery occlusive disease. J Vasc Surg 14:780–786, 786–788
8. Perko MJ, Just S, Schroeder TV (1997) Importance of diastolic velocities in the detection of celiac and mesenteric artery disease by duplex ultrasound. J Vasc Surg 26:288–293
9. Gentile AT, Moneta GL, Lee RW, et al. (1995) Usefulness of fasting and postprandial duplex ultrasound examinations for predicting high-grade superior mesenteric artery stenosis. Am J Surg 169:476–479
10. Meaney JF, Prince MR, Nostrant TT, et al. (1997) Gadolinium-enhanced MR angiography of visceral arteries in patients with suspected chronic mesenteric ischemia. J Magn Reson Imaging 7:171–176
11. Maki JH, Chenevert TL, Prince MR (1998) Contrast-enhanced MR angiography. Abdominal Imaging 23:469–484
12. Li KC, Dalman RL, Ch'en IY, et al. (1997) Chronic mesenteric ischemia: use of in vivo MR imaging measurements of blood oxygen saturation in the superior mesenteric vein for diagnosis. Radiology 204:71–77
13. McMillan WD, McCarthy WJ, Bresticker MR, et al. (1995) Mesenteric artery bypass: objective patency determination. J Vasc Surg 21:729–740

14. Nicoloff AD, Williamson WK, Moneta GL, et al. (1997) Duplex ultrasonography in evaluation of splanchnic artery stenosis. Surg Clin North Am 77:339–355
15. Stoney RJ, Ehrenfeld WK, Wylie EJ (1977) Revascularization methods in chronic visceral ischemia caused by atherosclerosis. Ann Surg 186:468–476
16. Cunningham CG, Reilly LM, Rapp JH, et al. (1991) Chronic visceral ischemia. Three decades of progress. Ann Surg 214:276–287
17. Hollier LH, Bernatz PE, Pairolero PC, et al. (1981) Surgical management of chronic intestinal ischemia: a reappraisal. Surgery 90:940–946
18. Moawad J, McKinsey JF, Wyble CW, et al. (1997) Current results of surgical therapy for chronic mesenteric ischemia. Arch Surg 132:613–618, 618–619
19. Johnston KW, Lindsay TF, Walker PM, et al. (1995) Mesenteric arterial bypass grafts: early and late results and suggested surgical approach for chronic and acute mesenteric ischemia. Surgery 118:1–7
20. Mateo RB, O'Hara PJ, Hertzer NR, et al. (1999) Elective surgical treatment of symptomatic chronic mesenteric occlusive disease: early results and late outcomes. J Vasc Surg 29:821–831, 832
21. McAfee MK, Cherry KJ Jr, Naessens JM, et al. (1992) Influence of complete revascularization on chronic mesenteric ischemia. Am J Surg 164:220–224
22. Calderon M, Reul GJ, Gregoric ID, et al. (1992) Long-term results of the surgical management of symptomatic chronic intestinal ischemia. J Cardiovasc Surg (Torino) 33:723–728
23. Cormier JM, Fichelle JM, Vennin J, et al. (1991) Atherosclerotic occlusive disease of the superior mesenteric artery: late results of reconstructive surgery. Ann Vasc Surg 5:510–518
24. Gentile AT, Moneta GL, Taylor LM Jr, et al. (1994) Isolated bypass to the superior mesenteric artery for intestinal ischemia. Arch Surg 129:926–931
25. Schneider DB, Nelken NA, Messina LM, et al. (1999) Isolated inferior mesenteric artery revascularization for chronic visceral ischemia. J Vasc Surg 30:51–58
26. Reilly LM, Ramos TK, Murray SP, et al. (1994) Optimal exposure of the proximal abdominal aorta: a critical appraisal of transabdominal medial visceral rotation [see comments]. J Vasc Surg 19:375–389, 389–390
27. Golden DA, Ring EJ, McLean GK, et al. (1982) Percutaneous transluminal angioplasty in the treatment of abdominal angina. Am J Roentgenol 139:247–249
28. Allen RC, Martin GH, Rees CR, et al. (1996) Mesenteric angioplasty in the treatment of chronic intestinal ischemia. J Vasc Surg 24:415–421
29. Hackworth CA, Leef JA (1997) Percutaneous transluminal mesenteric angioplasty. Surg Clin North Am 77:371–380
30. Maspes F, Mazzetti di Pietralata G, Gandini R, et al. (1998) Percutaneous transluminal angioplasty in the treatment of chronic mesenteric ischemia: results and 3 years of follow-up in 23 patients. Abdominal Imaging 23:358–363
31. Sheeran SR, Murphy TP, Khwaja A, et al. (1999) Stent placement for treatment of mesenteric artery stenoses or occlusions. J Vasc Intervent Radiol 10:861–867
32. Cavallaro A, di Marzo L, Cavallaro G, et al. (1998) Iliac-to-isolated hepatic artery bypass in the treatment of intestinal angina: two cases. J Vasc Surg 28:1115–1119

Ischemic Colitis

Christopher T. Smith · Donald L. Kaminski

Introduction

The disorder, ischemic colitis, is a relatively "new" disease process with the original description being produced in 1963 and the disease being somewhat misnamed in 1966 [1–3]. Over the years the disorder has come to be more widely recognized; however, it still remains poorly understood and controversial, both with regards to the etiology of the disorder as well as its diagnosis and management.

Our interest in ischemic colitis began in the early 1970s and has remained continuous with the accumulation of a large series of patients that has been periodically updated. The information presented in this chapter is based on our study of this disorder for many years and the patients with the disorder that we have treated [4–10].

Pathogenesis

The etiology of ischemic colitis is clearly unknown. Limited information exits regarding the cause of ischemic colitis and most theories related to the etiology of the disorder are not based on significant laboratory or clinical research. As indicated above the name of the disorder is generally inappropriate, as the disease does not seem to be associated with occlusive, embolic or thrombotic reduction of blood flow to the colon in the same sense that we recognize ischemic heart or peripheral vascular disease [3]. By definition, what the term "ischemic colitis" implies is that the blood supply to the colon is intact and that all or part of the colon has developed a necrotic process associated with an inflammatory response. The inflammatory response may be important regarding the etiology of the process as it tends to indicate that this does not represent some form of accelerated apoptosis [11]. The information concerning the likely presence of normal colonic blood supply has become so widely accepted that arteriograms are generally contraindicated in the evaluation of a patient with ischemic colitis [12].

While major vascular occlusion is not generally felt to be associated with ischemic colitis, local vascular changes in the wall of the colon may play a role. The vascular system in the colonic wall is extensive in the submucosal layers with arterial branches extending into each villous structure [13]. Vasoconstriction, produced by various associated processes involving the submucosal vessels or arteriovenous shunting, could result in an ischemic injury to the various layers of the bowel wall producing the disease process [14]. Some reports have suggested that patients with ischemic colitis may have fibrous hyperplasia and medial hypertrophy of the small terminal colonic arteries [15]; however, detailed arteriographic evaluation of the luminal blood supply of segments of colon with ischemic colitis generally appear to be hyperemic rather than vasospastic [3]. While it is possible that at the onset of the disease there is local ischemia produced by vasospasm and A-V shunts and that with the inflammatory process there is vasodilatation, there is little evidence available to support a sympathomimetic mediated vasospastic process as being the cause of ischemic colitis.

Information has accumulated that suggests that the development of ischemic colitis may be associated with cytokines or decreased blood flow induced stimulation of various mediators involved in reperfusion injury. Initially it was demonstrated that following 30 min of experimental colonic ischemia followed by reperfusion there was a burst of formation of markers of lipid peroxidation, even though histologic changes were not present [16]. Subsequently, considerable information has accumulated suggesting a relationship between platelet-activating factor and nitric oxide generation in the formation of oxygen-free radicals resulting in colonic tissue destruction [17, 18]. We have demonstrated that colonic tissue manifests platelet-activating factor receptors [19]. Theoretically a number of inciting events could stimulate this somewhat understood cascade including endotoxin, interleukins, as well as alterations in blood flow. Conceptually it may be beneficial in understanding what ischemic colitis is by pointing out that the disease is analogous to acute acalculous cholecystitis. Both disorders appear spontaneously in patients with no known precipitating cause [20, 21], both occur in acutely ill patients having experienced shock or trauma [22, 23] and both can progress to gangrene.

An interesting aspect of ischemic colitis is the isolated colonic involvement. There does not seem to be any analogous disorder affecting, for example, the small intestine where only occlusive mesenteric ischemia produces necrosis. There obviously could be numerous factors which contribute to the specific susceptibility of the colon, such as the bacterial flora in the colon or different patterns of cytokine production. A factor which may have some relevance to the susceptibility of the colon is the absence of the ability of the colon to autoregulate blood flow. In experimental studies in dogs, colonic blood flow progressively decreases with a decrease in blood pressure [24], while in the small intestine, auto-regulatory mechanisms maintain intestinal blood flow until a critically low perfusion pressure is reached around 40 mmHg [25, 26]. This inability of the colon to maintain satisfactory circulation in the presence of hypotension may incite the reperfusion injury in the colon while other parts of the gastrointestinal tract are unaffected.

Classification

There are generally two classification systems that are employed in delineating the spectrum of ischemic colitis. By definition the disorder is confined to the colon and by definition the process should be associated with the absence of occlusive vascular disease. A patient with sigmoid colon gangrene following treatment of an abdominal aortic aneurysm and ligation of the inferior mesenteric artery has colonic ischemia, not ischemic colitis. A patient that undergoes treatment of a ruptured abdominal aortic aneurysm with preoperative hypotension that develops gangrene of the right colon postoperatively has ischemic colitis.

The disease process has generally been recognized as being associated with varying depth of penetration. Transient mucosal involvement may or may not progress to partial thickness necrosis, which may recover with or without a stricture or progress to full thickness gangrene. The disease can involve any part of the colon and the rectum [27] and may involve the entire colon [10]. Distribution in one part of the colon may be patchy [28] and contiguous in another and although unusual the disease may begin in one part of the colon and subsequently progress to involve an adjacent area [28]. It does not seem practicable to engender any classification system based on the area of colon involved.

The disease as originally described and most frequently seen occurs spontaneously in patients with no associated acute condition, but who may have a variety of associated disease processes (Table 3). These patients are commonly seen and cared for by their physicians and frequently will not have progression of superficial mucosal involvement and not be seen by surgeons. Occasionally such

Table 3. Factors predisposing to the development of ischemic colitis

Spontaneous ischemic colitis	Shock-associated ischemic colitis
	Multiple trauma
Chronic obstructive lung disease	Cardiopulmonary bypass
Congestive heart failure	Ruptured ectopic pregnancy
Digitalis toxicity	Upper gastrointestinal hemorrhage
Collagen vascular disease	Pancreatitis
Hypercoagulable states	Cerebral vascular accident
Diabetes mellitus	Sepsis (renal, pulmonary)
Chronic renal failure	Cardiopulmonary arrest
	Status epilepticus

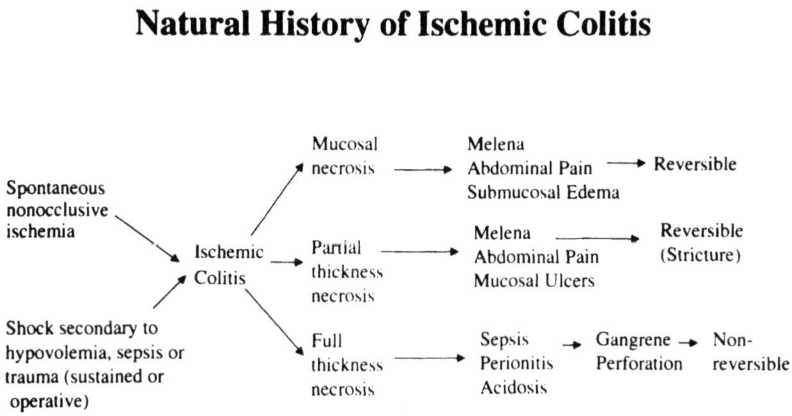

Fig. 1. Diagrammatic illustration of the classification of ischemic colitis

patients will have progression of their disease and develop a chronic ischemic stricture or full-thickness gangrene and require a colon resection.

In the early 1980s it came to be recognized that there was another patient cohort that developed a comparable colonic lesion. Patients were recognized that had experienced a severe systemic insult related to a variety of problems, frequently previously healthy young patients, who developed ischemic colitis [5]. This patient population was adjudged to have shock-associated ischemic colitis. The myriad clinical problems that we have seen associated with shock-associated ischemic colitis are presented in Table 3.

It is possible to combine the two different classification systems and to present a complete spectrum of the disease, which also provides a description of the natural history of ischemic colitis (Fig. 1). The variables depicted in Fig. 1 can be adjusted in various ways; however, the principle is that there are two clinical forms of the disease and the disease can be associated with varying degrees of involvement of the colonic wall. Presented in this manner the clinician can be mindful of the two patient populations that are susceptible to the disorder and be aware of the need to attempt to ascertain the depth of the colonic wall involved. While there is symmetry in Fig. 1, a patient with shock-associated ischemic colitis with mucosal necrosis only is rarely identified, while it is quite common in spontaneous ischemic colitis.

Diagnosis

A patient with spontaneous ischemic colitis presents typically with acute abdominal pain and melena. A patient with shock-associated ischemic colitis presents as a patient in the intensive care unit who is clinically deteriorating with signs suggesting that the patient's problem now may be intra-abdominal. The patient may have fever and leukocytosis and acidosis and lactic acidosis may suggest the presence of ischemia. A number of alternative tests are available to attempt to diagnose ischemic colitis, none of them uniformly satisfactory or applicable.

Abdominal radiographs may demonstrate an ileus, colonic dilation in the colon proximal to the area of ischemia or dilated ischemic colon, or free air [29]. Radionucleotide indium-labeled white blood cell studies have been reported to identify the ischemic area [30]. Nonspecific abnormalities may be seen on abdominal CT scans [31]. Arteriograms are generally not contributory to making a diagnosis of ischemic colitis [32].

Diagnosis is primarily made by contrast studies of the colon and endoscopy. Contrast studies of the colon will reveal the characteristic sub-mucosal edema referred to as thumb printing (Fig. 2). Patients with shock-associated ischemic colitis present unique problems. Endoscopy is the ideal method of diagnosis and in addition has some potential, when repeated, to follow the course of the disease. In some circumstances endoscopy may not succeed; for example, in a critically ill patient in the intensive care unit, the inability to prepare the colon may make examination of the entire colon impossible. Such a patient may also not be able to undergo a satisfactory contrast study of the colon. Ill patients in the intensive care unit can readily undergo abdominal CT scans. The findings on CT scan suggestive of ischemic colitis include colonic wall thickening indicative of sub-mucosal edema, fluid in the peritoneal cavity and pneumatosis coli [31]. A significant number of patients with shock-associated ischemic colitis will have the diagnosis made during an exploratory laparotomy for a suspected intra-abdominal septic process.

Patients with spontaneous ischemic colitis without evidence of peritonitis mandating emergency operative therapy would be best served by colonoscopic diagnosis and evaluation of the severity and extent of the disease. The patient should undergo repetitive endoscopy to evaluate the progression of the disease if clinically indicated. The endoscopic diagnosis of ischemic colitis based on clinical observation seems to be relatively straightforward with experienced endoscopists able to reliably identify the disease [33]. While a number of disorders need to be included in the endoscopic differential diagnosis (Table 4), pseudomembranous colitis seems to be the disorder producing the greatest degree of difficulty. Microbiologic data may be required to discriminate the two disorders [34]. Again, in spontaneous ischemic colitis, a surgeon may operate on a patient with an acute abdominal catastrophe to find colonic gangrene as the source of the problem.

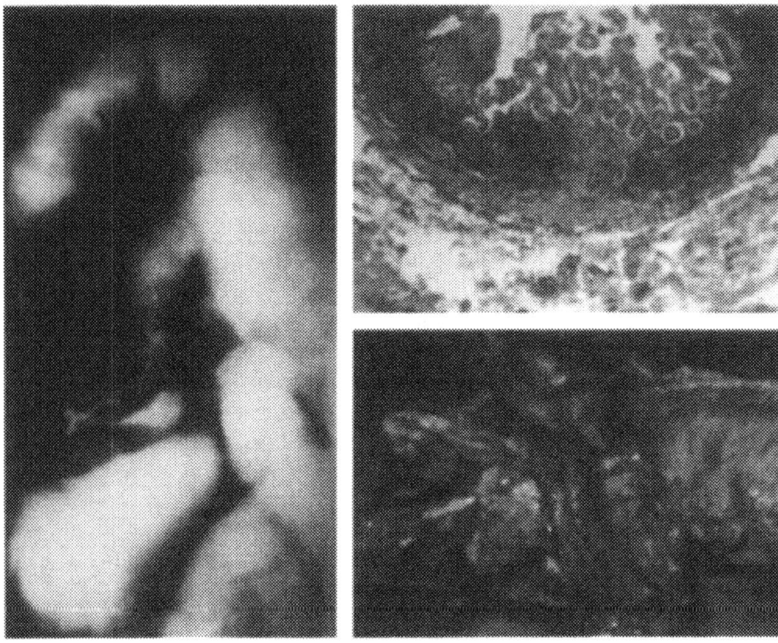

Fig. 2. Composite presentation of a patient with ischemic colitis involving the ascending colon. Contrast radiograph illustrates a segment of submucosal edema of the ascending colon. The gross pathology photograph illustrates the areas of full-thickness gangrene and the inflammatory process is demonstrated on the photograph of the histologic specimen

Table 4. Disease processes to be considered in the endoscopic differential diagnosis of ischemic colitis

Ischemic colitis vs.	Ulcerative colitis Crohn's disease Cancer Diverticulitis Pseudomembranous colitis Amebic colitis Bechet's disease Typhlitis Radiation colitis

Indications for Operation

The treatment of ischemic colitis is primarily symptomatic including naso-gastric decompression, intravenous fluids and parenteral antibiotics. Pharmacologic attempts to increase colonic blood flow have not been employed nor has intestinal antibiotic therapy. Observation of the patient continues to identify improvement or deterioration and the need for colectomy. The clinical condition of the patient will be the most important indication for operation and the standard indices will be employed including increasing abdominal pain, fever, leukocytosis, acidosis and increasing serum lactate levels.

Other modalities available include serial abdominal radiographs, endoscopy and CT scans. It was proposed that the area of colon that was involved with a superficial ischemic process would lose muscular function when the muscle became involved and would become dilated. This process could be observed with serial abdominal radiographs. Attempts to correlate full-thickness necrosis with distention were not successful and it was found that the viable colon proximal to the ischemic area was more frequently dilated [5]. Abdominal radiographs may reveal an increase in small bowel and colonic gas, suggesting the progressive development of ileus, or free intraperitoneal air. Serial CT scans can similarly demonstrate progressive thickening of the colonic wall and the development of intramural air or air in the portal system [31]. The endoscopist has the potential to evaluate the colon to ascertain whether the mucosal changes are improving [33]. If the area of involvement has patchy areas returning to more normal vascularity, the edema is decreasing or the area of involved colon is shrinking, the disease would be spontaneously resolving. If the opposite is present, the disease is progressing. The endoscopist may be able to detect areas of full-thickness involvement that balloon abnormally with air insufflation and aspiration.

Operative Treatment

The controversial aspect of operative management relates to the decision to perform a resection and stoma and mucous fistula or Hartman's pouch or resection and anastomosis. Patients with ischemia of their total abdominal colon with or without rectal involvement should not have an anastomosis performed at the time of resection [10], nor should patients with left-sided colonic involvement [5]. Ischemic colitis is recognized to uncommonly progress to another segment of the colon and by definition the ileum is not involved [28]. In selected patients with ischemic colitis isolated to the right colon an ileocolostomy can be performed with results not significantly different from those produced by treating patients with a resection and an ileostomy [5]. The distal colon should appear grossly normal and the mucosa at the level of transection should be healthy in appearance before an anastomosis is performed.

Patients undergoing colectomy and stoma formation should anticipate closure of the stoma in accordance with the usual guidelines employed by the surgeon. It is important to inform the patient with spontaneous ischemic colitis that there is a low incidence of recurrence in the remaining colon [35]. The mortality of operatively treated ischemic colitis has improved over the years but remains high. Segmental ischemic colitis requiring colectomy has recently been associated with 22% mortality, while total colonic ischemia requiring colectomy is associated with a 80% mortality [10].

References

1. Boley SJ, Schwartz S, Lash J, Sternhill V (1963) Reversible vascular occlusion of the colon. Surg Gynecol Obstet 116:53–60
2. Marston A, Pheils MT, Thomas ML, Morson BG (1966) Ischemic colitis. Gut 7:1–15
3. Williams LF, Wittenberg J (1975) Ischemic colitis: a useful clinical diagnosis, but is it ischemic? Ann Surg 182:439–446
4. Kaminski DL, Keltner RM, Willman VL (1973) Ischemic colitis. Arch Surg 106:558–563
5. Sakai L, Keltner RM, Kaminski DL (1980) Spontaneous and shock associated ischemic colitis. Am J Surg 140:755–760
6. Kaminski, DL, Herrmann VM (1986) Ischemic colitis. In: Cameron J (ed) Current surgical therapy, vol 2. Decker, Baltimore, p 110
7. Fitzgerald SF, Kaminski DL (1993) Ischemic colitis. Semin Colon Rectal Surg 4:222–228
8. Gandhi SK, Hanson MM, Vernava AM, Kaminski DL, Longo WE (1996) Ischemic colitis. Dis Colon Rectum 39:88–100
9. Gandhi SK, Longo WE, Kaminski DL (1998) Ischemic colitis. In: Longo WE, Peterson GJ, Jacobs DL (eds) Intestinal ischemia disorders. Quality Medical Publishers, St. Louis, p 221
10. Longo WE, Ward D, Vernava AM, Kaminski DL (1997) Outcome of patients with total colonic ischemia. Dis Colon Rectum 40:1448–1454
11. Kumar S (1999) Regulation of caspase activation in apoptosis: implications in pathogenesis and treatment of disease. Clin Exp Pharmacol Physiol 26:295–303
12. Toursarkissian B, Thompson RW (1997) Ischemic colitis. Surg Clin North Am 77:461–470
13. Marston A (1986) Applied anatomy of the intestinal circulation. In: Vascular diseases of the gastrointestinal tract. Baltimore, Williams and Wilkens, p 1
14. Bower TC (1993) Ischemic colitis. Surg Clin North Am 73:1037–1053
15. Williams LF, Bosniak MA, Wittenberg J, Mannel B, Grimes ET, Byrne JJ (1969) Ischemic colitis. Am J Surg 117:254–264
16. Douglas DM, Russell JC, Goren D, Dempsey S, Das DK (1989) Evidence of free radical (FR) involvement in ischemic colitis. Agents Actions 27:435–437
17. Nagahata Y, Azumi Y, Akimoto T, Nomura H, Ichihara T, Idei H, Kuroda Y (1999) Role of platelet activating factor on severity of ischemic colitis. Dis Colon Rectum 42:218–224
18. Wu Qu X, Rozenfeld RA, Huang W, Sun X, Di Tan X, Hsueh W (1999) Roles of nitric oxide synthases in platelet-activating factor-induced intestinal necrosis in rats. Crit Care Med 27:356–364
19. Longo WE, Carter JD, Chandel B, Niehoff M, Standeven J, Deshpande Y, Vernava AM, Polites G, Kulkarni AD, Kaminski DL (1995) WEB 2170 inhibition of PAF stimulated eicosanoid release: evidence for a PAF receptor. J Surg Res 58:12–18
20. Savoca PE, Longo WE, Zucker KA, McMillen MM, Modlin IM (1980) The increasing prevalence of acalculous cholecystitis in outpatients. Ann Surg 211:433–437
21. Longo WE, Ballantyne GH, Gusberg RJ (1992) Ischemic colitis: patterns and prognosis. Dis Colon Rectum 35:726–730
22. Shapiro MJ, Luchtefeld WB, Kurzweil S, Kaminski DL, Durham RM, Mazuski JE (1994) Acute acalculous cholecystitis in the critically ill. Am Surg 60:335–339
23. Levandoski G, Deitrick JE, Brotman S (1988) Necrosis of the colon as a complication of shock. Am Surg 45:621–626
24. Kvietys PR, Granger DN (1982) Regulation of colonic blood flow. Fed Proc 41:2106–2110
25. Johnson PC (1960) Autoregulation of intestinal blood flow. Am J Physiol 199:311–318
26. Kvietys PR, Granger DN (1984) Physiology, pharmacology, and pathology of the colonic circulation. In: Shepherd AP, Granger DN (eds) Physiology of the intestinal circulation. Raven Press, New York, p 131
27. Travis S, Davies DR, Creamer B (1991) Acute colorectal ischemia after anaphylactoid shock. Gut 32:443–446
28. Robert JH, Mentha G, Rohner A (1993) Ischaemic colitis: two distinct patterns of severity. Gut 34:4–6
29. Sherbon KJ (1970) The radiology of ischaemic colitis. Aust Radiol 14:46–55
30. Moallem AG, Gerard PS, Japanwalla M (1995) Positive In-111 WBC scan in a patient with ischemic ileocolitis and negative colonoscopies. Clin Nucl Med 20:483–485
31. Balthazar EJ, Yen BC, Gordon RB (1999) Ischemic colitis: CT evaluation of 54 cases. Radiology 211:381–388
32. Boley SJ (1990) Colon ischemia – 25 years later. Am J Gastroenterol 85:931–934

33. Habu Y, Tahashi Y, Kiyota K, Matsumura K, Hirota M, Inokuchi H, Kawai K (1996) Reevaluation of clinical features of ischemic colitis: analysis of 68 consecutive cases diagnosed by early colonoscopy. Scan J Gastroenterol 31:881–886
34. Dignan CR, Greenson JK (1997) Can ischemic colitis be differentiated from C Difficile colitis in biopsy specimens. Am J Surg Pathol 21:706–710
35. Saegesser F, Roenspies U, Robinson JWL (1979) Ischemic diseases of the large intestine. Pathobiol Ann 9:303–337

Invited Comment

Michael Klyachkin · John J. Ricotta

The management of mesenteric ischemia remains problematic for both the general and vascular surgeon. The articles included in this monograph deal very well with the current state of the art in diagnosis and management of this troubling spectrum of diseases. In the final analysis, however, contemporary results are not terribly improved over reports several decades ago, and these diseases continue to be associated with unacceptably high mortality and morbidity. While the reasons for this are manifold, two important ones are an increasingly aged and debilitated population, and a continuing delay in diagnosis, which often attends these disease processes. While we cannot control the former, we should strive to minimize the latter. Mesenteric ischemia should be included in the differential diagnosis of every patient who presents with abdominal pain. If this is done, delays in diagnosis will decrease, since the presentation is often characteristic in retrospect.

In the case of *acute mesenteric ischemia four etiologies are encountered*: arterial embolism, arterial thrombosis, venous thrombosis and nonocclusive mesenteric ischemia (NOMI). Each of these has a characteristic clinical presentation.

Patients with arterial emboli often present with atrial fibrillation, a history of prior embolic events or a recent myocardial infarction and those with arterial thrombosis have stigmata of systemic atherosclerosis and a history of abdominal pain. Venous occlusion is less common but often accompanied by dehydration, ascites and a history of venous thrombosis. Patients with NOMI are usually elderly with low cardiac output and vasoconstriction.

When the diagnosis of arterial insufficiency is suspected, arteriography should be performed unless an acute abdomen is present. Angiograms can usually be performed rapidly and with minimal morbidity. When the diagnosis is made at celiotomy, the surgeon must expose the superior mesenteric artery, either at the base of the mesentery or through the lesser sac by elevating the pancreas. Arterial perfusion should be restored by embolectomy or bypass. Embolectomy can be performed through the base of the mesentery at the first branch of the SMA. While large vessels can be approached through a transverse arteriotomy, we prefer a longitudinal incision with vein patch closure. In acute cases where bypass is required, we prefer single infrarenal bypass to the Superior Mesenteric Artery using saphenous vein. After restoration of flow intestinal viability is assessed as described by Drs. Lynch and Thompson. In cases of an embolization we restart heparin after 24 h, which allows us to minimize the risk of both recurrent embolization and postoperative hemorrhage. In patients who present with NOMI we catheterize the SMA transfemorally either before or after celiotomy for vasodilator infusion therapy.

Questions surrounding extent of resection and the indications for a "second look" celiotomy are thoroughly discussed by Drs. Lynch and Thompson and we follow the principles outlined in their manuscript. While some authors have advocated laparoscopy rather than laparotomy for "second-look" procedures, we do not agree. The increased time, increased intraabdominal pressure and potential limitation in assessment associated with laparoscopy are not balanced by any benefit in patients who already have a recent abdominal incision.

In addition to the forms of acute mesenteric ischemia noted above, vascular insufficiency can be associated with *acute aortic dissection*. Mortality in such cases is extremely high and management is difficult. Classically such cases are treated by proximal operative repair of the dissection with visceral revascularization added as required. Recently reports have surfaced on endovascular repair of acute aortic dissection, including patients with visceral complications. While the hospital mortality of these patients remains about 25% and the follow-up is limited, such an approach may offer benefits over standard operative therapy.

One additional comment is noteworthy. On occasion, *focal mesenteric ischemia* will be found on exploratory celiotomy for an acute abdomen. Many times a simple intestinal resection can be performed. We believe that it is mandatory in these cases to thoroughly evaluate the mesenteric circulation at the time of initial operation to exclude occult emboli or arterial stenosis. Furthermore, when the patient has recovered from operation a thorough evaluation for a source of ischemia is mandatory. This will include evaluation of the heart and thoracic aorta by transesophageal echography (TEE) as well as AP and lateral abdominal aortography. It is not unusual for the surgeon to focus on the initial ischemic process and its management rather than the underlying etiology. We believe that this is to be discouraged.

Chronic mesenteric ischemia and its management are well described by the vascular group at UC San Francisco. Again, vigilance is the cornerstone of expeditious diagnosis and management. Patients with unexplained abdominal pain and weight loss should have an aortogram if endoscopic and gastrointestinal imaging studies are inconclusive. This is particularly true in the case of patients with risk factors for or manifestations of atherosclerotic disease. We share the experience of others, that chronic ischemia is often overlooked by the treating physician for many months even when there is no established explanation of the patient's symptoms. We favor antegrade bypass whenever possible with revascularization of both the celiac and superior mesenteric arteries. Our experience with endarterectomy has been limited to middle-aged patients, many of them women. In the more typical elderly patient bypass is a less morbid procedure in our hands.

Mesenteric venous disease is a rare entity and difficult to differentiate from arterial problems other than by history or presentation (e.g., a middle-aged person without atherosclerosis and a history of venous thrombosis). Fortunately, contrast CT scan, a diagnostic study common in the evaluation of abdominal pain, can be diagnostic of this syndrome. We agree that whenever possible nonoperative treatment is preferable, since anticoagulation is part of the definitive management of these patients. Rudiger and Clavien's emphasis on the presence of peritoneal fluid as an indication for surgery and their suggestion that resection should include some normal bowel whenever clinically feasible are important clinical insights.

Ischemic colitis can be a catchall phrase which encompasses a wide variety of disease states. A high index of suspicion is again the key to management. We agree that early endoscopy is the key not only to diagnosis but appropriate management. Nontransmural ischemia is managed nonoperatively as long as the patient is stable, while evidence of peritoneal irritation or transmural necrosis on endoscopy calls for urgent operation. The majority of our experience has involved left-sided ischemic colitis after aneurysmectomy and we therefore prefer resection and colostomy to re-anastomosis. We would take exception to the assertion of Smith and Kaminski that arterial occlusion is by definition a different entity than "ischemic colitis." In the case of aortic aneurysm resection it is often a combination of hypotension and loss of the inferior mesenteric artery (IMA) that causes this problem. The observation that routine reimplantation of the IMA after aneurysmectomy can minimize postoperative ischemic colitis supports this point. While we have not adopted this policy we are increasingly liberal with IMA reimplantation. Unfortunately this is most difficult in the situation where it is needed most, i.e., ruptured AAA. Over the years we have become more sensitized to this diagnosis, which can be suggested by hematochezia, early (<24 h post operation) bowel movement, abdominal tenderness or persistent ileus, and have employed flexible sigmoidoscopy with increasing frequency.

The preceding articles present a comprehensive view of the various aspects of mesenteric ischemic disease. Each article contains important clinical points which should be considered for every patient who presents with abdominal pain. Since the general surgeon is the triage physician for most of these patients, it is of great importance that he/she have a thorough understanding of the pathophysiology as outlined in these articles and be prepared to expeditiously diagnose and treat these problems.

References

Ricotta JJ, d'Audiffret A (1998) Acute mesenteric occlusion. In: Cameron JL (ed) Current surgical therapy, pp 852–857

Testart J, Scotte M, Bokobza B, Leturgie C, Watelet J, Teniere P (1992) Is emergency aorto-superior mesenteric artery bypass worthwhile? Int Angiol 11:181–185

Slutzki S, Halpern Z, Negri M, Kais H, Halevy A (1996) The laparoscopic second look for ischemic bowel disease. Surg Endosc 10:729–731

Glattli A, Seiler C, Metzger A, Stirneman P, Baer HU (1994) Second look laparoscopy after mesenteric infarct. Langenbecks Arch Chir 379:66–69

Bradbury AW, Brittenden J, McBride K, Ruckley CV (1995) Mesenteric ischemia: a multidisciplinary approach. Br J Surg 82:1446–1459

Slonim SM, Miller DC, Mitchell RS, Semba CP, Razavi MK, Dake MD (1999) Percutaneous balloon fenestration and stenting for life-threatening ischemic complications in patients with acute aortic dissection. J Thoracic Cardiovasc Surg 117(6):1118–1126

Editorial Comment

The "publication-survival paradox" applies well to acute mesenteric ischemia: it means that the more is written about the management of a condition, the poorer are the results. Acute mesenteric ischemia still represents a virtually lethal condition. In a recent study from Scotland, 46 out of 57 (80%) patients suffering from acute mesenteric arterial ischemia died; only 18 (32%) patients were accurately diagnosed before operation or death [1]. A recent review of the results from our own teaching hospital in New York with acute mesenteric arterial ischemia shows a mortality rate of 90%. Clearly, much is known about the diagnosis and management of this condition but little is done in practice. Typically, each review or book chapter quotes the approach advocated more than 20 years ago by Boley et al. [2, 3] - including the use of early angiography and intra-arterial papaverine. We do not know of anybody else who published significant clinical experience with this method since.

What is the perceived reason behind the failure to improve results?

- Failure to suspect/consider ischemia before intestinal gangrene develops
- Failure to proceed with diagnostic/therapeutic angiography
- Failure to improve intestinal perfusion during laparotomy
- Failure to exteriorize the bowel or execute "second-look" operations

Notably, acute mesenteric ischemia is not an uncommon reason for malpractice claims, with an alleged failure to make a timely diagnosis, failure to provide anticoagulant protection, and failure to prevent nonocclusive ischemic infarction being the basis [4].

Drs. Smith and Kaminski writing about ischemic colitis did not allude to the classical studies by Fiddian-Green et al. who managed to predict and thus prevent colonic ischemia during aortic surgery by using indirect measurements of intramural pH in the colon [5].

Can we formulate a simple advice after reading all these truly excellent contributions? Well, be aggressive diagnostically and therapeutically in exactly those elderly-frail patients in whom you do not feel like being aggressive at all. Use CT early and liberally. The currently prevailing nihilism and procrastination will lead us to where we are now - at the abyss of bowel ischemia.

References

1. Mamode N, Pickford I, Leiberman P (1999) Failure to improve outcome in acute mesenteric ischaemia: seven-year review. Eur J Surg 165:203–208
2. Boley SJ, Feinstein FR, Sammartano R, Brandt LJ, Sprayregen S (1981) New concepts in the management of emboli of the superior mesenteric artery. Surg Gynecol Obstet 153:561–569
3. Boley SJ, Brandt J (ed) (1972) Intestinal ischemia. Surg Clin North Am 72
4. Fink S, Chaudhuri TK, Davis HH (2000) Acute mesenteric ischemia and malpractice claims. South Med J 93:210–214
5. Fiddian-Green RG, Amelin PM, Herrmann JB, Arous E, Cutler BS, Schiedler M, Wheeler HB, Baker S (1986) Prediction of the development of sigmoid ischemia on the day of aortic operations. Indirect measurements of intramural pH in the colon. Arch Surg 121:654–660

CHAPTER 9

Ascites

Nonoperative Management

Ramón Bataller · Vicente Arroyo

Bed Rest and Sodium Restriction in Patients with Ascites

In patients with cirrhosis and ascites, upright posture markedly activates sodium-retaining systems and impairs renal perfusion and sodium excretion [1]. Moreover, bed rest is associated with a greater response to diuretics in these patients [2]. For these reasons, bed rest has been traditionally recommended to cirrhotic patients with ascites. However, no clinical trials have specifically addressed whether bed rest improves the management of ascites in cirrhotic patients. At present, we think that bed rest should be only recommended to patients with a poor response to diuretics or with an impaired renal function.

Because the amount of fluid retention in the form of ascites or edema depends on the balance between sodium intake and excretion, the reduction in the quantity of sodium ingested with the diet facilitates the achievement of a negative sodium balance. However, studies assessing the impact of sodium intake restriction in the management of ascites do not support an important role of this maneuver in terms of response rate to medical treatment, diuretic drug dosage and costs [3]. Moreover, a moderate reduction in sodium intake (120 mmol/day) has proven to be equivalent to a low sodium diet (50 mmol/day) [4]. It should be taken into account that diets with severely reduced sodium content are unpalatable, thus leading to poor patient compliance. In addition, they may worsen the preexisting malnutrition. We recommend that dietary salt should be moderately restricted to 90 mmol/day and should be continued thereafter unless there is a spontaneous improvement of renal ability to excrete sodium. Once ascites and edema have disappeared or reduced markedly, sodium intake may be increased progressively in patients who had moderate sodium retention before treatment. By contrast, patients with marked baseline sodium retention usually have to be maintained on a sodium-restricted diet to prevent the recurrence of ascites.

Diuretic Treatment

The initial step in the treatment of mild or moderate ascites consists of the administration of diuretics (Fig. 1, p 197). The diuretic most commonly used is spironolactone (50–400 mg/day), which inhibits sodium reabsorption by blocking the effects of aldosterone (see Table 1) [5]. Spironolactone is frequently given alone or in combination with loop diuretics, especially furosemide (20–160 mg/day), which acts by inhibiting the Na^+-K^+-$2Cl^-$ cotransporter in the loop of Henle [6]. Diuretic dosage should be increased stepwise if there is insufficient diuretic response as defined by a weight loss of less than 1 kg in the first 7 days or 2 kg every 7 days thereafter – until ascites is adequately controlled. The response to diuretic therapy in cirrhotic patients should be evaluated regularly by measuring body weight, urine volume and sodium excretion. An inadequate sodium restriction is a common cause of failure to diuretic therapy. This situation should be suspected when body weight and ascites do not decrease despite a natriuresis higher than the prescribed sodium intake. Approximately 10–20% of patients with ascites either do not respond to diuretic therapy or develop diuretic-induced complications that prevent the use of high doses of these drugs. This condition is known as *refractory ascites* [7].

The most common complications of diuretic therapy in patients with cirrhosis include hepatic encephalopathy, hyponatremia, renal impairment, potassium disturbances, gynecomastia and muscle cramps [6, 8]. *Hepatic encephalopathy* occurs in up to one-fourth of hospitalized cirrhotic patients with ascites treated with diuretics, especially in those treated with higher doses. In cases of mild encephalopathy diuretics may be continued and this complication treated by conventional methods. For those with severe encephalopathy, diuretics should be stopped temporarily and their use reassessed.

A decrease in serum sodium is almost a universal finding in patients treated with diuretics. In most cases, only a minor reduction is observed. However, hyponatremia may develop or worsen in 30% of patients receiving diuretics. A reduction of more than 10 mmol/l to a level lower than 120–125 mmol/l usually constitutes an indication to stop therapy [7]. Treatment may be reintroduced when serum sodium increases.

The classical type of *renal dysfunction* during diuretic therapy is usually due to intravascular volume depletion, occurs in patients with positive response and is rapidly reversible after discontinuation of diuretics [9]. To avoid this complication, diuretic dosage should be adjusted to achieve a rate of weight loss less than an average of 500 g/day in patients without peripheral edema or 1 kg/day in those with edema.

Table 1. Response to furosemide and spironolactone in 40 nonazotemic cirrhotic patients with ascites (reproduced from Pérez-Ayuso et al. [5])

	Positive response	Negative response	Total
Furosemide	11	10 [a]	21 (80–160 mg/day)
Spironolactone	18	1 [b]	19 (150 mg/day)

[a] Nine cases responded later to spironolactone alone.
[b] This case did not respond later to furosemide alone.

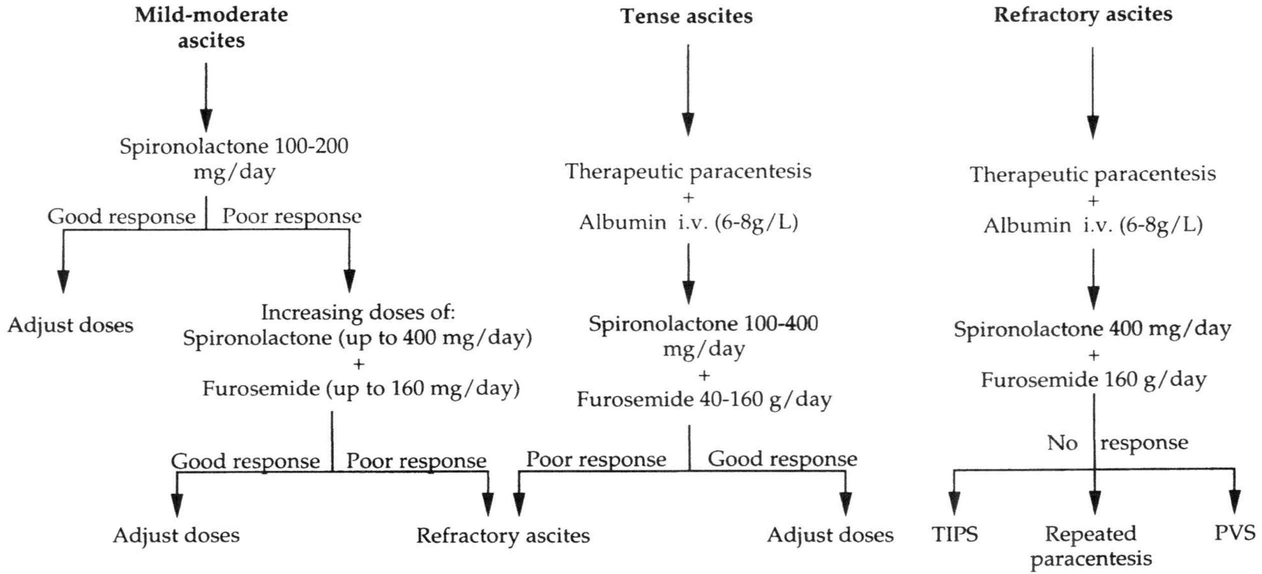

Fig. 1. Algorithm for treatment of ascites in cirrhotic patients (*TIPS* transjugular portosystemic shunt, *PVS* peritoneovenous shunt)

Severe hyperkalemia (greater than 6 mmol/l) is an uncommon complication of diuretics in patients with ascites without renal failure, but may develop when patients with renal failure are treated with moderate or high doses of spironolactone. Therefore, serum potassium should be monitored closely in patients with renal impairment (serum creatinine >1.2 mg/dl) treated with spironolactone. In cases of serum potassium levels over 5.5 mmol/l, the dosage of spironolactone should be reduced. In cases over 6.0 mmol/l, spironolactone should be stopped.

Hypokalemia occurs only in patients treated with loop diuretics alone not receiving oral potassium supplementation. *Gynecomastia* is a common complication of chronic spironolactone therapy and in some patients may be important enough to require the withdrawal of the drug. Amiloride may be an alternative therapy in these patients, but it is markedly less effective than spironolactone [10]. Finally, *muscle cramps* are frequent in patients treated with diuretics and may require the reduction of diuretic dosage. Quinidine (quinidine sulfate 400 mg/day) [11] or i.v. administration of albumin (25 g weekly) [12] have been shown to reduce the frequency and intensity of muscle cramps in cirrhotic patients with ascites treated with diuretics.

Therapeutic Paracentesis: Always Together with Plasma Volume Expansion?

Therapeutic paracentesis is now widely considered the treatment of choice in the management of large ascites in patients with cirrhosis. This is based on the results of several randomized comparative studies of paracentesis (either total removal of all ascitic fluid in a single tap or repeated taps of 4–6 l/day) together with plasma volume expansion vs. diuretic therapy in cirrhotic patients with large ascites [13, 14]. The results of these studies indicate that ascites is more rapidly and effectively removed using paracentesis than diuretics. Moreover, the removal of ascites by paracentesis is associated with lower number of complications compared with diuretic therapy (see Table 2). Finally, the use of paracentesis reduces the global cost of treatment because patients do not require prolonged hospitalization and can be treated as outpatients. Because paracentesis does not modify the preexist-

Table 2. Complications during the first hospital stay in patients treated with paracentesis plus intravenous albumin (group 1) and patients treated with diuretics (group 2) (reproduced from Ginès et al. [13])

	Group 1 ($n=58$)	Group 2 ($n=59$)	P
Patients with complications	10	36	<0.001
Hyponatremia	3	18	<0.001
Encephalopathy	6	17	<0.002
Renal impairment	2	16	<0.001
Hyperkalemia	1	7	n.s.
Gastrointestinal bleeding	2	6	n.s.
Peritonitis	0	4	n.s.
Bacteremia	2	0	n.s.
Others	0	4	n.s.

ing renal sodium retention, patients should be given diuretics after paracentesis to avoid positive sodium balance and reformation of ascites [15].

An important aspect of treatment of ascites with paracentesis is that this procedure should be performed in association with plasma volume expansion to prevent the side effects of paracentesis on circulatory function. Immediately after paracentesis there is an improvement of effective blood volume, with increased cardiac output, deactivation of vasoconstrictor and antinatriuretic systems (renin-angiotensin-aldosterone system and sympathetic nervous system) and increased plasma atrial natriuretic peptide levels. However, this early phase is rapidly followed by a circulatory dysfunction characterized by a reduction in effective blood volume [16, 17]. Once developed, this circulatory dysfunction is not spontaneously reversible and has a negative impact on the course of the disease, because patients who develop this abnormality require higher doses of diuretics to prevent ascites formation, have a greater risk of ascites reaccumulation and, most importantly, a shorter survival compared with patients who do not develop circulatory dysfunction. This post-paracentesis circulatory dysfunction may be prevented by the administration of plasma expanders. Albumin is more effective than the artificial plasma expanders, such as dextran-70 or polygeline [18]. In patients treated with albumin the risk of post-paracentesis circulatory dysfunction is low and independent of the volume of ascites removed. By contrast, in patients treated with other plasma expanders the risk of post-paracentesis circulatory dysfunction increases proportionally with the volume of ascitic fluid removed. When less than 5 l of ascites is removed, artificial plasma expanders and albumin are equally effective. However, when more than 5 l is removed, albumin is the plasma expander of choice. Albumin is administered at a dose of 8 g/l of ascites removed. Fifty percent of the total amount is given immediately after the procedure and 50% 2–4 h later. The recommended doses of dextran-70 and polygeline are 8 g and 150 ml per liter of ascites removed, respectively. The pathogenesis of circulatory dysfunction after paracentesis is not completely understood, but it does not seem to be secondary to a contraction of plasma volume, as classically believed, because plasma volume does not decrease in patients developing this complication [19]. More likely, circulatory dysfunction is related to an accentuation of the existent arterial vasodilatation that would cause a further impairment of the already reduced effective blood volume of cirrhotic patients with ascites [20].

Dilutional Hyponatremia in Cirrhosis: When and How Should It Be Treated?

Dilutional hyponatremia in cirrhosis is defined by a serum sodium concentration below 130 mmol/l in the presence of ascites and/or edema and is the clinical consequence of the impairment in water excretion [21]. This type of hyponatremia occurs in the setting of increased total body water and dilution of extracellular fluid volume. Dilutional hyponatremia is associated with sodium retention and increased total body sodium and should be distinguished from true hyponatremia due to sodium depletion that, although less common, may develop in cirrhotic patients who are maintained on excessive diuretic treatment and sodium restriction after complete disappearance of ascites and edema. In many patients, dilutional hyponatremia is asymptomatic, but in others it may be associated with clinical symptoms similar to those found in hyponatremia of other etiologies, including anorexia, headache, difficulty in mental concentration, sluggish thinking, lethargy, nausea, vomiting and, occasionally, seizures. An unanswered question is when dilutional hyponatremia should be treated. We recommend to treat this complication when it is associated with clinical symptoms or when serum sodium concentration is below 120 mmol/l.

At present, no pharmacological therapy exists for dilutional hyponatremia and the only therapeutic measure that may improve or stop the progression of hyponatremia is water restriction (500–1000 ml/day). Saline solutions are not recommended because they induce a markedly positive sodium balance with accumulation of ascites and edema. Recently, two types of drugs have been developed that selectively increase water excretion: antagonists of the V2 receptor of antidiuretic hormone and selective kappa opioid agonists [21]. The former group of drugs antagonizes selectively the water-retaining effect of antidiuretic hormone in the cortical collecting duct whereas the latter inhibit antidiuretic hormone release from the neurohypophysis and have also a direct tubular effect. Both groups of drugs, which are still not available for use in clinical practice, induce a dose-dependent increase in urine flow and free water excretion in normal animals as well as in healthy subjects [21]. The results of a randomized multicenter study showing that VPA-985, a specific V2 agonist, increases serum sodium concentration, urine output and free water clearance in cirrhotic patients with dilutional hyponatremia have recently been reported [22]. Further studies are required to delineate the precise indications of these drugs and to assess whether these new drugs also enhance the response to diuretics. Therefore, these compounds may offer a novel therapeutic approach for the treatment of dilutional hyponatremia in cirrhotic patients with ascites.

References

1. Bernardi M, Santini C, Trevisani F, et al. (1985) Renal function impairment induced by change in posture in patients with cirrhosis and ascites. Gut 26:629–635
2. Ring-Larsen H, Henriksen JH, Wilken C, et al. (1986) Diuretic treatment in decompensated cirrhosis and congestive heart failure: effect of posture. Br Med J 292:1351–1353
3. Gauthier A, Levy VG, Quinton A, et al. (1986) Salt or not salt in the treatment of cirrhotic ascites: a randomised study. Gut 27:705–709
4. Bernardi M, Laffi G, Salvagnini M, et al. (1993) Efficacy and safety of the stepped care medical treatment of ascites in liver cirrhosis: a randomized controlled clinical trial comparing two diets with different sodium content. Liver 13:156–162
5. Pérez-Ayuso RM, Arroyo V, Planas R, et al. (1983) Randomized comparative study of efficacy of furosemide versus spironolactone in nonazotemic cirrhosis with ascites. Relationship between the diuretic response and the activity of the renin-aldosterone system. Gastroenterology 84:961–968
6. Bataller R, Ginès P, Arroyo V (1997) Practical recommendations for the treatment of ascites and its complications. Drugs 54:571–580
7. Arroyo V, Ginès P, Gerbes A, et al. (1996) Definition and diagnostic criteria of refractory ascites and hepatorenal syndrome in cirrhosis. Hepatology 23:164–176
8. Sherlock S, Senewiratne B, Scott A, et al. (1966) Complications of diuretic therapy in hepatic cirrhosis. Lancet 1:1049–1052
9. Forns X, Ginès A, Ginès P, et al. (1994) The management of ascites and renal failure in cirrhosis. Semin Liver Dis 14:82–96

10. Angeli P, Pria MD, De Bei E, et al. (1994) Randomized clinical study of the efficacy of amiloride and potassium canreonate in nonazotemic cirrhotic patients with ascites. Hepatology 19:72–79
11. Lee FY, Lee SD, Tsai YT, et al. (1991) A randomized controlled trial of quinidine in the treatment of cirrhotic patients with muscle cramps. J Hepatol 12:236
12. Angeli P, Albino G, Carraro P, et al. (1996) Cirrhosis and muscle cramps: evidence of a causal relationship. Hepatology 23:264–270
13. Ginès P, Arroyo V, Quintero E, et al. (1987) Comparison of paracentesis and diuretics in the treatment of cirrhotics with tense ascites. Results of a randomized study. Gastroenterology 93:234–241
14. Salerno F, Badalamenti S, Incerti P, et al. (1987) Repeated paracentesis and i.v. albumin infusion to treat "tense" ascites in cirrhotic patients: a safe alternative therapy. J Hepatol 5:102–108
15. Fernández-Esparrach G, Guevara M, Sort P, et al. (1997) Diuretic requirements after therapeutic paracentesis in non-azotemic patients with cirrhosis. A randomized double-blind trial of spironolactone versus placebo. J Hepatol 26:614–620
16. Ginès P, Titó Ll, Arroyo V, et al. (1988) Randomized comparative study of therapeutic paracentesis with and without intravenous albumin in cirrhosis. Gastroenterology 94:1493–1502
17. Pozzi M, Osculati G, Boari G, et al. (1994) Time course of circulatory and humoral effects of rapid total paracentesis in cirrhotic patients with tense, refractory ascites. Gastroenterology 106:709–719
18. Ginès A, Fernández-Esparrach G, Monescillo A, et al. (1996) Randomized trial comparing albumin, dextran-70 and polygelin in cirrhotic patients with ascites treated by paracentesis. Gastroenterology 111:1002–1010
19. Saló J, Ginès A, Ginès P, et al. (1997) Effect of therapeutic paracentesis on plasma volume and transvascular escape rate of albumin in patients with cirrhosis. J Hepatol 27:645–653
20. Ruiz del Arbol L, Monescillo A, Jiménez W, et al. (1997) Paracentesis-induced circulatory dysfunction: mechanism and effect on hepatic hemodynamics in cirrhosis. Gastroenterology 113:579–587
21. Ginès P, Berl T, Bernardi M, et al. (1998) Hyponatremia in cirrhosis: from pathogenesis to treatment. Hepatology 28:851–864
22. Gerbes AL, Guelberg V, Grosshadern C (1999) VPA-895, an orally active vasopressin receptor antagonist, improves hyponatremia in patients with cirrhosis. A double-blind placebo controlled multicenter trial. Hepatology 30:419A

The Transjugular Intrahepatic Portosystemic Shunt Procedure

Gilles Pomier-Layrargues · Ziad Hassoun

Introduction

Ascites is a common major complication of cirrhosis and a sign of advanced liver disease. In the vast majority of patients, ascites can be controlled by dietary sodium restriction and diuretics. However, nearly 10% of patients with ascites later become resistant, being either unresponsive to medical treatment or developing complications related to large doses of diuretics (encephalopathy, hyponatremia, renal failure). Therapeutic options in this situation include repeated large volume paracentesis, continuous ultra filtration-reinfusion of ascitic fluid, peritoneojugular (Leveen) shunt, surgical portacaval shunt or liver transplantation [1]. Repeated large-volume paracentesis is the most widely used technique as it is rapid, safe and inexpensive; survival in patients treated by this method is similar to that observed after Leveen shunt [2, 3]. The surgical portacaval shunt is extremely efficient for clearing ascites but it is associated with a significant operative mortality, and chronic hepatic encephalopathy is a major problem during follow-up [4–5]. Transjugular intrahepatic portosystemic shunt (TIPS) is an equivalent of the surgical shunt, it is performed however without laparotomy or general anesthesia, and is associated with a low rate of complications (1%–2%). In addition, it induces only a partial diversion of portal flow in the majority of patients. Therefore, TIPS can combine the effectiveness of surgical shunting and the safety of a nonsurgical approach [6].

The clinical usefulness of TIPS in the treatment of refractory ascites is still difficult to evaluate but analysis of the literature can help determine the subset of cirrhotic patients who will likely benefit from this new therapeutic approach.

Analysis of the Literature

Seven studies published as full papers are now available involving 184 cirrhotic patients with refractory ascites [7–13]. Only one is a randomized controlled trial comparing TIPS and repeated paracentesis [13]. Criteria to define refractory ascites are quite variable which can explain some differences in the clinical evolution after treatment. Evaluation of the usefulness of TIPS in the treatment of refractory ascites should include the following end points: control of ascites, survival rate and incidence of hepatic encephalopathy. As shown in Table 3, all patients had moderate or severe liver failure (Pugh class B or C). Control of ascites was obtained in the vast majority of cirrhotic patients (mean 77.5%; range 50%–95%). This is not surprising given the well-demonstrated effects of the procedure on urinary sodium excretion as well as on hyperaldosteronism and renal function parameters [8, 9, 14, 15]. Noteworthy, the improvement in control of ascites is often delayed several days or weeks after TIPS placement; moreover a majority of patients still needs diuretic therapy during follow-up.

The 1-year survival rate is variable among different studies (mean 54%; range 29%–75%); this can be explained by differences in patient selection. However, the fact that half the patients with refractory ascites will die within 1 year emphasizes the poor prognosis associated with this complication and is a strong argument to consider liver transplantation in this situation.

Table 3. TIPS for refractory ascites: analysis of the literature

Author (reference)	Number of patients	Pugh class (B/C)	Control of ascites (1 year)	Survival (1 year)	Chronic encephalopathy (1 year)
Ferral [7]	14	6/8	50%	67%	?
Quiroga [8]	17	?	72%	75%	14%
Somberg [9]	19	11/8	74%	?	?
Ochs [10]	50	18/32	92%	55%	16%
Forrest [11]	18	?	95%	50%	11%
Deschênes [12]	53	35/18	90%	48%	26%
Lebrec [15]	13	9/4	70%	29%	15%

The true rate of hepatic encephalopathy is quite difficult to evaluate by analyzing the existing literature. However, the incidence of chronic disabling encephalopathy, which is the most important clinically relevant problem, varies between 10% and 25%, which represents a serious flaw of the TIPS procedure.

The occurrence of TIPS dysfunction during follow-up, as related to progressive stenosis of the shunt by intimal hyperplasia, is another major problem; this can be avoided by a careful monitoring of shunt function using Doppler ultrasonography and shunt catheterization with pressure measurement. Treatment of shunt dysfunction is usually very easy, consisting of dilatation using a balloon catheter, with insertion of a new stent in selected cases. Need for reintervention is frequent during the first year after TIPS placement but quite rare thereafter.

The ideal method to evaluate the effectiveness of TIPS in the treatment of refractory ascites would be to perform randomized controlled trials comparing this procedure with other techniques, such as the LeVeen shunt or large volume paracentesis. Two such studies are available in the literature. One has been published in abstract form and demonstrated that TIPS was more effective than paracentesis but that survival was similar for both groups [16]. The second one [13] involved small groups of cirrhotic patients (13 in the TIPS group and 12 in the paracentesis group). The authors confirmed that TIPS is more effective for ascites than paracentesis, but that survival was decreased in the Pugh class C patients. However, this study has several problems: (1) the sample size is small; (2) in the group of patients randomized to TIPS, the treatment could not be performed in 3/13 patients (23%), whereas the rate of failure of TIPS implantation in all centers experienced with this procedure is lower than 5%; and finally (3) two patients in the TIPS group died from massive GI hemorrhage which suggests that shunt stenosis has been missed during follow-up. This might be explained by a learning curve for this procedure.

Therefore existing data do not allow definite conclusions on the true usefulness of TIPS for patients with refractory ascites. Nonetheless, analysis of uncontrolled studies provides useful information to better select patients who might benefit from the TIPS procedure. The two largest published series demonstrated that the best predictor of response are age below 60 years and/or serum bilirubin lower than 1.3 mg/dl [10] or creatinine clearance higher than 36 ml/min [12].

As previously stated, the onset of refractory ascites is associated with a poor prognosis related to the severity of the underlying liver disease. Therefore, future comparative randomized clinical trials should evaluate not only survival, which will not likely be influenced by TIPS, but also quality of life and costs as main end-points.

Role of TIPS in the Therapeutic Strategy for Refractory Ascites

Occurrence of refractory ascites is associated with a 50% 1-year death rate. Survival after liver transplantation is in the 80% range after 1 year. Therefore, transplantation must be considered as the first therapeutic option. However, given the scarcity of donor organs, the waiting time is increasingly long. In these patients, TIPS might be used as a bridge to liver transplantation. If progressive liver failure occurs, transplantation can be performed on an emergency basis; if the patient develops chronic disabling encephalopathy, reduction of the size of the shunt [17] or even balloon occlusion might be performed [18]. In exceptional cases, TIPS might be so effective that the patient may be removed from the waiting list.

When a patient is not a good candidate for transplantation, the two options are repeated large volume paracentesis or TIPS. TIPS can be offered to patients with a Pugh score under 12 who judge that their quality of life is severely compromised by the need for repeated paracentesis, who have no contraindications for TIPS (cardiac failure, portal vein thrombosis) and have a renal function that is not too severely impaired.

Finally, several conditions are required for the optimal use of the TIPS procedure: availability of physicians experienced with the TIPS procedure and echo Doppler technology; need for a regular follow-up including clinical evaluation, echo Doppler examinations and shunt catheterization; and availability of surgeons experienced in hepatobiliary surgery and liver transplantation.

References

1. Olafson S, Blei AT (1995) Diagnosis and management of ascites in the age of TIPS. Am J Roentgenol 165:9–15
2. Gines P, Arroyo V, Vargas V, Planas R, Casafont F, Panes J, Hoyos M, Viladomiu L, Rimola A, Morillas R, Salmeron JM, Gines A, Esteban R, Rodes J (1991) Paracentesis with intravenous infusions of albumin as compared with peritoneovenous shunting in cirrhosis with refractory ascites. N Engl J Med 325:829–835
3. Stanley MM, Ochi S, Lee KK, Nemchausky BA, Greenlee HB, Allen JL, Allen MJ, Baum RA, Gadacz TR, Camara DS, Caruana JA, Schiff ER, Livingstone AS, Samanta AK, Najeh AZ, Glick ME, Juler GL, Adham N, Baker JD, Cain GD, Jordan PH, Wolf DC, Fulenwider JT, James KE, and the Veterans Administration Cooperative Study on the Treatment of Alcoholic Cirrhosis with Ascites (1989) Peritoneovenous shunting as compared with medical treatment in patients with alcoholic cirrhosis and massive ascites. N Engl J Med 321:1632–1638
4. Welch HF, Welch CS, Carter JH (1964) Prognosis after surgical treatment of ascites. Results of side-to-side shunt in 40 patients. Surgery 56:75–82
5. Franco D, Vons C, Traynor O, Smajda C (1988) Should portosystemic shunt be reconsidered in the treatment of untractable ascites in cirrhosis? Arch Surg 123:987–991
6. Schiffman ML, Jeffers L, Hoofnagle JH, Tralka TS (1995) The role of transjugular intrahepatic portosystemic shunt for treatment of portal hypertension and its complications: a conference sponsored by the National Digestive Diseases Advisory Board. Hepatology 22:1591–1597
7. Ferral HS, Bjarnason H, Wegryn SA, Rengel GJ, Mazarian GK, Rank JM, Tadavarthy SM, Hunter DW, Castaneda-Zuniga WR (1993) Refractory ascites: early experience in treatment with transjugular intrahepatic portosystemic shunt. Radiology 189:795–801
8. Quiroga J, Sangro B, Nunez M, Bilbao I, Longo J, Garcia-Villareal L, Zozaya JM, Betes M, Herrero JI, Prieto J (1995) Transjugular intrahepatic portal-systemic shunt in the treatment of refractory ascites: effect on clinical, renal, humoral and hemodynamic parameters. Hepatology 21:986–994
9. Somberg KA, Lake JR, Tomlanovich J, Laberge JM, Feldstein V, Bass N (1995) Transjugular intrahepatic portosystemic shunts for refractory ascites: assessment of clinical and hormonal response and renal function. Hepatology 21:709–716
10. Ochs A, Rossle M, Haag K, Hauenstein KH, Beibert P, Siegerstetter V, Huokner M, Langer M, Blum HE (1995) The transjugular intrahepatic portosytemic stent-shunt procedure for refractory ascites. N Engl J Med 332:1193–1197
11. Forrest EH, Stanley AJ, Redhead DN, McGilchrist AJ, Hayes PC (1996) Clinical response after transjugular intrahepatic portosystemic stent shunt insertion for refractory ascites in cirrhosis. Aliment Pharmacol Ther 10:801–806
12. Deschênes M, Dufresne MP, Bui B, Fenyves D, Spahr L, Roy L, Lafortune M, Pomier-Layrargues G (1999) Predictors of clinical response to transjugular intrahepatic portosystemic shunt (TIPS) in cirrhotic patients with refractory ascites. Am J Gastroenterol 94:1361–1365

13. Lebrec D, Giuily N, Hadengue A, Vilgrain V, Moreau R, Poynard T, Gadano A, Lassen C, Benhamou JP, Erlinger J, and a French group of clinicians and a group of biologists (1996) Transjugular intrahepatic portosystemic shunts: comparison with parecentesis in patients with cirrhosis and refractory ascites: a randomized trial. J Hepatol 25:135–144
14. Martinet JP, Legault L, Cernacek P, Roy L, Dufresne MP, Spahr L, Fenyves D, Pomier-Layrargues G (1996) Changes in plasma endothelin 1 and big endothelin 1 induced by transjugular intrahepatic shunt in cirrhotic patients with refractory ascites. J Hepatol 25:700–706
15. Wong F, Sniderman K, Liu P, Allidina Y, Sherman M, Blendis L (1995) Transjugular intrahepatic portosystemic stent shunt: effects on hemodynamics and sodium homeostasis in cirrhosis and refractory ascites. Ann Intern Med 122:816–822
16. Ochs A, Gerbes AL, Haag K, Holl J, Hauenstein KH, Waggershausen T, Reiser M, Paumgartner G, Blum HE, Rossle M (1995) TIPS and paracentesis in the treatment of refractory ascites (RA): interim analysis of a randomized controlled trial (abstract). Hepatology 22 (no. 4, part 2):297A
17. Hauenstein KH, Haag K, Ochs A, Langer M, Rossle M (1995) The reducing stent: treatment for transjugular intrahepatic portosystemic shunt induced refractory hepatic encephalopathy and liver failure. Radiology 194:175–179
18. Fenyves D, Dufresne MP, Raymond J, Lafortune M, Willems B, Pomier-Layrargues G (1994) Successful reversal of chronic incapacitating post-TIPS encephalopathy by balloon occlusion of the stent. Can J Gastroenterol 8:75–80

Operative Management

Dominique Franco

Patients with tense ascites who do not respond to medical measures may be treated by surgery. Two types of operations may be performed: portacaval shunt and peritoneovenous shunt.

Portocaval Shunt

Increased portal pressure is a determining factor in the pathogenesis of ascites, although not the only one. It was with the purpose of treating ascites that Eck in 1877 devised portacaval shunt in the dog – a procedure which lowers portacaval pressure gradient. Portacaval shunt was indeed very efficient on refractory ascites and associated renal failure [1–3]. Since ascites is produced both by abdominal peritoneum and the liver capsule, it was recommended to perform a side-to-side portacaval shunt [4, 5]. Results were plagued by a high operative mortality above 15%. This resulted from technical difficulties in dissecting the portal vein and the inferior vena cava from the thickened inflammatory peritoneum and from fluid and electrolyte imbalances. A better selection of patients, expertise in portal hypertensive surgery and improvement in fluid administration achieved a reduction in operative mortality to less than 5% [6, 7]. Above all, the rate of post-shunt encephalopathy was very high, averaging 50% at 2 years, higher than following shunting for variceal bleeding. This led to abandonment of portacaval shunting for refractory ascites. The Warren shunt or partial portal diversion, which is associated with less encephalopathy, does not decrease sinusoidal pressure as well as total shunts and therefore is much less efficient on ascites. Even though recent results with TIPS could urge again the use of surgical portacaval shunts in the treatment of ascites, we do believe that the operative risk, and that of encephalopathy, are strong arguments against this procedure.

Peritoneovenous Shunt

Twenty-five years ago, Harry LeVeen designed a barosensitive, unidirectional valve which could be easily implanted between the abdominal cavity and the superior vena cava [8]. It allowed permanent infusion of ascites, resulting in an increase in intravascular fluid volume, cardiac output, and ultimately in renal perfusion [9, 10]. Results in patients with intractable ascites were excellent. Patients would eliminate liters of urine during the first postoperative hours, loose weight and flatten their belly. After a short period of enthusiasm came a time of profound disillusion. In effect, the peritoneovenous shunt (PVS) was associated with a great number of postoperative complications and a high mortality rate. The most obvious were coagulation disorders [11] and acute cardiac failure [12], both resulting from the massive load of procoagulant factor-rich ascites into the general circulation. Infection was the next complication [13] and was related to the implantation of foreign material into ascites in an immunodepressed patient. The risk of postoperative infection was at its highest in patients with previous or unrecognized spontaneous bacterial peritonitis (SBP). The onset of one or the other of these complications triggered liver failure. Altogether the operative death rate averaged 18% [14]. The mortality rate was the highest in patients with advanced liver disease [13, 15].

Even in those patients who overcame the early postoperative period, there were still many complications to come. Severe infection was at risk as long as ascites had not completely disappeared. This may take several months. It should prompt removal of the shunt [16]. Above all there was a high incidence (about 50%) of shunt obstruction leading to recurrent ascites [17, 18]. This could be associated with thrombosis of the superior vena cava [19]. Finally chronic implantation of the LeVeen shunt specifically resulted in a very high (38%) rate of peritoneal fibrosis leading to intestinal obstruction in half of cases and to major operative difficulties in case of abdominal surgery and particularly of liver transplantation [20]. Other types of valve, such as the Denver shunt, which has a pumping device incorporated, were not better than the LeVeen shunt [21].

None of the six randomized studies comparing the efficacy of PVS to that of medical treatment in patients with tense ascites [22–27] showed a clear advantage of surgery but one (Table 4). In two of the five other studies the only benefit was a smaller number of readmissions in operated patients [25, 26]. It was therefore considered that the price to be paid after PVS was too high as compared to the benefit [15].

Would that definitely condemn PVS? We think not. It is possible to improve the results of PVS. Intraoperative drainage of ascites significantly decreases postoperative blood coagulation disorders. Together with diuretics it also decreases the intensity of postoperative hemodynamic changes and therefore the risk of cardiac failure [28]. Perioperative short-term administration of antibiotics diminishes the incidence of postoperative infection [29]. In addition, selection of patients – dis-

Table 4. Results of randomized prospective studies comparing peritoneovenous shunting (*PVS*) to medical treatment (*MT*) of refractory ascites

Authors, year	No. of patients	Operative mortality (%) PVS:MT	Readmissions for ascites (days) PVS:MT	Cumulative survival (%) PVS:MT
Wapnick et al. 1979 [22]	34	41:18	–	29:6 (2 years)
Bories et al. 1986 [23]	57	41:18	–	79:75 (1 year)
Stanley et al. 1989 [24]				
Good liver function	122	9.5:0	–	62:59 (2 years)
Moderate liver failure	144	8.7:10.7		33:33 (2 years)
Severe liver failure	33	50:47.4		36:21 (2 years)
Ring-Larsen et al. 1989 [25]	41	26:33	–	50:50 (6 months)
Gines et al. 1991 [26]	89	12:7	97:174	28:20 (3 years)
Gines et al. 1995 [27]	81	7.7:2.3	43:193	42:37 (2 years)

carding those with end-stage liver failure and those with previous recent SBP or uncontrolled variceal bleeding – decreases both the incidence of severe postoperative complications and the death toll from those complications [30, 31]. This brings operative mortality down to a very low level [30]. Improvement in the material used, and particularly the addition at the end of the venous catheter of a nonthrombogenic titanium tip, decreases the risk of late venous thrombosis [32]. Long-term antibiotics which have been advocated for prevention of SBP in patients with low ascitic protein concentration should also be given on a long range after peritoneovenous shunting. Altogether these measures lower the risk of late complications and increase survival rate without ascites to 71% at 2 years [30]. When the postoperative course is uneventful, patients regain a normal nutritional status within 6 months after surgery [33, 34]. Long-term success is observed mainly in patients with stable liver disease and above all in patients with alcoholic cirrhosis who stop drinking [35]. Interestingly patients surviving after 5 years seem to escape the risk of liver failure and die later on from other complications of chronic alcoholism such as throat or colonic cancers [35]. Clearly, PVS is a good treatment when it is correctly applied in a small group of cirrhotic patients with intractable tense ascites despite repeated large volume paracenteses and a stable liver disease.

However, although its effect on survival is not yet demonstrated [36], there is a clear trend towards liver transplantation in patients with cirrhosis, ascites and moderate (Child B) liver failure. Tense ascites per se may trigger liver transplantation. Since PVS may threaten the performance of the graft [20], it should be reserved to patients in whom liver transplantation is not contemplated. In those patients pleuroperitoneal shunting is also a good treatment of refractory hydrothorax [37]. In some patients double shunting by a pleuroperitoneal shunt combined with a PVS allows clearance of both intractable pleural effusion and ascites [38].

Clearly, PVS remains one piece in the armamentarium against ascites. Perhaps the direct saphenoperitoneal anastomosis which does not include any interposition of foreign material [39] will boost again the indication of peritoneovenous shunting in patients with tense ascites.

References

1. Barker HG, Reemtsma K (1960) The portacaval shunt operation in patients with cirrhosis and ascites. Surgery 48:142–154
2. Welch HF, Welch CS, Carter JH (1964) Prognosis after surgical treatment of ascites: results of side-to-side shunt in 40 patients. Surgery 56:75–82
3. Burchell AR, Rousselot LM, Panke WF (1968) A seven-year experience with side-to-side portacaval shunt for cirrhotic ascites. Ann Surg 168:655–670
4. Welch CS, Attarian E, Welch HF (1958) The treatment of ascites by side-to-side portacaval shunt. Bull NY Acad Med 34:249–255
5. Orloff MJ (1970) Pathogenesis and surgical treatment of intractable ascites associated with alcoholic cirrhosis. Ann NY Acad Sci 170:213–238
6. Franco D, Vons C, Traynor O, Smadja C (1988) Should portosystemic shunt be reconsidered in the treatment of intractable ascites in cirrhosis ? Arch Surg 123:987–991
7. Orloff MJ, Orloff MS, Orloff SL, Girard B (1997) Experimental, clinical, and metabolic results of side-to-side portacaval shunt for intractable cirrhotic ascites. J Am Coll Surg 184:557–570
8. Leveen HH, Christoudias G, Moon IP, Luft R, Falk G, Grosberg S (1974) Peritoneovenous shunting for ascites. Ann Surg 180:580–591
9. Blendis LM, Greig PD, Langer B, Baigrie RS, Ruse J, Taylor BR (1979) The renal and hemodynamic effects of the peritoneovenous shunt for intractable hepatic ascites. Gastroenterology 77:250–257
10. Vons C, Hadengue A, Lee SS, Smadja C, Franco D, Lebrec D (1991) Splanchnic and systemic hemodynamics in cirrhotic patients with refractory ascites. Effect of peritoneovenous shunting. HPB Surg 3:259–269
11. Ragni MV, Lewis JH, Spero JA (1983) Ascites-induced LeVeen shunt coagulopathy. Ann Surg 198:91–95
12. Darsee JR, Fulenwider JT, Rikkers LF, et al. (1981) Hemodynamics of LeVeen shunt pulmonary edema. Ann Surg 194:189–192
13. Smadja C, Franco D (1985) The LeVeen shunt in the elective treatment of intractable ascites in cirrhosis. A prospective study on 140 patients. Ann Surg 201:488–496
14. Moskovitz M (1990) The peritoneovenous shunt: expectations and reality. Am J Gastroenterol 85:917–929
15. Zervos EE, McCormick J, Goode SE, Rosemurgy AS (1997) Peritoneovenous shunts in patients with intractable ascites: palliation at what price? Am Surg 63:157–162
16. Prokesch RC, Rimland D (1983) Infectious complications of the peritoneovenous shunt. Am J Gastroenterol 78:235–240
17. Smadja C, Tridard D, Franco D (1986) Recurrent ascites due to central venous thrombosis after peritoneojugular (LeVeen) shunt. Surgery 100:535–540
18. Schwartzentruber DJ, Leapnan SB, Filo RS, Madura JA (1987) Thrombofibrinous sheath occlusion of peritoneovenous shunts. Surgery 102:534–539
19. Eckhauser FE, Strodel WE, Knol JA, Turcotte JG (1979) Superior vena caval obstruction associated with long-term peritoneovenous shunting. Ann Surg 190:758–760
20. Stanley MM, Reyes CV, Greenlee HB, Nemchausky B, Reinhardt GF (1996) Peritoneal fibrosis in cirrhotics treated with peritoneovenous shunting for ascites. An autopsy study with clinical correlations. Dig Dis Sci 41:571–577
21. Fulenwider JT, Galambos JD, Smith RB, Henderson JM, Warren WD (1986) LeVeen vs. Denver peritoneovenous shunts for intractable ascites in cirrhosis. Arch Surg 121:351–355
22. Wapnick S, Grosberg SJ, Evans MI (1979) Randomized prospective matched pair study comparing peritoneovenous shunt and conventional therapy in massive ascites. Br J Surg 66:667–670
23. Bories P, Garcia-Compean D, Michel H, et al. (1986) The treatment of refractory ascites by the LeVeen shunt: a multi-centre controlled trial (57 patients). J Hepatol 3:212–218
24. Stanley MM, Ochi S, Lee KK, et al. (1989) Peritoneovenous shunting as compared with medical treatment in patients with alcoholic cirrhosis and massive ascites. N Engl J Med 321:1632–1638
25. Ring-Larsen H, Siemssen O, Krintel JJ, Stadager C, Henriksen JH (1989) Denver shunt in the treatment of refractory ascites in cirrhosis. A randomized control trial. Gastroenterology 96:A649
26. Gines P, Arroyo V, Vargas V, et al. (1991) Paracentesis with intravenous infusion of albumin as compared with peritoneovenous shunting in cirrhosis with refractory ascites. N Engl J Med 325:829–835

27. Gines A, Planas R, Angeli P, et al. (1995) Treatment of patients with cirrhosis and refractory ascites using LeVeen shunt with titanium tip: comparison with therapeutic paracentesis. Hepatology 22:124-131
28. Hillaire S, Labianca M, Smadja C, Grange D, Franco D (1998) La dérivation péritonéoveineuse dans la cirrhose: résultats d'une étude prospective sur les facteurs d'amélioration du pronostic. Gastroentérol Clin Biol 12:681-686
29. Meakins JL, Hillaire S, Vons C, Smadja C, Franco D (1989) Perioperative antibiotics (two doses) control early but not late infectious complications of peritoneovenous shunt. Surg Res Commun 5:55-58
30. Hillaire S, Labianca M, Borgonovo G, Smadja C, Grange D, Franco D (1993) Peritoneovenous shunting of intractable ascites in cirrhotic patients: improving results and predictive factors of failure. Surgery 113:373-379
31. Guardiola J, Xiol W, Escriba JM, et al. (1995) Prognosis assessment of cirrhotic patients with refractory ascites treated with a peritoneovenous shunt. Am J Gastroenterol 90:2097-2102
32. Franco D, Labianca M, Smadja C, Fragoso J (1998) A titanium catheter tip for peritoneovenous shunts. Artif Organs 12:81-82
33. Franco D, Charra M, Jeambrun P, Belghiti J, Cortesse A, Sossler C (1983) Nutrition and immunity after peritoneovenous drainage of intractable ascites in cirrhotic patients. Am J Surg 146:652-657
34. Blendis LM, Harrison JE, Russel DM, et al. (1986) Effects of peritoneovenous shunting on body composition. Gastroenterology 90:127-134
35. Franco D, Meakins JL, Wu A, et al. (1989) Long-term results (>5 years) in patients with peritoneovenous shunting for intractable ascites: liver function and cancer mortality. HPB Surg 1:185-194
36. Poynard T, Naveau S, Doffoel M, et al. (1999) Evaluation of efficacy of liver transplantation in alcoholic cirrhosis using matched and simulated controls: 5-year survival. Multi-centre group. J Hepatol 30:1130-1137
37. Yiou R, Vons C, Franco D (1997) Traitement de l'hydrothorax du cirrhotique par une valve de dérivation pleuro-péritonéale. Gastroentérol Clin Biol 20:1135
38. Montanari M, Orsi P, Pugliano G (1996) Hepatic hydrothorax without diaphragmatic defect. An original surgical treatment. J Cardiovasc Surg 37:425-427
39. Vadeyar HJ, Doran JD, Charnley R, Ryder SD (1999) Saphenoperitoneal shunts for patients with intractable ascites associated with chronic liver disease. Br J Surg 86:882-885

Invited Comment

Sheila Sherlock

The development of ascites in a patient with cirrhosis is a serious event implying a 5-year survival of 50%. Moreover, if the ascites proves resistant to diuretic therapy, the 5-year outlook is only 20%. Ascites therefore predicts liver failure and, for surgeons particularly, the "when," "where" and "if" of liver transplant must be considered.

The section by Bataller and Arroyo from the Barcelona Group gives comprehensive, largely standard textbook, account of the *medical management of ascites.* Figure 1 provides a good algorithm of medical management. An important discussion concerns the use of drugs which selectively increase water excretion and are of value in the dilutional hyponatremia developing with diuretic therapy. These selectively increased water excretion by acting on anti-diuretic hormone in the cortical collecting ducts or by inhibiting ADH release from the neurohypophysis [1]. Other reports are awaited.

Paracentesis abdominis, whether acute or chronic, is easy and gives satisfaction to both the operator and the patient. However, it has to be combined with intravenous albumin replacement, the gold standard. No other fluid replacement is as satisfactory. However, cost limits its use [2]. In the United States, albumin costs $5 to $25 per gram and at least 175 g are probably required for a 70-kg patient [3].

Infections are common in cirrhotic patients, with or without ascites. They are largely derived from bacterial toxins with endotoxemia.

This symposium does not discuss the early diagnosis and treatment of *spontaneous bacterial infection* of the ascites or of infections generally in cirrhotic patients [4]. Infections are particularly important when TIPS have been inserted or LeVeen shunts used. How did the authors propose to prevent this occurrence? The long-term use of antibiotics such as norfloxacin is followed by the development of bacterial resistance [5]. What other antibiotic regimes do the authors suggest?

TIPS is a noninvasive portal-systemic venous shunt administered by radiologists. It has all the complications of surgical shunts. This lowers the portal hypertension and improves renal sodium excretion [6]. Its use is limited to patients with no underlying cardiopulmonary disease, good renal function (creatinine lower than 250), serum bilirubin level less than 300, and no encephalopathy or sepsis. The improved renal function is of particular value in obtaining better hepatic transplant results. Indeed in some patients, the improved quality of life after TIPS results in the transplant becoming delayed or indeed unnecessary. In most instances, however, TIPS should be regarded as a pretransplant procedure. The present chapter by Pomier-Layrargues and Hassoun from Montreal gives a good comprehensive review of results. It is difficult to decipher the author's personal views.

Dominique Franco from Paris discusses *operative management.* A case can be made for the occasional use of side-to-side surgical porta-caval anastomosis [7] to select better risk patients who will stand surgical operative techniques. It may be of use in centers which cannot offer TIPS and transplant. Franco believes, as I do, that surgical risk and postoperative encephalopathy rates are strong arguments against this treatment of ascites.

In 1974, LeVeen [8] introduced the *peritonejugular shunt.* Complications are many, particularly coagulation disorders, acute heart failure and severe infection. However, improved techniques such as initial operative drainage of ascites, antibiotics and diuretics improve the results. Occasional successes are seen in stable cirrhotics, particularly alcoholic patients who stop drinking. I wonder how often the LeVeen shunt is used today. It has been overtaken by TIPS and by hepatic transplantation.

These contributions are largely routine and noncontroversial. What a pity that spontaneous bacterial peritonitis and infections generally, the hepatorenal syndrome and especially hepatic transplantation were not discussed in more detail.

References

1. Gerbes AL, Guelberg V, Grosshadren C (1999) VPA-895, an orally active Vasopressin receptor antagonist, improves hyponatremia in patients with cirrhosis. A double-blind placebo controlled multicenter trial. Hepatology 30:419A
2. Runyon BA (1998) Management of adult patients with ascites caused by cirrhosis. Hepatology 27:264–272

3. Sort P, Navasa M, Arroyo V, et al. (1999) Effect of intravenous albumin on renal impairment and mortality in patients with cirrhosis and spontaneous bacterial peritonitis. N Engl J Med 341:403–409
4. Goulis J, Patch D, Burroughs AK (1999) Bacterial infection in the pathogenesis of variceal bleeding. Lancet 353:139–142
5. Aparicio JR, Such J, Pascual S, et al. (1999) Development of quinolone-resistant strains of *Escherichia coli* in stools of patients with cirrhosis undergoing norfloxacin prophylaxis: clinical consequences. J Hepatol 31:277–283
6. Wong F, Blendis L (1995) Transjugular intrahepatic portosystemic shunt for refractory ascites: tipping the sodium balance. Hepatology 22:358–364
7. Orloff MJ, Orloff MS, Orloff SL, et al. (1997) Experimental, clinical and metabolic results of side-to-side porta-caval shunt for intractable cirrhotic ascites. J Am Coll Surg 184:557–570
8. Le Veen HH, Christoudias G, Moon IP, et al. (1974) Peritoneovenous shunting for ascites. Ann Surg 180:580–591

Editorial Comment

Drs. Bataller and Arroyo outline the modern conservative management of ascites, Drs. Pomier-Layragues and Hassoun discuss the somewhat limited role of the TIPS procedure and Dr. Franco the very limited role of the peritoneovenous shunt. Sheila Sherlock – the Dame of Hepatology – asserts that the above contributions are "largely routine and noncontroversial" and is disappointed that the role of hepatic transplantation, the management of the hepatorenal syndrome and spontaneous bacterial peritonitis were not discussed in more detail. The role of hepatic transplantation in patients with end-stage portal hypertension was, however, discussed in a previous volume of this series [1, 2] and the others will be included in future volumes.

None of the contributors to this chapter mentioned that the adverse physiological effects of ascites, and the benefits of its successful treatment, are "mediated," at least partially, through mechanisms related to the increased intra-abdominal pressure (IAP). Tense ascites in cirrhotics represents an acute on chronic abdominal compartment syndrome [3]; IAP, when measured noninvasively via a bladder catheter, is an accurate and useful parameter to follow manipulation of ascitic fluid pressure quantitatively in order to optimize the hemodynamics and renal function [4, 5].

Recently, Rossle, et al. [6] randomized 60 patients with cirrhosis and refractory or recurrent ascites (Child-Pugh class B in 42 patients and class C in 18 patients) to treatment with TIPS (29 patients) or large-volume paracentesis (31 patients). The primary outcome measured was survival without liver transplantation. In the TIPS group, 15 died and one underwent liver transplantation during the study period, as compared with 23 patients and 2 patients, respectively, in the paracentesis group. The probability of survival without liver transplantation was 69% at 1 year and 58% at 2 years in the TIPS group, as compared with 52% and 32% in the paracentesis group ($P=0.11$). In a multivariate analysis, treatment with TIPS was independently associated with survival without the need for transplantation ($P=0.02$). At 3 months, 61% of the patients in the TIPS group and 18% of those in the paracentesis group had no ascites ($P=0.006$). The frequency of hepatic encephalopathy was similar in the two groups. The authors concluded that in comparison with large-volume paracentesis, the creation of TIPS could improve the chance of survival without liver transplantation in patients with refractory or recurrent ascites.

Other forms of ascites - malignant or pancreatic - are "another story" and a subject for future chapters.

References

1. Adam R, Bismuth H (1997) The role of hepatic transplantation - the French view. In: Schein M, Wise L (eds) Crucial controversies in surgery. Karger Landes Systems, Basel, p 159
2. Knechte SJ, Rikkers LF (1997) The role of hepatic transplantation - the American view. In: Schein M, Wise L (eds) Crucial controversies in surgery. Karger Landes Systems, Basel, p 166
3. Schein M, Wittmann DH, Aprahamian CC, Condon RE (1995) The abdominal compartment syndrome: the physiological and clinical consequences of elevated intra-abdominal pressure. J Am Coll Surg 180:745–753
4. Savino JA, Cerabona T, Agarwal N, Byrne D (1988) Manipulation of ascitic fluid pressure in cirrhotics to optimize hemodynamic and renal function. Ann Surg 208:504–511
5. Luca A, Cirera I, Garcia-Pagan JC, Feu F, Pizcueta P, Bosch J, Rodes J (1993) Hemodynamic effects of acute changes in intra-abdominal pressure in patients with cirrhosis. Gastroenterology 104:222–227
6. Rossle M, Ochs A, Gulberg V, et al. (2000) A comparison of paracentesis and transjugular intrahepatic portosystemic shunting in patients with ascites. N Engl J Med 342:1701–1707

CHAPTER 10

Surgical Intensive Care Unit

Ventilation Strategies in the Surgical Intensive Care Unit

Philip S. Barie

"Less is more" characterizes the trends in ventilation strategies. The minimalist approach is to avoid intubating the airway at all. Noninvasive positive pressure ventilation (NPPV) uses a gas-tight facemask to deliver volume- or pressure-controlled mechanical ventilator breaths, bi-level positive airway pressure (BIPAP), or continuous positive airway pressure (CPAP) [1]. Several studies suggest that NPPV may avoid intubation and decrease the risk of nosocomial pneumonia in patients with acute exacerbations of chronic obstructive pulmonary disease (COPD), and limited data suggest that NPPV may be used for other causes of acute respiratory failure [2], and as an adjunct to weaning [3].

Data are quite limited for the use of NPPV in surgical units, and circumspection is warranted. The mask is cumbersome, and an ill-fitting mask diminishes the effectiveness markedly. Noninvasive PPV should not be used in obtunded patients, and should be used with care in patients with copious airway secretions. Extra effort must be made to ensure airway patency, because routine suctioning during NPPV requires that the facial seal of the mask be disrupted. For tenuous postextubation airways, NPPV will occasionally stave off reintubation. For the stridorous airway, ventilation with heliox (a 60% He:40% O_2 mixture) [4] may be beneficial whether NPPV or a conventional face mask is used, owing to less viscosity and favorable air flow characteristics compared with N_2:O_2 mixtures.

Protective Ventilation

Protective ventilation strategies for intubated patients are rapidly becoming accepted after a prolonged period of controversy. One way to characterize the acute respiratory distress syndrome (ARDS) is by loss of lung volume and decreased functional residual capacity (FRC) as a result of alveolar collapse [5]. The controversy centered around whether the lungs should be ventilated with a high tidal volume (V_T) and level of positive end-expiratory pressure (PEEP) to maximize alveolar recruitment and thereby reduce ventilation–perfusion inequality and shunt, while maximizing lung volume and FRC. The counter-argument states that the use of high-V_T, high-PEEP ventilation would overdistend and injure the remaining small population of distensible alveoli, producing alveolar injury by barotrauma or volutrauma. By ventilating at lower V_T, (6–7 ml/kg), mean airway pressure (PAW_{mean}) and plateau pressure (P_{plat}) would be decreased and the propensity for iatrogenic lung injury thereby minimized. The latter approach has been validated by a major multicenter study of 861 patients [6] that was closed prematurely by its safety board for unequivocal evidence of efficacy. Patients with acute lung injury/ARDS who were ventilated with a V_T of 6 ml/kg had significantly fewer ventilator-free days and lower P_{plat} and mortality (30% vs. 40%) as compared with patients ventilated with a V_T of 12 ml/kg. This is the only randomized, controlled trial of any kind to show a mortality benefit in ARDS, and the low-V_T strategy is worthy of widespread incorporation into practice.

The low-V_T strategy calls into question whether other ventilator strategies are truly valuable [7] (e.g., inverse-ratio ventilation, which increases PAW_{mean} because of breath-stacking or auto-PEEP that results from insufficient time for exhalation). The controversy of how to determine the "best" level of PEEP for a patient persists [7]. The latest fad is to set the level of PEEP just above the lower inflection point on the inspiratory pressure–volume curve, in the belief that it reflects the lowest alveolar distending pressure sufficient to prevent cyclical alveolar collapse during the ventilatory cycle and consequent alveolar damage. In actuality, the pressure–volume curve is difficult to interpret and the lower inflection point is often impossible to discern.

Inhaled Nitric Oxide

Nitric oxide ($NO^\bullet$) has been heralded as therapy for cardiopulmonary disorders characterized by pulmonary hypertension, taking advantage of a potent but short-lived vasodilator response. Therapy must therefore be given as a continuous inhalation. Under pathologic conditions associated with excess concentrations of reactive oxygen species (ROS), $NO^\bullet$ and superoxide (O_2^-) react readily to form peroxynitrite (^-OONO). The actions of ^-OONO upon biomolecules such as lipids, proteins, and DNA include oxidation, peroxidation, and nitration [8]. Tyrosine phosphorylation is inhibited, surfactant function is impaired, and mitochondrial respiratory enzymes are inhibited by ^-OONO. The balance of oxidant versus antioxidant (scavenging of ROS) effects depends on the concentrations of the various species; therefore the inhaled [$NO^\bullet$] must be regulated carefully (5–40 ppm). Given these effects, it was rational to hypothesize that inhaled $NO^\bullet$ would be effective therapy for ARDS, which is characterized by pulmonary hypertension, the need for ventilation at an increased F_IO_2, and evidence of ROS generation, oxidant injury to lung tissue, and impaired surfactant function. Unfortunately, enthusiasm developed to a degree disproportionate to the modest findings of initial studies (reviewed in [9]).

Although inhaled $NO^\bullet$ in low doses (1–10 ppm) reduces mean pulmonary artery pressure effectively in a majority of patients (55%–70%) [10], the response abates rapidly as soon as the inhalation is stopped. Improved oxygenation has also been described [10, 11], but is similarly short-lasting. Published clinical trials have failed to demonstrate reduced mortality or a decreased duration of mechanical ventilation in ARDS [10, 12], possibly because overall organ dysfunction, not gas exchange, is the primary determinant of outcome in ARDS [9]. It is also possible that the toxicity offsets the benefit, or that the therapeutic index is too narrow for safe use. Regardless, inhaled NO• currently has no therapeutic role in ARDS outside of formal scientific studies, even as salvage therapy.

Weaning from Mechanical Ventilation

Although modern microprocessor-controlled mechanical ventilators are versatile tools for the management of patients with respiratory failure, ventilator support must be withdrawn as soon as possible to avoid nosocomial complications, increased expense, and frustration for patients, families, and caregivers. The process of withdrawal of mechanical ventilation presupposes that the underlying cause of respiratory failure has been corrected, and that no iatrogenic abnormalities (e.g., inappropriate ventilator settings, compromised airway patency) persist [13]. The patient should have stable hemodynamics and causes of excessive respiratory muscle loads [minute ventilation (V_E) >20 l/min] – e.g., bronchospasm, increased dead space ventilation – should be reversed before beginning the weaning process because excessive loads are the most common causes of unsuccessful weaning.

Numerous assessment tools have been championed to determine whether the patient is ready to breathe unassisted. Weaning parameters – V_T, vital capacity (VC), maximal inspiratory pressure (PI_{max}, sometimes referred to as negative inspiratory force-NIF) – are popular but depend on a cooperative patient making a maximal effort, which may not be possible in a given circumstance. A PI_{max} greater than 25 cm/H_2O is often used as a criterion, but studies in surgical patients showed poor specificity and an area under the receiver-operator characteristic (ROC) curve of only 0.68 (0.50 equals a chance event, whereas 1.00 demonstrates perfect discrimination for a dichotomous event) [14]. No data whatsoever support use of either V_T or VC as a predictor. Nor is there much support for the use of estimates of respiratory muscle load, e.g., V_E, static respiratory system compliance (Crs_{stat}), and airway resistance, to predict success, despite its importance for successful weaning. A V_E of less than 10 l/min has been associated with weaning success, but the ROC area was only 0.54 [14]. The discrimination of Crs_{stat} is somewhat better (ROC area 0.68) [15], but still below the 0.80 threshold for meaningful clinical utility. No studies have examined whether there is a value of airway resistance that precludes successful weaning [13]. In aggregate, these studies may be helpful to diagnose a reversible cause in the patient who has failed a trial of spontaneous breathing (see below).

Several integrative indices have been described for predictive purposes, incorporating several different parameters. The CROP Index (compliance, rate, oxygenation, pressure) uses the equation:

$$CROP = Crs_{dynamic} \times Pi_{max} \times (PaO_2/P_AO_2)/frequency \quad (1)$$

to predict weaning success. In one study, a CROP greater than 13 had a ROC curve area of 0.78 [14], but its cumbersome nature has precluded widespread adoption. In contrast, the Rapid Shallow Breathing Index (RVR, f/VT, "Tobin Index") [14, 15] is simple and quite accurate (ROC area 0.89), performing better than V_E and PI_{max} in comparative studies [14]. The threshold that best predicts weaning outcome is a respiratory rate: V_T ratio less than 105 breaths per minute per liter, but RVR may be proportional to endotracheal tube diameter and higher in females [16]. Therefore, specificity is low and false-positives are possible, so an RVR less than 105 should prompt a 30–120-min trial of spontaneous ventilation prior to extubation. Although the RVR appears to be the single best predictor, and worthy of general adoption, the obligation to ensure that the patient is ready for weaning and extubation remains [17]. Before assessing the RVR, any sedative/narcotic effects should be allowed to wear off, and the patient should trigger more than 2–3 breaths/min above the set ventilator rate.

The choice of whether to rely upon inspiratory pressure support [18], CPAP, or T-piece trials to test patient readiness remains a matter of physician preference, as controlled studies show similar rates of failure [19]. For patients who fail, elevated respiratory load, neuromuscular competence, cardiovascular stability, ventilator/breathing circuit integrity, and psychological status should be evaluated. The writer prefers to wean patients using intermittent mandatory ventilation (IMV) if the trial of spontaneous ventilation has failed. Pressure support may be used as a stand-alone modality, but there is no backup mode, so that strategy should be avoided in patients predisposed to apnea. However, pressure support, which augments inspiratory gas flow and decreases the work of breathing, can be used in conjunction with IMV, although IMV itself remains controversial [20]. If conversion to IMV causes agitation or tachypnea, it is usually manageable with the addition of pressure support (10–20 cm H_2O), which is titrated to produce the desired exhaled V_T and then weaned as tolerated.

Most ventilator weaning decisions are made by physicians, with one result being that incremental steps are taken only when rounds are made or the physician is present on the unit. The net result may be a conservative (and slow) approach, wherein weaning never occurs at "off" hours, and mechanical ventilation is prolonged. Several studies [21, 22] indicate that protocol-directed weaning has advantages compared with conventional physician-directed weaning. In protocol-directed weaning, incremental progress is made when the patient reaches specified, predefined milestones in the weaning process, regardless of the time of day. Weaning can be managed by the bedside nurse or the respiratory therapist without physician input at each step. In a randomized, controlled trial [21], protocolized weaning led to extubation more often, sooner, and with equal safety. Similar results were obtained in a before–after comparison trial [22], wherein the duration of mechanical ventilation was reduced by a mean of 58 h, the ICU stay was reduced by 1.77 days, and cost was reduced by more than $600,000. In the writer's opinion, protocol-directed weaning is a genuine advance that should be implemented in every ICU as part of an overall process improvement program.

Tracheostomy

The timing of tracheostomy and the optimal method to establish a surgical airway remain controversial. Tracheostomy facilitates pulmonary toilet, and decreases the work of breathing. Because the work of breathing is decreased, weaning may be facilitated, so it may be shortsighted to reserve tracheostomy until several attempts at weaning have failed. It is unresolved whether tracheostomy increases or decreases the risk of nosocomial pneumonia, because it has been difficult to distinguish the role of the airway from prolonged ventilator dependence, itself a known risk factor for pneumonia. The issue of timing remains important despite the fact that improved endotracheal tube technology has decreased the risk of occlusion balloon-related complications. Especially for patients who primarily need airway protection to reduce the risk of aspiration (e.g., neurosurgical patients), early tracheostomy may shorten ICU length of stay and thereby decrease cost. If pneumonia is avoidable, then the benefit of early tracheostomy (within 3–5 days) would accrue to many more patients. Unfortunately, a randomized, controlled trial designed to answer these questions failed because of poor patient accrual [23]. Physician bias limited entry into the study, and statistical power was inadequate to assess the primary endpoints of ICU length of stay, pneumonia, or death.

Percutaneous tracheostomy is gaining favor as a bedside procedure, but debate continues regarding its safety and the optimum technique to be used (e.g., with fiberoptic bronchoscopic guidance). More than 30 trials have now been published and reviewed by the technique of meta-analysis [24]. Percutaneous tracheostomy is associated with a statistically higher incidence of insertion-related and early postoperative complications, including cardiorespiratory arrests and death, but the difference between the techniques is less than 2%. In contrast, late postoperative complications are significantly more likely after open tracheostomy [24]. On balance, the writer favors early percutaneous tracheostomy under bronchoscopic control.

References

1. Rabatin JT, Gay PC (1999) Noninvasive ventilation. Mayo Clin Proc 74:817–820
2. Martin TJ, Hovis JD, Costantino JP, et al. (2000) A randomized, prospective evaluation of noninvasive ventilation for acute respiratory failure. Am J Respir Crit Care Med 161:807–813
3. Nava S, Ambrosino N, Clini E, et al. (1988) Noninvasive mechanical ventilation in the weaning of patients with respiratory failure due to chronic obstructive pulmonary disease. A randomized controlled trial. Ann Intern Med 128:721–728
4. Jolliet P, Tassaux D, Thouret JM, Chevrolet JC (1999) Beneficial effects of helium:oxygen versus air:oxygen noninvasive pressure support in patients with decompensated chronic obstructive pulmonary disease. Crit Care Med 27:2422–2429
5. Sandur S, Stoller JK (1999) Pulmonary complications of mechanical ventilation. Clin Chest Med 20:223–247
6. The Acute Respiratory Distress Syndrome Network. (2000) Ventilation with lower tidal volumes as compared with traditional tidal volumes for acute lung injury and the acute respiratory distress syndrome. N Engl J Med 342:1301–1308
7. Hirvela ER (2000) Advances in the management of acute respiratory distress syndrome. Protective ventilation. Arch Surg 135:126–135
8. Szabo C (1996) The pathophysiological role of peroxynitrite in shock, inflammation, and ischemia-reperfusion injury. Shock 6:79–88
9. Steudel W, Hurford WE, Zapol WM (1999) Inhaled nitric oxide. Basic biology and clinical applications. Anesthesiology 91:1090–1121
10. Dellinger EP, Zimmerman JL, Taylor RW, et al. (1998) Effects of inhaled nitric oxide in patients with acute respiratory distress syndrome: results of a randomized Phase II trial. Crit Care Med 26:15–23
11. Gerlach H, Rossaint R, Pappert D, Falke KJ (1993) Time-course and dose-response of nitric oxide inhalation for systemic oxygenation and pulmonary hypertension in patients with adult respiratory distress syndrome. Eur J Clin Invest 23:499–502

12. Troncy E, Collet JP, Shapiro S, et al. (1998) Inhaled nitric oxide in acute respiratory distress syndrome. Crit Care Med 157:1483–1488
13. Manthous CA, Schmidt GA, Hall JB (1998) Liberation from mechanical ventilation. A decade of progress. Chest 114:886–901
14. Jacob B, Chatila W, Manthous CA (1996) The unassisted respiratory rate:tidal volume ratio accurately predicts weaning outcome. Crit Care Med 101:61–67
15. Yang KL, Tobin MJ (1991) A prospective study of indexes predicting the outcome of trials of weaning from mechanical ventilation. N Engl J Med 324:1445–1450
16. Epstein SK, Ciubotaru RL (1996) Influence of gender and endotracheal tube size on preextubation breathing pattern. Am J Respir Crit Care Med 154:1647–1652
17. Johannigman JA, Davis K Jr, Campbell RS, et al. (1997) Use of the rapid shallow breathing index as an indicator of patient work of breathing during pressure support ventilation. Surgery 122:737–740
18. Dekel B, Segal E, Perel A (1996) Pressure support ventilation. Arch Intern Med 156:369–373
19. Esteban A, Alia A, Gardo F, et al. (1997) Extubation outcome after spontaneous breathing trials with T-tube or pressure support ventilation. Am J Respir Crit Care Med 156:459–465
20. Dries DJ (1997) Weaning from mechanical ventilation. J Trauma 43:372–384
21. Kollef MH, Shapiro SD, Silver P, et al. (1997) A randomized, controlled trial of protocol-directed versus physician-directed weaning from mechanical ventilation. Crit Care Med 25:567–574
22. Horst HM, Mouro D, Hall-Jenssens RA, Pamukov N (1998) Decrease in ventilation time with a standardized weaning process. Arch Surg 133:483–488
23. Sugerman HJ, Wolfe L, Pasquale MD, et al. (1997) Multicenter, randomized prospective trial of early tracheostomy. J Trauma 43:741–747
24. Dulgerov P, Gysin C, Pergener TV, Chevrolet JC (1999) Percutaneous or surgical tracheostomy: a meta-analysis. Crit Care Med 27:1617–1625

Hemodynamic Monitoring and Support

David T. Harrington · William G. Cioffi

Hemodynamic Monitoring

In a landmark 1996 article, Connors et al. concluded that pulmonary artery catheters (PAC) are potentially dangerous and were responsible for added mortality in the critically ill population they studied [7]. Though this was not the first critical assessment of PACs, the large number of patients analyzed in this paper (n=5735) lead to the authors' bold assertion of added mortality and served as a scathing criticism of the prevailing management of critically ill patients. In the wake of this article old and new questions arise as to the ideal method to manage the hemodynamic status of the intensive care patient. We will address four questions in this article:

- Do pulmonary artery catheters improve patient outcomes?
- Should pulmonary artery catheters be used to maximize oxygen delivery?
- Are MvO_2 (mixed venous saturation), RVEDV (right ventricular end-diastolic volume), and CCO (continuous cardiac output) catheters superior to the standard pulmonary artery catheter?
- Will the monitoring of individual tissue beds replace global indexes of perfusion in the modern ICU?

Do Pulmonary Artery Catheters Improve Patient Outcomes?

Yes. PACs are an accurate and vital tool in the management of the critically ill patient, providing two critical pieces of information: pre-load and cardiac output. The ability of the clinician to assess these parameters is no better than a flip of a coin without a PAC, especially in the patient with respiratory failure [8, 12, 13, 24, 33]. While the information from a PAC may not improve outcomes in all patients, it has been shown that several high-risk populations such as patients with myocardial infarction complicated by cardiogenic shock, high-risk vascular patients undergoing peripheral vascular or aortic surgery, and trauma patients have better outcomes when a PAC is used [1, 3, 20, 28, 36]. The catheters are safe with reported morbidity, such as pneumothorax, hemothorax, and line infection, occurring in less than 5% of patients [27, 37].

No. Though the PAC may be an accurate tool, clinicians cannot reliably interpret the PAC waveforms [23, 30]. Data supporting improved outcomes in patients managed with PAC are not from well-powered, randomized and prospective trials and, therefore, cannot be used to prove the clinical utility of PAC. Furthermore, several trials - some retrospective, others prospective - have suggested that PAC may actually increase morbidity [16, 17, 19]. The largest and best powered of these trials was reported in the 1996 JAMA article by Connors. Using a "propensity score" (propensity to receive a PAC) and performing a case-matching analysis to control for comorbidities and acute illness, Connors prospectively analyzed 5,735 ICU patients and found statistically increased mortality in the patients managed with a PAC in the first 24 h of their intensive care unit stay compared to their matched cohorts who did not receive a PAC [7]. Sources of the excess mortality were not clearly elucidated, but could include a direct morbidity from the catheter in terms of bleeding or infection, reflect the misinterpretation of data from the PAC by the clinician, or reflect an aggressive style of management (over-resuscitation or supranormal cardiac output) by the clinician that was not tolerated by the patient. In addition to the added morbidity of the catheter, PAC increases length of stay, the use of inotropic drugs, and hospital costs [32, 34].

Conclusion. Though the Connors study design was thoughtful and thorough, it was not a randomized control trial and, therefore, did not control for who received a PAC or in what manner the PAC data were used. Multiple obstacles prevent appropriate assessment of the clinical impact of the PAC: different population groups (sepsis, elderly, cardiac, and trauma patients), therapeutic plans (resuscitation, supranormal cardiac output), confounding variables (sedation/paralysis regimes, ventilatory management, and nutritional support), and ethical issues of randomization. Since it is unlikely that the clinical impact of the PAC can be measured, what is the role of the PAC in the year 2000? Since clinical assessment does not reliably reflect the hemodynamic status of the patient, PAC should be used when conventional data are equivocal or conflicting or in the high-risk perioperative patient. The PAC should not be used only for pulmonary artery occlusion pressure (PAOP) and cardiac output, but also for other important data, such as mixed venous oxygen saturation, oxygen consumption, and oxygen extraction ratio, which should be used to direct therapy. Finally, to ensure that accurate information is obtained, ICUs should educate their staff and enforce standards for the interpretation and use of PACs.

Should Pulmonary Artery Catheters Be Used to Maximize Oxygen Delivery?

Yes. Multiple patient series have shown that low cardiac output and oxygen delivery states are risk factors for organ failure and mortality [3, 31]. Two prospective randomized trials have shown that driving oxygen delivery index (DO_2I) to above 600 ml/min per square meter leads to improved survival [2, 35]. Though critics state that this technique only reduces morbidity in patients with normal cardiac function, early identification of nonresponders may lead to further therapeutic interventions.

No. Good medical care is often the difference between what can be done and what should be done. Intensive treatment of non-Q wave myocardial infarction with stress tests, angiography/angioplasty and coronary artery bypass grafting and intensive suppressive therapy of cardiac arrhythmias with flecainide/encainide was shown to increase mortality when compared to standard treatment in randomized, prospective trials [4, 10]. While increasing cardiac output and oxygen delivery and consumption may be possible, it is not clear that this improves outcome. Blind application of any approach to all patients with a particular disease will result in an increased morbidity [14, 19].

Conclusion. The majority of patients who end up with a PAC do not have unisystem failure and may be intolerant of volume loading necessary for supranormal oxygen delivery because of pulmonary dysfunction and widened A-aO_2 gradients. Many of these patients will require inotropic therapy to achieve the predetermined endpoints. The morbidity associated with this approach may partially explain the increased mortality associated with PAC in Connors' paper [7]. An individualized approach is warranted in which patients with evidence of a mounting O_2 debt should be treated in a manner to maximize O_2 delivery and consumption. Although this is a difficult diagnosis to make, this represents a perfect example of how a single measurement or test cannot totally replace clinical judgment. It should also be noted that in the trials of supranormal versus standard therapy, the excess mortality occurred in the patients who were not capable of mounting this response either on their own or iatrogenically [2, 35]. Supranormal oxygen delivery should not be used as a treatment regimen for all patients.

Are RVEDV, MvO_2, and CCO Catheters Superior to the Standard Pulmonary Artery Catheter?

Yes. RVEDV catheters, by the use of a more efficient dispersion of the thermal bolus and integrated EKG monitoring, can calculate an RVEDV and eliminate the error inherent in standard PAC, which assumes that the pressure–volume relationship of the ventricle remains constant and that PAOP equals left atrial pressure (LAP), which equals left ventricular end-diastolic pressure (LVEDP), which equals left ventricular end-diastolic volume (LVEDV) [11, 15, 22]. RVEDV more closely estimates LVEDV than PAOP and allows accurate guiding of fluid resuscitative strategies [8, 9]. Further, RVEDV catheters can measure right ventricular ejection fraction (RVEF), which can be a sensitive marker of RV failure and an early indicator of the failure of volume loading [30]. MvO_2 and CCO catheters provide rapid, invaluable data that facilitates the monitoring of trends and titration of therapies in critically ill patients [38].

No. The RVEDV catheters calculate RVEDV and RVEF by analyzing the exponential decay of the thermodilution curve, which is related to cardiac output. The stronger statistical relationship of RVEDV versus PAOP to changes in cardiac output is based on the RVEDV's mathematical coupling to cardiac output, not its inherently superior accuracy. Furthermore, RVEF does not necessarily reflect right ventricular function, for RVEF is more influenced by pulmonary artery pressure than right ventricular contractility. These catheters add more data points to the ICU flow sheet but do not improve outcomes.

Conclusion. These catheters provide valuable data on the critically ill patient, data not obtainable with a standard PAC. Pressure and volume are not linearly related, which at least partially explains why RVEDV and not PAOP more accurately predicts response to volume loading [8]. The continuous nature of the data provided by MvO_2 and CCO catheters appears advantageous since these catheters allow for minute-to-minute titration of therapy. The cost of these catheters, which is 2–4 times the cost of the standard PAC, demands that they be used only in patients for whom a standard PAC is deemed inadequate.

Will Monitoring of Individual Tissue Beds Such as the Gut or Skeletal Muscle Replace Global Indexes of Perfusion in the Modern ICU?

Yes. The gut and splanchnic circulation have been identified as the engine of the systemic inflammatory response syndrome [29]. Skeletal muscle appears to suffer from prolonged ischemia following shock, perhaps allowing for significant loss of vital protein stores [26]. Global O_2 utilization indicators such as MvO_2 and oxygen extraction ratios do not accurately describe the state of these vital tissue beds [6]. To address these key sources of critical illness, we must develop monitoring systems such as gastrointestinal tonometry, laser Doppler probes and near-infrared spectroscopy so that treatment can be tailored to protect these organs [5, 18, 21, 25].

No. Even the standard PAC provides clinical data that cannot be accurately assessed by physical examination: volume status, cardiac output, and O_2 consumption. Treatments based on this information have been shown to improve outcomes in high-risk patients [1, 3, 20, 28, 36]. Though gut tonometry is a potentially useful monitoring tool, it is labor intensive and often unreliable, and to date treatments based on optimizing mucosal pH have not been shown to improve outcomes.

Conclusion. Monitoring of global indexes and tissue beds will exist side by side in the modern ICU. Much of the improved outcomes in surgery over the last three decades reflect better perioperative monitoring and careful resuscitation. However, further improvements in care will be manifested not as a dramatic reduction of already low mortality rates, but as an improvement in functional outcomes. Recognizing the importance of vital tissue beds and techniques to monitor and treat them will be the challenge of the next generation. Patients in whom tissue ischemia is recognized will likely be the ones who will benefit from attempts to achieve supranormal hemodynamic function.

References

1. Berlauk JF, Abrams JH, Gilmour IJ, et al. (1991) Preoperative optimization of cardiovascular hemodynamics improves outcome in peripheral vascular surgery: a prospective, randomized clinical trial. Ann Surg 214:289–297
2. Bishop MH, Shoemaker WC, Appel PL, et al. (1995) Prospective, randomized trial of survivor values of cardiac index, oxygen delivery, and oxygen consumption as resuscitation endpoints in severe trauma. J Trauma 38:780–787
3. Bishop MH, Shoemaker WC, Appel PL, et al. (1993) Relationship between supranormal circulatory values, time delays, and outcome in severely traumatized patients. Crit Care Med 21:56–63
4. Boden WE, O'Rourke RA, Crawford MH, et al. (1998) Outcomes in patients with acute non-Q-wave myocardial infarction randomly assigned to an invasive as compared with a conservative management strategy. N Engl J Med 338:1785–1792
5. Chang MC, Cheatham ML, Nelson LD, et al. (1994) Gastric tonometry supplements information provided by systemic indicators of oxygen transport. J Trauma 37:488–494
6. Chang MC, Meredith JW (1997) Cardiac preload, splanchnic perfusion, and their relationship during resuscitation in trauma patients. J Trauma 42:577–582
7. Connors AF, Speroff T, Dawson N, et al. (1996) The effectiveness of right heart catheterization in the initial care of critically ill patients. JAMA 276:889–897
8. Diebel LN, Wilson RF, Tagett MG, et al. (1992) End-diastolic volume: better indicators of preload in the critically ill. Arch Surg 127:817–822
9. Durham R, Neunaber K, Vogler G, et al. (1995) Right ventricular end-diastolic volume as a measure of preload. J Trauma 39:218–223
10. Echt DS, Liebson PR, Mitchell LB, et al. (1991) Mortality and morbidity in patients receiving encainide, flecainide, or placebo. The Cardiac Arrhythmia Suppression Trial. N Engl J Med 324:781–788
11. Eddy AC, Rice CL, Anardi DM (1988) Right ventricular dysfunction in multiple trauma victims. Am J Surg 155:712–715
12. Eisenberg PR, Jaffe AS, Schuster DP (1984) Clinical evaluation compared to pulmonary artery catheterization in the hemodynamic assessment of critically ill patients. Crit Care Med 12:549–553
13. Fein AM, Goldberg, SK, Walkenstein MD, et al. (1984) Is pulmonary artery catheterization necessary for the diagnosis of pulmonary edema? Am Rev Respir Dis 129:1006–1009
14. Gattinoni L, Brazzi L, Pelosi P, et al. (1995) A trial of goal-oriented hemodynamic therapy in critically ill patients: SvO_2 Collaborative Group. N Engl J Med 333:1025–1032
15. Glantz SA, Parmley WW (1978) Factors which affect the diastolic pressure-volume curve. Circ Res 42:171–180
16. Gore JM, Goldberg RJ, Spodick DH, et al. (1987) A community-wide assessment of the use of pulmonary artery catheters in patients with acute myocardial infarction. Chest 92:721–727
17. Guyatt G (1991) A randomized control trial of right-heart catheterization in critically ill patients. Ontario Intensive Care Study Group. J Intensive Care Med 6:91–95
18. Hamilton-Davies C, Mythen MG, Salmon JB, et al. (1997) Comparison of commonly used indicators of hypovolaemia with gastrointestinal tonometry. Intensive Care Med 23:276–281
19. Hayes MA, Timmins AC, Yau EH, et al. (1994) Elevation of systemic oxygen delivery in the treatment of critically ill patients. N Engl J Med 330:1717–1722
20. Hochman JS, Boland J, Sleeper LA, et al. (1995) Current spectrum of cardiogenic shock and effect of early revascularization on mortality: results of an International Registry, SHOCK Registry Investigators. Circulation 91:873–881
21. Ivatury RR, Simon RJ, Havriliak D, et al. (1995) Gastric mucosal pH and oxygen delivery and oxygen consumption indices in the assessment of adequacy of resuscitation after trauma: A prospective, randomized study. J Trauma 39:128–134

22. Janicki JS, Weber KT (1980) Factors influencing the diastolic pressure-volume relation of the cardiac ventricles. Fed Proc 39:133–140
23. Komadina KH, Schenk DA, LaVeau P, et al. (1991) Interobserver variability in the interpretation of pulmonary artery catheter pressure tracings. Chest 100:1647–1654
24. Lappas D, Lell WA, Gabel, et al. (1973) Indirect measurement of left-atrial pressure in surgical patients – pulmonary-capillary wedge and pulmonary-artery diastolic pressures compared with left-atrial pressure. Anesthesiology 38:394–397
25. Madan AK, UyBarreta VV, Aliabadi-Wahle S, et al. (1999) Esophageal Doppler ultrasound monitor versus pulmonary artery catheter in the hemodynamic management of critically ill surgical patients. J Trauma 46:607–611
26. McKinley BA, Butler BD (1999) Comparison of skeletal muscle PO_2, PCO_2, and pH with gastric tonometric $P(CO_2)$ and pH in hemorrhagic shock. Crit Care Med 27:1869–1877
27. Miller JA, Singireddy S, Maldjian P, et al. (1999) A reevaluation of the radiographically detectable complications of percutaneous venous access lines inserted by four subcutaneous approaches. Am Surg 65:125–130
28. Mimoz O, Rauss A, Rekik N, et al. (1994) Pulmonary artery catheterization in critically ill patients: A prospective analysis of outcome changes associated with catheter-prompted changes in therapy. Crit Care Med 22:573–579
29. Moore EE, Moore FA, Franciose RJ, et al. (1994) The post-ischemic gut serves as a priming bed for circulating neutrophils that provoke multiple organ failure. J Trauma 37:881–887
30. Moore FA, Chang M, Cryer HG, et al. (1998) Symposium: Monitoring in the SICU: Current controversies in the use of pulmonary artery catheters. Contemporary Surg 53:213–228
31. Moore FA, Haenel JB, Moore EE, et al. (1992) Incommensurate oxygen consumption in response to maximal oxygen availability predicts postinjury multiple organ failure. J Trauma 33:58–65
32. Shoemaker WC (1990) Use and abuse of the balloon tip pulmonary artery (Swan-Ganz) catheter: Are patients getting their money's worth? Crit Care Med 18:1294–1296
33. Steingrub JS, Celoria G, Vickers-Lahti M, et al. (1991) Therapeutic impact of pulmonary artery catheterization in a medical/surgical ICU. Chest 99:1451–1455
34. Tuman KJ, McCarthy RJ, Spiess BD, et al. (1989) Effect of pulmonary artery catheterization on outcome in patients undergoing coronary artery surgery. Anesthesiology 70:199–206
35. Shoemaker WC, Appel PL, Kram HB, et al. (1988) Prospective trial of supranormal values of survivors of therapeutic goals in high-risk surgical patients. Chest 94:1176–1186
36. Whittemore AD, Clowes AW, Hechtman HB, et al (1980) Aortic aneurysm repair: reduced operative mortality associated with maintenance of optimal cardiac performance. Ann Surg 192:414–421
37. Yilmazlar A, Bilgin H, Korfali G, et al. (1997) Complications of 1303 central venous cannulations. J R Soc Med 90:319–321
38. Zollner C, Polasek J, Kilger E, et al. (1999) Evaluation of a new continuous thermodilution cardiac output monitor in cardiac surgical patients: a prospective criterion standard study. Crit Care Med 27:293–299

Renal Support

Bashar Fahoum

During the last 50 years, morbidity and mortality from renal failure have been declining but are still as high as 77% and 58%, respectively, in the setting of critical illness [1].

Etiology

Renal failure could result from the original insult or as a complication of treatment.

- Injury related: This includes shock, increased intra-abdominal pressure (IAP) [2], direct renal parenchymal injury, and crush injury leading to rhabdomyolysis.
- During treatment: This results from inadequate volume replacement or by adding nephrotoxic agents to an already injured kidney (e.g., contrast material, amimoglycosides).
- After treatment: This occurs within a few days to weeks after the initial insult and is usually due to an acquired insult during the course of treatment (e.g., multi-organ failure, increased IAP).

During the initial insult the proximal tubule is the first to be harmed because it is the most active portion of the nephron. If the insult is reversed early on, high output renal failure may develop; if it continues, a more extensive injury occurs causing an oliguric failure.

Pathophysiology

- Hypoperfusion: This is the most common mechanism. When renal blood flow is severely reduced, oxygen delivery is diminished, causing tubular swelling and necrosis [3].
- Sepsis: The damaging mechanism is hypovolemia, endotoxemia, and re-perfusion injury.
- Contrast media: This is a direct toxic effect on the tubular cells [4].
- Drugs: Aminoglycosides are the most common nephrotoxic drugs, acting through a direct insult to the mitochondria.

Assessment of Renal Function

Creatinine clearance remains the most accurate renal function test. Other tests include BUN, urine and serum electrolytes, and serum pH (metabolic acidosis).

Renal Support

Ensuring adequate oxygen delivery to the kidneys is the single most important factor to prevent renal injury in the critical-care setting. A few adjunctive modalities for renal support are available:

Diuretics. Diuretics have a role only after ensuring adequate renal blood flow. Brater has suggested that all diuretics except spironolactone must reach the lumen or urinary side of the nephron to exert their effects [5]. Thus, in settings of decreased renal function, doses must be high in order to deliver more diuretic into the urine. In edematous conditions such as cirrhosis and congestive heart failure, there is a diminished response due to unknown mechanisms, and combinations of diuretics, rather than large doses of a single diuretic, may be more effective in this setting. Others contend, however, that high doses of loop diuretics are the drugs of choice [6]. Diuretics decrease smooth muscle swelling and tubular destruction, but Epstein and Prasad pointed out that this occurs more in young subjects [7]. This has been attributed to a decline in renal prostaglandin production with increasing age. Shilliday et al. conducted a prospective, randomized, placebo-controlled, double-blind study and concluded that although diuretics given to patients with acute renal failure result in diuresis, there is no evidence that they alter outcome [8]. Furthermore, Lassnigg and coworkers concluded their prospective randomized study with the notion that diuretics have a detrimental effect in patients with renal dysfunction after cardiac surgery [9]. We therefore conclude, like others [10], that the protective role of loop diuretics in developing or established acute renal failure is unknown.

Dopamine. Dopamine, when administered in small does (1–5 μg/kg per minute) has a unique ability to increase renal blood flow by stimulation of dopamine receptors (D3) without any cardiac effects [11]. It has been suggested that this action is due to preferential postglomerular vasoconstriction [12], but other investigators have shown that the mechanism is mainly related to a direct tubular effect of dopamine [13]. Clark et al. attribute the diuretic effects of dopamine to the stimulation of alpha-adrenoceptors [14], and to opposing the effects of anti-natriuretic factors such as angiotensin II [15].

A few randomized trials assessing the value of dopamine in acute renal failure have been done. A limited study showed a renal-protective effect of low-dose dopamine (2 μg/kg per minute) during vigorous diuresis for congestive heart failure, associated with mild or moderate renal insufficiency [16]. Another study demonstrated an increased creatinine clearance with prolonged low-dose dopamine infusion [17]. These effects reached a maximum during 8 h of dopamine infusion but despite a slight persistent increase in diuresis the improvement in creatinine clearance disappeared after 48 h. The authors concluded that it is likely that tolerance develops to dopamine-receptor agonists in critically ill patients at risk of developing acute renal failure. Others arrived at identical conclusions suggesting dopamine-receptor desensitization [18].

It has become a common practice in critical care units to add "renal dose" dopamine to patients already receiving "vasopressors." One randomized trial concluded that the addition of dopamine (3 μg/kg per minute) to pressor doses of norepinephrine normalized renal blood flow in healthy volunteers; this however was not reflected in urine output and glomerular filtration rate [19]. In a similar study in healthy volunteers it was found that concomitant dopamine administration prevents the pressor-generated decrease in renal plasma flow, increases sodium excretion, and also attenuates the norepinephrine-induced systemic blood pressure increase [20]. Ichai et al. showed that a 4-h infusion of dopamine significantly increased creatinine clearance, diuresis, and the fractional excretion of sodium in stable critically ill patients. They suggested that although the level of mean arterial pressure might partially contribute to the improvement in renal variables, it is more likely that the activation of renal dopamine receptors played a prominent role [21]. Notably, cardiac side effects of low-dose dopamine, like arrhythmias, do occur, explained by the change of catecholamine receptor affinity to dopamine due to various factors including the serum pH.

So what is the verdict on dopamine? It is widely used to protect the kidney in intensive care units, but is it effective? Despite the aforementioned studies which suggested a transient benefit in terms of diuresis, no reliable evidence exists that "renal-dose dopamine" prevents or ameliorates renal function and modifies patient outcome. Therefore, I agree with Perdue et al. [22], who after an exhaustive review concluded that the routine use of prophylactic "renal dose dopamine" in surgical patients is not recommended. To promote diuresis dopamine should be used only in normovolemic patients with no cardiac irritability.

Atrial Natriuretic Peptide. This peptide is produced in the right atrium and increases the glomerular filtration rate and renal blood flow, and has been studied as a possible treatment for acute renal failure. A prospective randomized trial concluded that parenteral atrial natriuretic peptide (ANP) increases creatinine clearance and reduces the need for dialysis in patients with established acute renal failure, not changing, however, the rate of survival [23]. The clinical role of ANP remains under investigation.

Dialysis

The timing and frequency of dialysis depend on the indication.

- Absolute indications: Fluid overload with hypoxemia, drug overdose, uncontrolled hyperkalemia, and pericarditis.
- Relative indications: There are no magical levels of BUN/creatinine but most physicians agree the BUN >100 mg, or platelet dysfunction with bleeding are relative indications for dialysis.

Continuous Arteriovenous Hemofiltration

Critically ill patients who require dialysis but are hemodynamically unstable can undergo continuous arteriovenous hemofiltration (CAVH). CAVH does not require a pump but uses the patient's own blood pressure to pump the blood through a balanced electrolyte solution; solutes are removed via ultrafiltration [24]. It does require arterial and venous access, and heparin to minimize blood clotting. It has been shown that continuous venovenous hemodialysis (CVVHD) is safer and effective in hemodynamically unstable patients and has the advantage of requiring only one venous access [25]. CVVHD is well tolerated but the survival rate depends more on the severity of illness and the primary diagnosis than on the method of dialysis.

Conclusions

It appears that current pharmacological modalities used to protect acutely compromised kidneys are more a myth than a reality and, at best, remain controversial [26, 27]. Clearly, maintenance of renal perfusion by adequate volume replacement, timely management of remote infections, combating any factor, which may contribute to systemic inflammatory response syndrome, and avoidance of nephrotoxic agents, are the mainstay of renal support to prevent acute renal failure.

References

1. Morris JA, Mucha P., Ross SE, et al. (1991) Acute posttraumatic renal failure: a multi-central prospective. J Trauma 31:1584–1590
2. Harman PK, Kron IL, McLachlan HD, et al. (1982) Elevated intra-abdominal pressure and renal failure. Ann Surg 196:594–597
3. Klausner JM, Paterson IS, Goldman G, et al. (1989) Post ischemic renal injury. Am J Physiol 256:F794–802
4. Mudge GH (1980) Nephrotoxcity of urographic contrast drugs. Kidney Int 18:540–552
5. Brater DC (2000) Pharmacology of diuretics. Am J Med Sci 319:38–50
6. Risler T, Kramer B, Muller GA (1991) The efficacy of diuretics in acute and chronic renal failure. Focus on torasemide. Drugs 41[Suppl 3]:69–79
7. Epstein FH, Prasad P (2000) Effects of furosemide on medullary oxygenation in younger and older subjects. Kidney Int 57:2080–2083
8. Shilliday IR, Quinn KJ, Allison ME (1997) Loop diuretics in the management of acute renal failure: a prospective, double-blind, placebo-controlled, randomized study. Nephrol Dial Transplant 2:2592–2596
9. Lassnigg A, Donner E, Grubhofer G, et al. (2000) Lack of renoprotective effects of dopamine and furosemide during cardiac surgery. J Am Soc Nephrol 11:97–104
10. Allison ME, Shilliday I (1993) Loop diuretic therapy in acute and chronic renal failure. J Cardiovasc Pharmacol 22[Suppl 3]:S59–70
11. Chertow GM, Sayegh MH, Allgren, et al. (1996) Is the administration of dopamine associated with adverse or favorable outcomes in acute renal failure? Am J Med 101:49–53
12. Luippold G, Schneider S, Vallon V, et al. (2000) Postglomerular vasoconstriction induced by dopamine D(3) receptor activation in anesthetized rats. Am J Physol Renal Physiol 278:F570–575
13. Benmalek F, Behforouz N, Benoist J, et al. (1999) Renal effects of low-dose dopamine during vasopressor therapy for posttraumatic intracranial hypertension. Intensive Care Med 25:399–405
14. Clark KL, Robertson MJ, Drew GM (1991) Do renal tubular dopamine receptors mediate dopamine-induced diuresis in the anesthetized cat? J Cardiovasc Pharmacol 17:267–276
15. Aperia AC (2000) Intrarenal dopamine: a key signal in the interactive regulation of sodium metabolism. Annu Rev Physiol 62:621–647
16. Varriale P, Mossavi A (1997) The benefit of low-dose dopamine during vigorous diuresis for congestive heart failure associated with renal insufficiency: does it protect renal function? Clin Cardiol 20:627–630
17. Ichai C, Passeron C, Carles M, et al. (2000) Prolonged low-dose dopamine infusion induces a transient improvement in renal function in hemodynamically stable, critically ill patients: a single-blind, prospective, controlled study. Crit Care Med 28:1329–1335
18. Lherm T, Troche G, Rossignol M et al. (1996) Renal effects of low-dose dopamine in patients with sepsis syndrome or septic shock treated with catecholamines. Intensive Care Med 22:213–219
19. Richer M, Robert S, Lebel M (1996) Renal hemodynamics during norepinephrine and low-dose dopamine infusions in man. Crit Care Med 24:1150–1156
20. Hoogenberg K, Smit AJ, Girbes AR (1998) Effects of low-dose dopamine on renal and systemic hemodynamics during incremental morepinephrine infusion in healthy volunteers. Crit Care Med 26:260–266
21. Ichai C, Soubielle J, Carles M, et al. (2000) Comparison of the renal effects of low to high doses of dopamine and dobutamine in critically ill patients: a single-blind randomized study. Crit Care Med 28:921–928
22. Perdue PW, Baiser JR, Lipsett PA, et al. (1998) Renal dose dopamine in surgical patients: dogma vs science. Ann Surg 227:470–473
23. Rahman SN, Kim GE, Matthew AS, et al. (1994) Effect s of atrial natriuretic peptide in clinical renal failure. Kidney Int 45:1731–1738
24. Mehta RL (1994) Therapeutic alternatives to renal replacement for critically ill patients in acute renal failure. Sem in Neph 146–8 14; 64–82

25. Bellomo R, Farmer M, Boyce N (1995) A prospective study of continuous venovenous hemodiafiltration in critically ill patients with acute renal failure. J Intensive Care Med 10:187–192
26. Cosentino F (1995) Drugs for the prevention and treatment of acute renal failure. Cleve Clin J Med 62:248–53
27. Galley HF (2000) Can acute renal failure be prevented? J R Coll Surg Edinb 45:44–50

The Gut

Charles A. Adams Jr. · Edwin A. Deitch

Introduction

Over the past decade, new information regarding the role of the gut in critical illness has emerged, driving changes in the clinical management of critically ill patients. Today, the gut is viewed as both an indicator of systemic stress as well as a potential contributor to the systemic stress response in ICU patients. In the past, the role of the gut in critical illness could be summarized by the simple belief that if there was no ileus and stress, ulcer bleeding could be prevented, "all was well." Subsequently, the concept of "well" changed, as we became aware that the gut was capable of multiple functions (immune, endocrine, and metabolic) that could modulate and even contribute to a patient's disease state. The development of total parenteral nutrition (TPN) during the 1970s revolutionized the way patients in the surgical intensive care unit (SICU) were treated. However, with time, this initial enthusiasm for TPN progressively waned. Currently, there is a wealth of clinical and experimental evidence documenting that the enteral route of feeding is superior to parenteral nutrition in patients with a working gut. Specifically, enteral feeding is associated with fewer infections [1, 3], decreased financial costs [2], and better outcomes [1, 3, 4]. Thus, in this regard, the question of whether ICU patients should receive enteral versus parenteral nutrition is no longer controversial; however, many aspects regarding enteral nutrition (EN) remain debatable.

Controversies

Of the many possible unresolved controversies revolving around the gut in the SICU, we chose to focus on two areas. The first dispute is not whether to feed the gut, but how to feed it. Should feeding be given by continuous infusion or intermittently? Should the feeds be delivered into the stomach or the small bowel? When should feeds be started? What type of enteral access is best? These seemingly simple questions frequently invoke widely divergent responses reflecting strongly held beliefs, but these beliefs are largely based on tradition and anecdotal observations. Thus, while these questions appear simple, the true answers to these questions are anything but simple. The second controversy concerns the potential role of the gut as a cause of the multiple organ dysfunction syndrome (MODS) and whether MODS can be modified by gut-directed resuscitation and special enteral diets. While experimental evidence has shown that under certain circumstances, the gut can directly [5, 6] and indirectly [7, 8] contribute to distant organ injury, this topic is still in the early stages of investigation and remains unsettled.

Controversy 1: How to Feed the Gut

While some still debate the pros and cons of EN in the SICU, studies show that it can improve immune function [9–12], hasten wound healing [13, 14], attenuate burn injury-induced catabolism [15, 16], and improve patient outcomes after abdominal trauma [1, 3], liver transplantation [17], major surgery [18, 19], pancreatitis [20], peritonitis [21], as well as in critically ill or injured adults [22] and children [23]. These observations prompted Frost [24] to remark that "enteral feeding should be an obsession in the ICU! Failure to feed the patient via an intact small bowel is failure to deliver high-quality intensive care." Thus, the current controversies center not on giving EN, but on the methods of administering EN. There is a perception among many surgeons that feeding the small bowel is safer than feeding the stomach. Some small clinical studies do cite increased aspiration and pneumonia rates in critically ill patients fed into the stomach [25, 26]. However, the bulk of the literature on feeding through nasogastric and jejunal tubes indicates that aspiration rates are similar with both types of tubes [27–32]. Thus, the perception that feeding into the jejunum is safer appears to be based largely on anecdotes, not data.

While the rate of aspiration is similar between gastric and postpyloric feeding, there is a trend in the literature suggesting that reduced time is required to reach nutritional targets with jejunal feeding compared to gastric feeding [25, 33]. This apparent "pro" must be balanced against the fact that gastric feeding has been shown to be an effective prophylaxis against stress ulceration [34–36] since it effectively raises the gastric pH to levels equivalent to antacid or H_2 blocker therapy [37]. However, the fact that both gastric and postpyloric feeding result in colonization of the stomach and hypopharynx with enteric bacteria [37, 38] may explain why studies comparing these two feeding methods have failed to detect a difference in the incidence of pneumonia [25, 33]. In an attempt to prevent bacterial overgrowth of the stomach, interrupted enteral feeding (IEF), defined as 16 h of continuous feeding followed by an 8-h fast, has been evaluated as a way of allowing gastric pH to "recover" its acidity. Unfortunately, results with IEF have been mixed. Two studies showed a reduction in the incidence of pneumonia [39, 40] while another did not [41]. It should be noted that the latter study was nonrandomized, used historical controls, and did not control for the usage of pH altering drugs. Thus, on balance, it appears that IEF can offer some benefit by reducing gastric bacterial overgrowth and subsequent nosocomial pneumonia.

The "fear" of ileus causes many surgeons to be hesitant to embrace the policy of early EN after injury or surgery. While it is true that ileus often follows major surgery or trauma, its effects are primarily on the stomach and colon, leaving small bowel function intact [42]. "Bowel sounds" are notoriously bad predictors of small bowel function and are frequently absent in the intubated patient who is not swallowing air [43]. Thus, the small bowel can be fed even in the face of the most severe surgical or traumatic stress [44, 45]. Postpyloric feeding is thought to be desirable in these situations, since gastric emptying can be erratic at best; but this begs the question of how postpyloric enteral access should be achieved. In the case of a trauma laparotomy, a small-bore feeding tube (FT) passed transnasally can be guided postpylorically with a minimal time investment; but what of the postoperative or nonoperative SICU patient? It is hard to justify the risk of moving a critically ill patient to the fluoroscopy suite for FT placement, so bedside procedures are desirable. The panoply of techniques ranging from ultrasound [46] and endoscopic [47] guidance to manual "corkscrew" techniques [48, 49], promotility regimens [50–52], air insufflation [53, 54], and even magnets [55] attest to the difficulty of inserting a postpyloric FT.

Since the ultimate goal is to feed the gut of the critically injured patient as soon as possible and many studies show that enterally fed patients often receive only a fraction of their calculated nutritional needs, we offer a simple, pragmatic approach. The nasogastric tube (NGT) inserted at the time of admission to the OR, ER, or trauma area can be used for feeding once the patient is hemodynamically stable. NGTs are easily inserted, more readily identified on radiographs [31], facilitate more accurate assessments of gastric residuals [56] (the most common indicator of feeding intolerance), and have aspiration rates equivalent to small-bore FTs [31]. An intermittent feeding schedule should be followed and although data are lacking, a bolus pattern of feeding may be beneficial in reducing gastric and pharyngeal colonization and pneumonia [39, 40]. Bolus feeding closely resembles normal enteral intake and does have favorable effects on visceral protein synthesis [57]. With this approach, the use of promotility agents and/or bedside techniques to place postpyloric feeding tubes can be initiated on an as-needed basis and used only in the subgroup of patients with persistently high gastric residuals.

Controversy 2: Role of the Gut in MODS

MODS remains the leading cause of death in SICU patients. In light of this, efforts have been made to identify those patients at greatest risk of developing the syndrome so that resuscitative and supportive measures can be maximized. Several clinical trials comparing intramucosal pH (pHi), as assessed by gastric tonometry, to global oxygen delivery indices have shown that pHi is a better predictor of patients likely to develop MODS [58–63]. These observations suggested that strategies directed at improving gut perfusion might be clinically beneficial. Hence, the concept of gut-directed resuscitation has been offered both as a sensitive indicator of the adequacy of cardiovascular resuscitative efforts as well as a potential strategy for decreasing the incidence of MODS. Likewise, specialized enteral diets have been developed to optimally support gut function and bolster the immune response.

Enteral, "immune-enhancing, gut-protective" diets have shown beneficial clinical effects in the critically ill patients studied, in 12 of 13 prospective, randomized clinical trials [22, 44, 45, 65–74] reported. Although the exact composition of these diets varied slightly among the studies, they typically contained factors that have been shown experimentally to optimally support the intestinal mucosa and/or limit gut injury (arginine, glutamine, cysteine, nucleotides, omega-3 fatty acids, fiber, and antioxidants). Some might argue that the additional costs of these immune-enhancing, gut-protective diets are not justified, since in none of these studies was mortality decreased. We believe that the savings, both in dollars and in patient discomfort, reaped by their ability to reduce morbidity, justifies their use [44, 45]. In fact, in one prospective study, trauma patients fed an immune-enhancing diet did not develop organ failure or abdominal sepsis while a significant number of those fed a standard formula did ($P = 0.023$) [44].

The use of antioxidants to treat and/or prevent MODS has been less successful. To date, only one prospective, controlled clinical trial has been performed looking at the ability of oral antioxidants (vitamins C, E, and the glutathione precursor, *N*-acetylcysteine) to affect the outcome of severely injured patients [75]. The rationale behind this study was the notion that, by giving oral antioxidants, ischemia–reperfusion-mediated gut injury could be reduced, thereby reducing infectious complications and organ dysfunction. The results of this study support this hypothesis, since the group of patients receiving the antioxidant mixture had fewer infectious complications and no organ failure. However, due to the small number of patients enrolled, the study was not adequately powered to unequivocally establish the benefits of therapy. Similar encouraging results have been seen when a diet rich in fish oil and antioxidants was fed to patients with the acute respiratory distress syndrome (ARDS). In that study, the patients who were fed the modified diet exhibited a significant improvement of their respiratory status compared to those receiving the control diet [76]. Consequently, it appears that the development of organ dysfunction following a critical insult can be reduced by manipulating the gut through the administration of diets enriched with antioxidants and omega-3 fatty acids. However, studies with larger numbers of patients are needed to verify these results.

Until more information is amassed, the debate on whether the gut plays a major role in the pathogenesis of the immuno-inflammatory cascade leading up to MODS will continue. However, while this debate continues, we believe it is prudent to feed high-risk SICU patients with immune-enhancing, gut-protective diets and strive to maintain optimal gut perfusion.

References

1. Moore FA, Moore EE, Jones TN, et al. (1989) TEN vs. TPN following major abdominal trauma: reduced septic morbidity. J Trauma 29:916–923
2. Lipman TO (1998) Grains or veins: Is enteral nutrition really better than parenteral nutrition? A look at the evidence. JPEN 22:167–182
3. Kudsk KA, Croce MA, Fabian TC, et al. (1992) Enteral feeding versus parenteral feeding. Ann Surg 215:503–513
4. Kudsk KA, Stone JM, Carpenter G, et al. (1983) Enteral and parenteral feeding influences mortality after hemoglobin-E. coli peritonitis in rats. J Trauma 23:605–609
5. Magnotti LJ, Upperman JS, Xu D, Lu Q, Deitch EA (1998) Gut-derived mesenteric lymph but not portal blood increases endothelial cell permeability and potentiates lung injury following hemorrhagic shock. Ann Surg 228:518–527
6. Upperman JS, Deitch EA, Guo W, Lu Q, Xu D (1998) Post-hemorrhagic shock mesenteric lymph is cytotoxic to endothelial cells and activates neutrophils. Shock 10:407–414
7. Moore EE, Moore FA, Franciose RJ, Kim FJ, et al. (1994) The postischemic gut serves as a priming bed for circulating neutrophils that provoke multiple organ failure. J Trauma 37:881–887
8. Koike K, Moore EE, Moore FA, Kim FJ, et al. (1995) Gut phospholipase A2 mediates neutrophil priming and lung injury after mesenteric ischemia-reperfusion. Am J Physiol 268:G397–G403

9. DeWitt RC, Kudsk KA (1999) The gut's role in metabolism, mucosal barrier function, and gut immunology. Inf Dis Clin N Amer 13:465–481
10. Meyer J, Yurt RW, Duhaney R, Hesse DG, et al. (1988) Differential neutrophil activation before and after endotoxin infusion in enterally versus parenterally fed volunteers. Surg Gynecol Obstet 167:504–509
11. Lowry SF (1990) The route of feeding influences injury response. J Trauma 30 (12 Suppl):S10–15
12. Alverdy J, Chi HS, Sheldon G (1985) The effect of parenteral nutrition on gastrointestinal immunity: the importance of enteral immunity. Ann Surg 202:681–684
13. Demetriades H, Botsios D, Kazantzidou D, et al. (1999) Effects of early postoperative enteral feeding on the healing of colonic anastomoses in rats. Eur Surg Res 31:57–63
14. Kiyama T, Witte MB, Thornton FJ, Barbul A (1998) The route of nutrition support affects the early phase of wound healing. JPEN 22:276–279
15. Mochizuki H, Trocki O, Dominoni L, et al. (1984) Mechanism of prevention of postburn hypermetabolism and catabolism by early enteral feeding. Ann Surg 200: 297–310
16. Chiarelli A, Enzi G, Casadei A, et al. (1990) Very early nutrition supplementation in burned patients Am J Clin Nutr 51:1035–1039
17. Hasse JM, Blue LS, Liepa GU, et al. (1995) Early enteral nutrition support in patients undergoing liver transplantation. JPEN 19:437–443
18. Sand J, Luostarinen M, Matikainen M (1997) Enteral or parenteral feeding after total gastrectomy: prospective randomised pilot study. Eur J Surg 163:761–766
19. Stewart BT, Woods RJ, Collopy BT, et al. (1998) Early feeding after elective open colorectal resections: a prospective randomized trial. Aust NZ J Surg 68:125–128
20. Kalfarentzos F, Kehagias J, Kokkinis K, et al. (1997) Enteral nutrition is superior to parenteral nutrition in severe acute pancreatitis: results of a randomized prospective trial. Br J Surg 84:1665–1669
21. Singh G, Ram RP, Khanna SK (1998) Early postoperative enteral feedings in patients with nontraumatic intestinal perforation and peritonitis. J Am Coll Surg 187:142 146
22. Atkinson S, Sieffert E, Bihari D (1998) A prospective, randomized, double-blind, controlled clinical trial of enteral immunonutrition in the critically ill. Guy's Hospital Intensive Care Group. Crit Care Med 26:1164–1172
23. Chellis MJ, Sanders SV, Webster H, et al. (1996) Early enteral feeding in the pediatric intensive care unit. JPEN 20:71–73
24. Frost P, Edwards N, Bihari D (1997) Gastric emptying in the critically ill: the way forward? Int Care Med 23:243–245
25. Montecalvo MA, Steger KA, Farber HW, et al. (1992) Nutritional outcome and pneumonia in critical care patients randomized to gastric or jejunal tube feedings. Crit Care Med 20:1377–1387
26. Weltz CR, Morris JB, Mullen JL (1992) Surgical jejunostomy in aspiration risk patients Ann Surg 215:140–145
27. Lazarus BA, Murphy JB, Culpepper L (1990) Aspiration associated with long-term gastric versus jejunal feeding: a critical analysis of the literature. Arch Phys Med Rehab 71:46–53
28. DiSario JA, Foutch PG, Sanowski RA (1990) Poor results with percutaneous endoscopic jejunostomy. Gastroint Endos 36:257–260
29. Spain DA, DeWeese RC, Reynolds MA, et al. (1995) Transpyloric passage of feeding tubes in patients with head injuries does not decrease complications. J Trauma 39:1100–1102
30. Strong RM, Condon SC, Solinger MR, et al. (1992) Equal aspiration rates from postpylorus and intragastric-placed small-bore nasoenteric feeding tubes: a randomized, prospective study. JPEN 16:59–63
31. Sands JA (1991) Incidence of pulmonary aspiration in intubated patients receiving enteral nutrition through wide- and narrow-bore nasogastric feeding tubes Heart Lung 20:75–80
32. Ciocon JO, et al. (1992) Continuous compared with intermittent tube feeding in the elderly. JPEN 16:525–528
33. Kortbeek JB, Haigh PI, Doig C (1999) Duodenal versus gastric feeding in ventilated blunt trauma patients: a randomized controlled trial. J Trauma 46:992–998
34. Solem LD, Strate RG, Fischer RP (1979) Antacid therapy and nutritional supplementation in the prevention of Curling's ulcer. Surg Gynecol Obstet 148:3767–3780
35. Choctaw WT, Fujita C, Zawacki BE (1980) Prevention of upper gastrointestinal bleeding in burn patients. Arch Surg 115:1073–1076
36. Pingleton SK, Hadzima SK (1983) Enteral alimentation and gastrointestinal bleeding in mechanically ventilated patients. Crit Care Med 11:13–16
37. Heyland D, Bradley C, Mandell LA (1992) Effect of acidified enteral feedings on gastric colonization in the critically ill patient. Crit Care Med 20:1388–1394

38. Pingleton SK, Hinthorn DR, Liu C (1986) Enteral nutrition in patients receiving mechanical ventilation. Am J Med 80:827–832
39. Lee B, Chang RWS, Jacobs S (1990) Intermittent nasogastric feeding: a simple and effective method to reduce pneumonia among ventilated ICU patients. Clin Intens Care 1:100–102
40. Skiest DJ, Khan N, Feld R (1996) The role of enteral feeding in gastric colonization: a randomized controlled trial comparing continuous to intermittent enteral feeding in mechanically ventilated patients. Clin Intens Care 7:138–143
41. Spilker CA, Hinthorn DR, Pingleton SK (1996) Intermittent enteral feeding in mechanically ventilated patients. Chest 110:243–248
42. Tinckler LF, Kulke W (1963) Post-operative absorption of water from the small intestine. Gut 4:8–12
43. Raper S, Maynard N (1992) Feeding the critically ill patient. Br J Nursing 1:273–279
44. Moore FA, Moore EE, Kudsk KA, et al. (1994) Clinical benefits of an immune-enhancing diet for early postinjury enteral feeding. J Trauma 40:37607–37615
45. Kudsk KA, Minard G, Croce MA, et al. (1996) A randomized trial of isonitrogenous enteral diets after severe trauma: an immune enhancing diet reduces septic complications. Ann Surg 224:531–543
46. Hernandez-Scorro CR, Marin J, Ruiz-Santana S, et al. (1996) Bedside sonographic-guided versus blind nasoenteric feeding tube placement in critically ill patients. Crit Care Med 24:1690–1694
47. Napolitano LM, Wagle M, Heard S (1998) Endoscopic placement of nasoenteric feeding tubes in critically ill patients: a reliable alternative. J Laparoendo Adv Surg Tech 8:395–400
48. Zaloga GP (1991) Bedside method for placing small-bore feeding tubes in critically ill patients. A prospective study. Chest 100:1643–1646
49. Thurlow PM (1986) Bedside enteral feeding tube placement into duodenum and jejunum. JPEN 10:104–105
50. Stern MA, Wolf DC (1994) Erythromycin as a prokinetic agent: a prospective, randomized, controlled study of efficacy in nasoenteric tube placement. Am J Gastroenterol 89:2011–2013
51. Kalifas S, Choban PS, Ziegler D, et al. (1996) Erythromycin facilitates postpyloric placement of nasoduodenal feeding tubes in intensive care unit patients: randomized, double-blinded, placebo-controlled trial. JPEN 20:385–388
52. Kittinger JW, Sandler RS, Heizer WD (1987) Efficacy of metoclopramide as an adjunct to duodenal placement of small-bore feeding tubes: a randomized, placebo-controlled, double-blind study. JPEN 11:33–37
53. Salasidis R, Fleiszer T, Johnston R (1998) Air insufflation technique of enteral tube insertion: a randomized, controlled trial. Crit Care Med 26:1036–1039
54. Ugo PJ, Mohler PA, Wilson GL (1992) Bedside postpyloric placement of weighted feeding tubes. Nutr Clin Pract 7:284–287
55. Gabriel SA, Ackermann RJ, Castresana MR (1997) A new technique for placement of nasoenteral feeding tubes using external magnetic guidance. Crit Care Med 25:641–645
56. Metheny NA (1986) Aspiration pneumonia in patients fed through nasoenteral tubes. Heart Lung 15:256–261
57. Pinchcofsky-Devin GD, Kaminski MV (1992) Visceral protein increase associated with interrupt versus continuous enteral hyperalimentation. JPEN 16:525–528
58. Ivatury RR, Simon RJ, Islam S, et al. (1996) A prospective randomized study of end points of resuscitation after major trauma: global oxygen transport indices versus organ-specific gastric mucosal pH. J Am Coll Surg 183:145–154
59. Chang MC, Cheatham ML, Nelson LD, et al. (1994) Gastric tonometry supplements information provided by systemic indicators of oxygen transport. J Trauma 37:488–494
60. Kirton OC, Windsor J, Wedderburn R, et al. (1998) Failure of splanchnic resuscitation in the acutely injured trauma patient correlates with multiple organ system failure and length of stay in the ICU. Chest 113:1064–1069
61. Marik PE (1993) Gastric intramucosal pH. A better predictor of multiorgan dysfunction and death than oxygen-derived variables in patients with sepsis. Chest 104:225–229
62. Toninelli A, Agapiti C, Terenghi P, et al. (1995) Gastric intramucosal pH in trauma patients: an index for organ failure risk? Minerva Anestesiol 61:9–14
63. Barquist E, Kirton O, Windsor J, et al. (1998) The impact of antioxidant and splanchnic-directed therapy on persistent uncorrected gastric mucosal pH in the critically injured trauma patient. J Trauma 44:355–360
64. Gottschlich MM, Jenkins M, Warden GD, et al. (1990) Differential effects of three enteral dietary regimens on selected outcome variables in burn patients. JPEN 14:225–236

65. Daly JM, Lieberman MD, Goldfine J, et al. (1992) Enteral nutrition with supplemental arginine, RNA, and omega-3 fatty acids in patients after operation: immunologic, metabolic, and clinical outcome. Surgery 112:56–67
66. Chlebowski RT, Beall G, Grosvenor M, et al. (1993) Long-term effects of early nutritional support with new enterotropic peptide-based formula vs. standard formula in HIV-infected patients: randomized prospective trial. Nutrition 9:507–512
67. Brown RO, Hunt H, Mowatt-Larssen CA, et al. (1994) Comparison of specialized and standard enteral formulas in trauma patients. Pharmacotherapy 14:314–320
68. Bower RH, Cerra FB, Bershadsky B, et al. (1995) Early enteral administration of a formula (Impact®) supplemented with arginine, nucleotides, and fish oil in intensive care patients: results of a multicenter, prospective randomized clinical trial. Crit Care Med 23:436–449
69. Daly JM, Weintraub FN, Shou J, et al. (1995) Enteral nutrition during multimodality therapy in upper gastrointestinal cancer patients. Ann Surg 221:327–338
70. Mendez C, Jurkovich GJ, Garcia I, et al. (1997) Effects of an immune-enhancing diet in critically injured patients. J Trauma 42:933–941
71. Senkal M, Mumme A, Eickhoff U, et al. (1997) Early postoperative enteral immunonutrition: clinical outcome and cost-comparison analysis in surgical patients. Crit Care Med 25:1489–1496
72. Braga M, Gianotti L, Vignali A, et al. (1998) Artificial nutrition after major abdominal surgery: impact of route administration and composition of the diet. Crit Care Med 26:24–30
73. Galban C, Celaya S, Marco P, et al. (1998) An immune-enhancing enteral diet reduces mortality and episodes of bacteremia in septic ICU patients (abstract). JPEN 22:S13
74. Zaloga GP, Roberts PR (1997) Early enteral feeding improves outcome. In: Vincent JL (ed.) Yearbook of Intensive Care and Emergency Medicine. Berlin, Springer, pp 701–714
75. Porter JM, Ivatury RR, Azimuddin KA, et al. (1999) Antioxidant therapy in the prevention of organ dysfunction syndrome and infectious complications after trauma: early results of a prospective randomized study. Amer Surg 65:478–483
76. Gadek JE, DeMichele SJ, Karlstad MD, et al. (1999) Effect of enteral feeding with eicosapentaenoic acid, gamma-linolenic acid, and antioxidants in patients with acute respiratory distress syndrome. Enteral Nutrition in ARDS Study Group. Crit Care Med 27:1409–1420

Ethics in the Surgical Intensive Care Unit: Medical Futility

Avery B. Nathens

The availability of advanced technologies to prolong life in the surgical intensive care unit (SICU) has resulted in a number of controversies centered on their appropriate use. The controversies have developed under the guise of the *technological imperative,* implying that the availability of a particular technology requires that this technology be used. To counter the technological imperative, physicians have invoked the concept of futility to limit its inappropriate use. Unfortunately, a clear understanding of futility has proved elusive, resulting in confusion and at times, conflict when caring for critically ill patients. Many physicians view futility the way one judge viewed pornography – they may not be able to define it, but they know it when they see it [1].

In the strictest sense, true medical futility occurs rarely and signifies interventions that simply should not be offered. For example, we do not offer ongoing medical care to a patient who is clinically brain dead. The majority of therapies that physicians judge to be futile are not truly futile. They are more accurately termed inadvisable or inappropriate because the chances of achieving the intended goal are exceedingly low, their benefits are controversial, or their costs are excessively great [2]. Implicit in this definition is a clear understanding of the real or perceived therapeutic endpoint, i.e., it is meaningless to say an intervention is futile without specifying the goal of the intended therapy. Conflicts arise when there are disagreements about the intended goal, whether the desired goal is appropriate, and whether the probability of success is sufficiently great. In this sense, there are both qualitative (value-driven) and quantitative (probabilistic) aspects to the understanding and application of futility in the SICU [3, 4].

Qualitative Aspects of Futility

Futility judgments should not be made without agreeing upon the goal of therapy. Clearly, a reasonable goal is open to interpretation. Two cases highlight the potential problems that may arise:

> A five-year old boy fell two stories, developed respiratory distress, was intubated, and was transferred to the pediatric ICU. Despite maximal ventilatory support, adequate oxygenation could not be maintained and extracorporeal membrane oxygenation (ECMO) was proposed as a heroic measure to support the child until the pulmonary status improved. The family agreed to a 2-week trial of ECMO. While receiving ECMO, the patient developed renal failure and hepatic dysfunction. On day 13, a trial of conventional mechanical ventilation was attempted but failed after 20 s due to profound hypoxemia and bradycardia. Having failed a trial of ECMO, the parents were informed that there was no indication of improvement and ECMO would be discontinued. The parents threatened to bring a malpractice suit against the hospital and physicians if the therapy was withdrawn [5].
>
> At Hennepin County Medical Center, Minnesota, an 86-year-old ventilator-dependent woman was in a persistent vegetative state for over a year. The controversy that resulted pitted her husband and children, who wanted her maintained on a ventilator, against her physicians who wanted to discontinue ventilatory support because they felt this to be inappropriate treatment. The family argued that life should be maintained as long as possible and that the patient shared this belief. On the other hand, several citizens complained to the county claiming that the patient was receiving expensive therapy paid for by people who had not consented to underwrite a level of medical care whose appropriateness was defined by family demands [6, 7].

In both cases the interpretation by the patient's surrogate of the goals of treatment differed from their physicians' interpretation. In the first case, the physicians' purpose for instituting ECMO was to support the patient for a defined period of time. ECMO was clearly used only as a heroic measure to buy time until pulmonary function returned. In the absence of improved pulmonary function and with progressive multiple organ failure the chances of recovery were remote. In effect, they felt that continued support with ECMO was futile because it could not achieve the intended goal, i.e., return of pulmonary function in a defined period of time. In the eyes of the child's parents, this intervention was not futile therapy as it was clearly accomplishing its purpose by supporting gas exchange and in so doing, keeping their child alive.

The second case presented a different dilemma. In this setting mechanical ventilation was futile in the eyes of the physicians as it was incapable of restoring an adequate quality of life. By contrast, the patient's family believed that maintenance of biologic life represented the goal and continuation of mechanical ventilation was the only possible method of doing so. These differing interpretations of what constitutes futility resulted in a conflict between patient autonomy and the physicians' moral and ethical obligation to the patient.

Until recently, patient autonomy had been considered an inviolate right in medical bioethics. This principle was extrapolated from the right of patients to refuse therapy to the authority of patients and their families to demand the right to whatever life-sustaining intervention they desired. The case at Hennepin County Medical Center was brought to court and the judge decided in favor of the family. However, the supremacy of patient autonomy in this clinical setting has been questioned. Although the second case never went to trial, the hospital attorney counseled the physicians to discontinue therapy, as there was no legal obligation to seek court authorization for the discontinuation of a therapy that had failed to achieve an agreed-upon therapeutic goal [5]. In a consensus paper on this issue, the Society of Critical Care Medicine supports the contention that any intervention derives its justification from the scientific evidence that it provides a diagnostic or therapeutic benefit. Further, when that benefit has been achieved or can no longer be reasonably expected, the treatment loses its justification and may be withdrawn [2].

In cases where the value of the benefit remains contentious, there is clearly precedent for the support of physicians. In another judgment, a court ruled that physicians should not be compelled to act contrary to their moral and ethical principles when these are recognized and accepted by a large segment of the medical profession [8]. In the minds of many people, the right to demand treatment has been confused with the right to refuse care. The latter has been well supported in the courts and has its basis in the constitutional rights of privacy, liberty, and religious choice or the common law right against battery [9]. The right to insist upon an intervention that counters the professional standards and ethics of the treating physician(s) simply does not exist.

Quantitative Aspects of Futility

The last two decades have spawned the development of a number of objective severity of illness measures to evaluate and compare outcomes in large groups of patients. Although these scoring systems were not devised to predict outcome and thus guide the institution or withdrawal of therapy for individual patients, there has been some effort on the part of investigators to adapt these measures for this purpose. In effect, if the anticipated survival is below a certain threshold, the intervention, whether it is access to ICU resources or implementation of a costly therapeutic regimen, might be considered futile or inadvisable and not instituted.

There are several problems with this conceptually appealing approach. All of these measures predict outcome in patients who have received ICU care and therefore should not be used to determine whether admission to an ICU is futile. This approach might result in a significant misappropriation of resources. Further, estimates of survival probability are derived not for individual patients but for populations of patients with similar characteristics. The resultant imprecision makes application of these prognostic scoring systems dangerous for the purpose of guiding therapy. Finally, the surgeon needs to know whether an individual patient will live or die with some degree of accuracy, rather than a predicted risk of death. In essence, a binary prediction model optimized to ensure maximal concordance between predicted and observed outcomes for individual patients is required [10]. Satisfactory binary prediction models do not yet exist. Further, adaptation of currently available aggregate measures of outcome for the purposes of binary prediction are notoriously inaccurate, incorrectly classifying as many as 20% of all patients [10].

Declarations of futility based on probability have the additional disadvantage of becoming self-fulfilling prophecies. The pronouncement of futility for every case appearing hopeless mitigates the discovery of unique circumstances allowing survival or new therapeutic modalities that may alter survival. For example, the survival of patients with metastatic cancer suffering in-hospital cardiopulmonary arrest was unprecedented in the late 1980s, leading to several reports suggesting that CPR in this patient population was futile and should not be offered as a therapeutic option [11, 12]. By 1991, a report of a series of patients with metastatic cancer suffering cardiac arrest was published, claiming an 11% survival to hospital discharge, emphasizing that generalizations from insufficient data and failure to recognize advances in treatment can lead to erroneous futility judgments [9, 13].

Can Declarations of Futility Be Used for Resource Allocation?

The current emphasis on futility may represent an indirect response to the rising costs of healthcare. One argument for the declaration of futility in critically ill patients is to reduce cost and improve resource allocation by changing the way care is provided to terminally ill patients. Clearly, one such strategy is to eliminate futile care of these patients by withdrawing care in the ICU or by transferring these patients to standard ward care. Directing resources, or rationing, is often cited as a reason for making futility judgments. In the current sociopolitical climate, discussions on rationing are often avoided, leading many physicians to cloak this subject in the "objective" language of medical science, i.e., futility.

There are problems with using futility judgments to ration care. As described above, the science behind the declaration of futility from a probabilistic standpoint is presently inadequate. Even if our predictive abilities were greatly improved, futility judgments may be too infrequent to have a significant impact on global resource utilization. To evaluate the prevalence of futility, Halevy classified a cohort of patients admitted to an ICU into three operational definitions of futility: imminent demise, qualitative, and lethal condition futility [14]. *Imminent demise* futility was considered to be imminent death, regardless of intervention. Using the APACHE II prognostic model, these patients were then classified into predicted mortalities of 90%, 95%, and 99%. The percentage of total ICU bed days used by patients who met this operational definition with a predicted mortality of over 90% was only 0.3%. There were no bed days in the higher mortality strata. Only 3.6% of bed days were used for patients fulfilling criteria for *qualitative* futility, an unacceptable quality of life due to a persistent vegetative state or anoxic brain injury precluding meaningful survival. Just over 16% of bed days were used by patients fulfilling criteria for *lethal condition* futility in whom long-term survival was not anticipated because of underlying chronic disease. Whether this last cohort can be considered futile by any means is debatable as over 40% of these patients survived to discharge and one-third remained alive at 1 year. These data suggest that judgments of medical futility, both at the quantitative and qualitative level, are made relatively infrequently. In view of their rarity, society is unlikely to use futility arguments to drive the rationing of medical resources.

A Practical Approach to Futility in the SICU

Surgeons use the term futility in multiple and contradictory ways, creating a relationship strained by confusion, and at times distrust between the patient (or their proxy) and the surgical team. Inappropriate declarations of futility are common; we rarely if ever can predict with absolute certainty whether a patient will survive their ICU stay. In effect, we are offering opinions colored by our own values, not objective data. These tendencies to frame value judgments as medical decisions based on such data are inappropriate. Therapeutic interventions should be directed not toward eliciting a desired physiologic effect, but towards an agreed upon goal that is consistent with the wishes of the patient while maintaining professional integrity. Failure to achieve that goal renders the treatment futile.

The Society of Critical Care Medicine advocates developing hospital policies on the issue of futile care [2]. Policies may be definitional or procedural. A definitional policy is one in which an intervention is considered futile if it leads to success in a sufficiently small number of cases. Most have found these operational definitions to be unworkable because of the lack of data available for most clinical scenarios and the inability to predict outcomes for individual patients. The preferred alternative is a procedural policy wherein each case is treated individually and the steps to conflict resolution are clearly delineated [15]. Using this approach an intervention might be considered inadvisable after consensus is reached among all interested parties as to the goals of treatment. In this scenario, the probability of success is relevant but not necessarily determinative.

References

1. Jacobellis v. State of Ohio (1964) 84 S Ct 1676.
2. Ethics Committee of the Society of Critical Care Medicine (1997) Consensus statement of the Society of Critical Care Medicine's Ethics Committee regarding futile and other possibly inadvisable treatments. Crit Care Med 25:887–891
3. Schneiderman LJ, Jecker NS, Jonsen AR (1990) Medical futility: its meaning and ethical implications. Ann Intern Med 112:949–954
4. Truog RD, Brett AS, Frader J (1992) The problem with futility. N Engl J Med 326:1560–1564
5. Paris JJ, Schreiber MD, Statter M, Arensman R, Siegler M (1993) Beyond autonomy – physicians' refusal to use life-prolonging extracorporeal membrane oxygenation. N Engl J Med 329: 354–357
6. Angell M (1991) The case of Helga Wanglie: a new kind of right to die case. N Engl J Med 325:511–512

7. Miles SH (1991) Informed demand for "non-beneficial" medical treatment. N Engl J Med 325: 512–515
8. Brophy v. New England Sinai Hospital (1986) 389 Mass. 497 NE 2d 626
9. Youngner SJ (1996) Medical futility. Crit Care Clin 12:165–178
10. Lemeshow S, Klar J, Teres D (1995) Outcome prediction for individual intensive care patients: useful, misused, or abused. Intensive Care Med 21:770–776
11. Blackhall LJ (1987) Must we always use CPR? N Engl J Med 317:1285
12. Faber-Longendoen K (1991) Resuscitation of patients with metastatic cancer: Is transient benefit still futile? Arch Intern Med 151:235–239
13. Vitelli CE, Cooper K, Rogatko A, et al. (1991) Cardiopulmonary resuscitation and the patient with cancer. J Clin Oncol 9:111–115
14. Halevy A, Neal RC, Brody BA (1996) The low frequency of futility in an adult intensive care unit setting. Arch Intern Med 156:100–104
15. Halevy A, Brody BA (1996) A multi-institution collaborative policy on medical futility. JAMA 276:571–574

Invited Comment

Larry M. Gentilello

The preceding chapters on critical care are well written, thoroughly updated, and supportive randomized, prospective trials are cited as appropriate. However, certain topics remain controversial.

Ventilation

The most obvious example is low tidal volume ventilator support, summarized by Barie as "less is more." The multicenter trial that compared low tidal volumes (4–6 ml/kg) with traditional tidal volumes (10–12 ml/kg) demonstrated a 22% reduction in mortality (31.0% vs. 39.8%, $P=0.007$) in the low tidal volume group [1]. This was attributed to a decrease in plateau pressure (25 vs. 34 cm H_2O, $P=0.001$), and to the associated risk of volutrauma.

The surgeon should keep in mind that only a minority of patients in the study were surgical patients (roughly 30%) and only 8% were trauma patients. Differences in physiology may limit the advisability of using low-pressure ventilation in some surgical patients. Alveolar overdistension is a function of transpulmonary pressure, not plateau pressure. In most medical patients a normal pleural pressure (-5 cm H_2O) is assumed, and a plateau pressure of 25 cm H_2O results in a transpulmonary pressure of 30 cm H_2O [25–(–5) = 30 cm H_2O].

Surgical, and especially trauma patients may develop elevated intra-abdominal pressure. In an experiment to determine the relationship between abdominal pressure and pleural pressure, an abdominal pressure of 25 mmHg resulted in a pleural pressure of 24 cm H_2O [2]. If pleural pressure is 24 cm H_2O a plateau pressure of 54 cm H_2O is required to reach a transpulmonary pressure of 30 cm H_2O (54–24 = 30 cm H_2O) and the same risk of volutrauma as the low tidal volume group. This is analogous to playing the trumpet, which produces a pulmonary pressure as high as 180 cm H_2O without lung injury because the accompanying Valsalva maneuver increases pleural pressure and prevents alveolar overdistension.

It is also important to consider abdominal pressure when using PEEP. If the level of PEEP (e.g., 10 cm H_2O) is less than pleural pressure (e.g., 25 cm H_2O) the patient has negative end-expiratory pressure (NEEP = 15 cm H_2O), not PEEP. Thoughtless application of low-pressure ventilation in surgical patients with abdominal distension, chest wall edema, undrained pleural fluid, or other factors that increase pleural pressure may lead to inadvertent hypoventilation, a decreased V/Q ratio, and progressive pulmonary shunt.

The information on weaning provided in this chapter cannot be overemphasized. Physicians generally underestimate the potential of patients to be extubated, resulting in increased costs and complications. Two studies to determine which ventilator mode is most effective at reducing the duration of mechanical ventilation used a 2-h T-piece trial to confirm ventilator dependence as part of entry criteria [3, 4]. Amazingly, 77% and 88% of patients passed the T-piece trial and were extubated at the time of study entry!

Hemodynamic Monitoring and Support

Pulmonary artery catheters (PAC) are controversial due to a lack of prospective data demonstrating a beneficial effect on outcome. Retrospective studies, though controlled, do not explain why physicians placed a PAC in some patients but not in others with the same severity of illness. I agree with the authors that some patients most likely failed to respond to resuscitation (a poor prognostic sign) despite similar severity characteristics as their case-control, which prompted invasive monitoring, accounting for the outcome differences between groups.

The authors of this chapter indicate that right ventricular end-diastolic volume (RVEDV) is superior to wedge pressure as a method for titrating volume resuscitation because RVEDV has a stronger correlation with cardiac output. However, variability in ventricular compliance explains the poor correlation between wedge pressure and cardiac output. Ventricular volume, and therefore contractility, is a function of intraventricular (wedge) pressure, and myocardial compliance. A compliant heart may have an RVEDVI of 135 ml with a wedge pressure of 15 mmHg (compliance=135 ml/15 mmHg=9 ml/mmHg).

Older patients, those with hypertrophic ventricles, ischemic hearts or elevated pleural pressure require a higher wedge pressure to attain the same RVEDVI. A patient with a wedge pressure of 20 mmHg and an RVEDVI of 80 ml (compliance=4 ml/mmHg) would require a wedge pressure of 30 mmHg to attain an RVEDVI of 120 ml, assuming linear ventricular compliance. Since wedge pressure correlates with pulmonary capillary pressure, using RVEDVI without consideration of the wedge pressure required to achieve it may place the patient at increased risk for pulmonary edema.

A wedge pressure that is elevated due to high pleural pressures is not inaccurate; that external pressure is transmitted to the heart, decreasing its compliance and reducing venous return, resulting in a low RVEDVI despite the high wedge. The low RVEDVI will correlate with the low cardiac output, not the high wedge pressure. The high wedge pressure will correlate with pulmonary capillary pressure and the risk of pulmonary edema that is associated with trying to increase the RVEDVI.

Proper use of volumetric catheters requires knowledge of the interdependence between RVEDV and wedge pressure (compliance), not exclusive reliance on one or the other. This may avoid the argument I have often seen in our ICU. The nurse says "this patients needs a diuretic; the wedge pressure is 30 mmHg!" The resident's response is "no, the patient needs more fluid; the RVEDVI is only 80!"

Renal Support

As with respiratory failure, treatment of renal failure is merely supportive, and management consists of avoiding stressors that predispose the nephron to injury. Pathologic reduction in the glomerular filtration rate (GFR)is the sine qua non of renal failure; thus, the goal of the clinician is to avoid factors that have a deleterious effect on GFR. Autoregulation, the renin-angiotensin-aldosterone system, antidiuretic hormone, renal prostaglandin production, and extrinsic pressure on the kidney and renal vein are the primary factors that may adversely affect GFR in critically ill patients. The intensivist can manipulate these factors by paying strict attention to arterial and renal venous pressure, and renovascular resistance.

As blood pressure decreases, GFR is maintained by autoregulation. The safe pressure range depends on the patient's chronic blood pressure. Mere avoidance of hypotension may not keep the elderly, chronically hypertensive patient within their safe autoregulatory range, resulting in ischemia unless a higher blood pressure is maintained. "Damage control" is an important new surgical approach to treating unstable patients. It consists of a series of operations performed at intervals in accordance with the patient's physiologic tolerance. Bleeding is often reduced but not stopped, the need for abdominal packing is common, and increased abdominal pressure is a frequent result. A pressure greater than 30 mmHg is invariably associated with oliguria due to decreased renal blood flow associated with increased renal venous pressure and a calculated increase in renovascular resistance [5]. A decrease in urine output or an increase in serum creatinine should prompt transcystic measurement of abdominal pressure and decompressive celiotomy in such patients.

The most potent effectors of renovascular resistance are not exogenously administered drugs, but are endogenously secreted. Decreased pressure at the juxtaglomerular apparatus causes renin secretion, and intense angiotension-mediated renal vasoconstriction. Antidiuretic hormone (ADH) is another potent endogenous renovasoconstrictor. In addition to hypovolemia, other potent ADH secretory stimuli include hyperosmolarity and hypernatremia, both of which should be corrected in the patient with evidence of failing kidneys. Nonsteroidal anti-inflammatory medications are being prescribed with increasing frequency for pain control, or routinely after repair of vascular injuries. The resultant loss of vasodilatory prostaglandins may have profound effects on renovascular esistance, particularly in the elderly patient.

Atrial natriuretic polypeptide also has important renovascular modulatory effects. Given the intensity of the endogenously mediated renovasoconstriction that occurs as a result of hypotension, it is not surprising that norepinephrine has been given a "new look" as a potential treatment for incipient renal failure. Despite its vasoconstrictive properties, the resultant increase in systemic arterial pressure may shut down the kidney's own secretion of the even more potent endogenous factors that decrease GFR, with a net beneficial on renal function. In a study of 24 patients with septic shock, early renal dysfunction and oliguria, norepinephrine administration resulted in normalization of hemodynamics, and was followed by reestablishment of urine flow, decrease in serum creatinine, and an increase in creatinine clearance [6]. Only four patients remained oliguric, two of whom died, and two of whom developed renal failure.

The Gut

Enteral feeding has a well-established place in critical care, and is associated with a decreased risk of infection. However, the mechanism is still controversial. There are two frequently unmentioned possibilities to explain the decrease in infection rate. Enteral feedings are often not tolerated or only partially tolerated, and only 50% of patients meet their caloric requirements by the third to fourth day. Because full caloric support is quickly obtained with TPN it is associated with a higher risk of hyperglycemia, a well-known risk factor for infection [7]. The reduced infection risk with enteral feedings may be due to failure to control for hyperglycemia in TPN patients, and not due to a protective role of the gut.

Inadvertent underfeeding is common with tube feedings. Anorexia is part of the response to critical illness and short-term diminished caloric intake may be beneficial. Underfeeding diminishes the cytokine response to endotoxin challenge and decreases release of IL-1 [8, 9]. Compared with reduced intake, normal nutrient intake during TNF infusion in animals diminishes TNF clearance, increases multisystem organ dysfunction, and decreases survival after endotoxin administration, and after intraperitoneal injection of *Salmonella*, *Pseudomonas*, *Escherichia coli*, or *S. aureus* [10–18]. Anorexia may have evolved as a feedback mechanism to blunt exaggerated cytokine responses during serious illness, and the association between enteral feeding and improved outcome may be fortuitously related to the difficulties associated with establishing full nutritional support through the gut.

Ethics

With respect to ethical dilemmas related to futility, courts have reached a consensus regarding protecting patient–family autonomy to refuse or withdraw care, while insulating physicians who act reasonably and in good faith from legal liability. Conflicts arise when families insist on continuance of treatment when the physician feels that such care is futile and wastes scarce, expensive ICU resources. Families may not see support as futile if it is keeping the patient alive. Physicians, however, claim the right to declare futility because they feel they can make informed decisions based on their knowledge, experience, and understanding of life-support systems.

In actual practice, this remains a hazy dilemma because the declaration of futility is a clinical judgment that is susceptible to human error, and it is naive to believe that such an ill-defined concept as futility is not subject to physician bias, personal experience, training, and commitment to an individual patient. Physicians working in the same intensive care unit often have different opinions about when treatment is futile. Physicians must ask themselves "Is an illegal worker without friends or family visitors, and who has no financial resources likely to receive the same extent of care as a similarly ill patient with higher social status and concerned family members, one of whom is an attorney?"

As the author of this chapter states, "physicians view futility the way some judges view pornography; they may not be able to define it, but they know it when they see it." Yet, the definition of pornography varies from jurist to jurist and from state to state. Matters of life and death should be held to a higher degree of precision, and a definition of futility should be preestablished and agreed upon beforehand so that it can be applied equally to all hospital admissions. Is the line drawn at 10%, 5%, 1%, or 0.1% chance of survival? Society should decide beforehand if they wish to pay for unsuccessful treatment for 9, 95, 99, or 999 patients in order to save the life of someone who would otherwise have lived if care were not withdrawn. Such a process is already underway in Denver, where a consortium of hospitals is developing the GUIDe: Guidelines for the Use of Intensive Care in Denver.

Physicians frequently cite the costs of utilizing expensive resources on a single patient that may be used to benefit a greater number of patients; however, our society traditionally focuses on individual rights over the rights of the "masses." Also many families consider this issue from the perspective of sanctity of life, which is beyond monetary value. Indeed, our laws are based on this principle. Under this premise even a substantially diminished quality of life is acceptable.

Physicians who cite cost issues have very little data on the costs of "futile" treatment. While patients who die spend twice as long in the ICU as patients who live, physicians base their declaration of futility on the development of severe organ failure or deteriorating physiology that are typically not present until shortly before death occurs, resulting in the use of only a very small percentage of bed days. Cost control is more likely to be achieved by decreasing expenditures in all patients throughout the ICU stay by eliminating unnecessary tests, using preestablished protocols or clinical pathways, and by avoidance of the latest, but still unproven technology. Changing current wasteful practices appears to be a challenge that physicians are reluctant to take on.

Fortunately, public debate about these issues has led to greater and greater agreement between families and physicians regarding when life-support should be withdrawn. However, continued improvements in technology will keep this issue alive despite the statement by George Bernard Shaw in his "Preface" to the *Doctor's Dilemma*: "Do not try to live forever. You will not succeed."

References

1. The Acute Respiratory Distress Network (2000) Ventilation with lower tidal volumes as compared with traditional tidal volumes for acute lung injury and the respiratory distress syndrome. N Eng J Med 242:1301–1321
2. Ridings PC, Bloomfield GL, Blocher CR, Sugerman H (1995) Cardiopulmonary effects of raised intra-abdominal pressure before and after intravascular expansion. J Trauma 39:1071–1075

3. Brochard L, Rauss A, Benito S, et al. (1994) Comparison of three methods of gradual withdrawal from ventilatory support during weaning from mechanical ventilation. Am J Respir Crit Care Med 150:896–903
4. Esteban A, Frutos F, Tobin MJ, et al. (1995) A comparison of four methods of weaning patients from mechanical ventilation. N Eng J Med 332:345–350
5. Harman PK, Kron IL, McLachlan HD, Freedlender AE, Nolan ST (1982) Elevated intra-abdominal pressure and renal function. Ann Surg 196:594–597
6. Marin C, Eon B, Saux P, Aknin P, Gouin F (1990) Renal effects of norepinephrine used to treat septic shock patients. Crit Care Med 18:282–285
7. Khaodhiar L, McCowen K, Bistrian B (1999) Perioperative hyperglycemia, infection or risk? Curr Opin Clin Nutr Metab Care 2:79–82
8. Elsasser TH, Kahl S, Steele NC, et al. (1997) Nutritional modulation of somatotrophic axis-cytokine relationships in cattle: a brief review. Comp Biochem Physiol 116:209–221
9. Grimble RF (1994) Malnutrition and the immune response. 2. Impact of nutrients on cytokine biology in infection. Trans R Soc Trop Med Hyg 88:615–619
10. Clouva-Molyvdas P, Peck MD, et al. (1990) Short-term dietary protein manipulation does not affect survival from intraperitoneal pseudomonas infection in mice. J Parentr Entr Nutr 14:366–370
11. Bhuyan UN, Ramalingaswami V (1972) Responses of the protein deficient rabbit to Staphylococcal bacteremia. Am J Pathol 69:359–366
12. Jakab GJ, Warr GA, Astry CL (1981) Alterations of pulmonary defense mechanisms by protein depletion diet. Infect Immun 34:610–622
13. Peck MD, Alexander JW, Gonce SJ, et al. (1989) Low protein diets improve survival from peritonitis in guinea pigs. Ann Surg 209:448
14. Peck MD, Babcock GF, Alexander JW (1992) The role of protein and calorie restriction in outcome from Salmonella infection in mice. J Parentr Entr Nutr 16:561–565
15. Alexander JW, Gonce SJ, Miskell PW, et al. (1989) A new model for studying nutrition in peritonitis: the adverse effect of overfeeding. Ann Surg 209:334–340
16. Matsui J, Cameron RG, Kurian R, et al. (1993) Nutritional, hepatic and metabolic effects of cachectin/tumor necrosis factor in rats receiving total parenteral nutrition. Gastroenterology 104:235–243
17. Keith ME, Norwich KH, Jeejeebhoy KN (1995) Nutrition support affects the distribution and organ uptake of cachectin/tumor necrosis factor in rats. J Parentr Etr Nutr 19:341–350
18. Zaloga GP (1999) Full Nutritional Support in the Critically Ill. In: Technique and Technology. Society of Critical Care Medicine Symposium Syllabus, Anaheim, CA

Editorial Comment

In this chapter, Drs. Barrie, Harrington and Cioffi, Fahoum, Adams and Deitch, and Nathens, discuss the controversies surroundings specific fields in surgical critical care. Dr. Gentilello then eloquently provides his own perspective.

The immense biophysiological complexity and "chaos" associated with any critical illness has to be appreciated and reemphasized. Of course it is much easier for us to "conceptualize patients" in clear, linear fashion (e.g., "low BP is bad, high BP is good" or "starvation is bad so feeding is good"). But the disease processes in ill surgical patients do not follow these simple, linear lines. Instead, they involve numerous "pro" and "contra" mediators, amplifying and downgrading each other in numerous positive and negative feedback loops [1]. Thus, it is naive to hope that one new magic bullet can change events. It is also naive to believe that, in general, "more is better." For example let us look at the issue of postoperative feeding. Dr. Gentilelo suggested above that enteral nutrition in the SICU might improve survival through "forced starvation." But without including unfed arms in randomized studies we will never know for sure whether the current obsession with overfeeding is damaging or not. We must also be suspicious of "novel therapies"; see for instance anabolic hormones in critically ill patients - the hitherto promising use of growth hormone not only did not improve results but also worsened it [2].

A witty but wise and refreshing collection of "100 thoughts for the critical care practitioner in the new millennium" has been recently amassed by Franklin [3]. We recommend that you read it.

References

1. Seely AJ, Christou NV (2000) Multiple organ dysfunction syndrome: exploring the paradigm of complex nonlinear systems. Crit Care Med 28:2193–2200
2. Takala J, Ruokonen E, Webster NR, et al. (1999) Increased mortality associated with growth hormone treatment in critically ill adults. N Engl J Med 341:785–792
3. Franklin C (2000) 100 thoughts for the critical care practitioner in the new millennium. Crit Care Med 28:3050–3052

CHAPTER 11

Advanced Laparoscopic Surgery

Antireflux Surgery

Joaquin A. Rodriguez · Ronald A. Hinder

Introduction

Since its introduction to the United States in 1991, laparoscopic antireflux surgery (LARS) has created renewed interest in the surgical treatment of gastroesophageal reflux disease (GERD). Acceptance of the reliability of the laparoscopic procedure combined with the attraction to both patients and physicians of shorter recovery and hospital stay and decreased pain has led to a dramatic increase in the numbers of these procedures being performed. We will discuss controversies in indications for surgery, necessary preoperative work-up and technical aspects of antireflux surgery.

Changing Indications

Before minimally invasive antireflux surgery was offered, only patients with the most severe form of GERD whose medical therapy had failed were offered a surgical procedure. With the advent of laparoscopic antireflux procedures, more patients are being offered surgical therapy and indications have changed. In order to understand which patients will benefit most from a surgical approach we must first understand the natural history of GERD. GERD is a debilitating and chronic disease. In a study from Switzerland [1], 750 patients with grades I–III esophagitis were given empiric therapy and followed by endoscopy. Of these, 45% never required further therapy, 32% had recurrent episodes without progression of their disease, and 23% had progressive disease with one-half of these going on to develop strictures or esophageal ulcerations. It has also been reported that up to 80% of patients will relapse within 6–8 months of cessation of medical therapy and up to 25% of patients on proton pump inhibitors will relapse within 12 months [2]. This has led to increasing interest in durable antireflux surgery. Interesting new considerations for surgery are noncompliance with medications, intolerance of medical therapy, burden of cost of medication, and requirement of escalating doses of proton pump inhibitors to control symptoms. Special consideration should be given to younger patients who face potential lifelong medical therapy. A recent study on cost-effectiveness showed that the cost of surgical therapy was less than the lifetime cost of medical management in men and women younger than 49 and 56 years old, respectively [3]. Kahrilas [4] disagrees, stating that not all surgical series have demonstrated good outcome, that health resources continue to be required after LARS, and that the use of LARS in uncomplicated reflux disease is not indicated. We believe that patients with complicated GERD are effectively treated by surgical therapy. This is because medical therapy decreases the acidity of the juices bathing the esophagus but does little to alter lower esophageal sphincter (LES) pressure or reduce herniation. Klingler et al. showed that in patients on medical therapy for esophageal strictures, the mean rate of dilations was decreased from 5.3 per patient in the 26 months preceding surgery to 1.8 per patient in the 25-month postoperative period [5]. The incidence of frequent pneumonias prior to surgery decreased from 13.5% to 0% in the postoperative period in the same group of patients. Wetscher et al. showed that respiratory symptoms improved in 85% of patients treated with surgery compared with only 14.5% in patients treated medically [6].

Preoperative Testing

The continuing success of laparoscopic antireflux surgery depends on selecting appropriate candidates for surgery. Campos et al. [7] recently demonstrated that a history typical of GERD symptoms and a significant response to acid suppression are two of three factors that were predictive of a successful outcome after fundoplication. The third predictor of a successful outcome was an abnormal 24-h esophageal pH study. However, in patients with a typical history and a good response to histamine receptor blocker or PPI (proton pump inhibitor) therapy, this test can be avoided. If the diagnosis is in doubt because of atypical symptoms or poor response to medication, the pH study is valuable in determining the appropriateness of surgery. Gastric emptying studies are only required in patients in whom gastroparesis is felt to be present. This is likely in diabetic patients and those who have had previous upper GI surgery or have retained food on endoscopic evaluation. In patients who have recurrent symptoms after fundoplication, the 24-h esophageal pH documents whether the symptoms are in fact due to acid reflux and the barium esophagogram provides information regarding the status of the wrap and presence of a diaphragmatic hernia. A barium esophagogram should also be performed in all cases of large hiatal hernia or esophageal stricture to assess esophageal length. The two mandatory tests in all patients are esophagogastroduodenoscopy and esophageal manometry. Endoscopy corroborates the history of reflux with esophagitis and allows for the identification of patients with Barrett's esophagus, malignancy, strictures, peptic ulcer disease, and Schatzki's ring which may be contributing factors to the patient's symptoms. Manometry characterizes the LES pressure and length and overall esophageal body motility allowing for tailoring of the wrap to the amount of esophageal "squeeze" present. Patients found to have esophageal body dysmotility, characterized by greater than 30% nontransmitted waves or less than 30 mmHg of amplitude of waves in response to a wet swallow in the distal esophagus, should have a partial rather than a complete wrap. Manometry's greatest value is in diagnosing unsuspected esophageal spasm, scleroderma, nutcracker esophagus or achalasia where a wrap would be poorly tolerated.

Fundus Mobilization

It has been learned from past variations of surgical technique that small changes in surgical technique can have profound effects on postoperative results. Through trial and error it was discovered that a fundoplication greater than 3 cm has a significantly increased incidence of dysphagia. Similarly we are beginning to understand the role of complete fundal mobilization by division of the short gastric vessels. Some have presented good results with the Rosetti-Nissen modification in which the short gastric vessels are not divided and the anterior gastric wall is used for the wrap, but recent reports of increased dysphagia with this technique have surfaced. In his initial experience with the laparoscopic Nissen fundoplication, Jamieson [8] did not divide the short gastric vessels and experienced a combined 8% incidence of persistent dysphagia and reoperation for dysphagia. Recently, Hunter [9] presented his data comparing laparoscopic Rosetti-Nissen with intact short gastric vessels, the laparoscopic Toupet partial fundoplication with intact short gastric vessels, and laparoscopic Nissen fundoplication with the short gastric vessels divided. He found that new onset solid-food dysphagia was seen in 54% of the Rosetti-Nissen group compared to 16% in the Nissen and Toupet groups. At 3 months, 11% of the Rosetti-Nissen group still had dysphagia compared with 2% in the Nissen and Toupet groups [9]. A report from Laycock [10] also found a significantly greater incidence of short-term and persistent dysphagia in patients who did not undergo division of their short gastric vessels. The rationale for these differences is explained by Hunter who feels that when the anterior wall of the stomach is used for the fundoplication rather than the fundus, less tissue is available for creation of the nipple valve. The likelihood of a tension-free or floppy Nissen fundoplication is thus decreased. Furthermore, tension on the fundus tethered by short gastric vessels can result in a counterclockwise axial twisting of the esophagus. This creates a narrow spiral valve causing dysphagia. This type of "anatomic" defect is refractory to postoperative dilation since dilators uncurl the spiral which reforms upon removal of the dilator. It appears that the partial wrap is more tolerant of leaving the short gastric vessels intact by providing less resistance to esophageal flow. The fears of some surgeons that fundal mobilization would lead to increased bleeding, increased rates of splenectomy and significantly prolonged operative times have not been validated.

Intraoperative Use of Dilators

Many surgeons use intraoperative esophageal dilators when performing a laparoscopic fundoplication. The rationale for their use is to size the crural closure and fundal wrap to prevent dysphagia. However, the use of dilators is not without risk. Lowham et al. found that the incidence of esophageal or gastric perforation with size 56-60 Hurst Maloney dilators was 0.8% [11]. In most of these instances the operator noted no increase in resistance with the passage of the dilator. It is postulated that the anterior esophageal angulation created by hiatal closure combined with the loss of manual feedback with the laparoscopic approach is the predominant mechanism for distal esophageal and gastric perforations. Similar findings were reported by Schauer et al. who identified that incorrect traction on the stomach during passage of the dilator resulted in severe angulation of the distal esophagus in 5 out of 17 of their perforations [12]. They reported two more patients in whom the presence of the bougie in the esophageal lumen during posterior dissection of the esophagus contributed to the perforation. Although the incidence of less than 1% is low, the mortality of 26% for this complication is high. Thus we advocate not using a dilator during laparoscopic antireflux procedures especially if preexistent esophageal pathology such as a diverticulum is present. Instead we rely on visual assessment and full mobilization of the fundus to create a loose, less than 2-cm wrap that prevents reflux without causing dysphagia

Crural Closure

Crural closure is a controversial step in antireflux procedures. Some question its value and do not perform it routinely for fear of increasing the incidence of postoperative dysphagia. We believe that plication of the diaphragmatic hiatus with a nonabsorbable suture is a crucial component of the antireflux operation. The crural diaphragm is 2 cm in length and normally encircles the proximal 2 cm of the LES. Both the LES and crural diaphragm contribute to the esophagogastric junction intraluminal pressure. Approximation of the crura supports the effect of the fundal wrap in preventing reflux by augmenting LES pressure, especially under straining conditions. Furthermore, crural repair helps maintain the fundoplication in the abdomen where higher intra-abdominal pressures will transmit a higher pressure to the LES. In an early series of 198 patients with laparoscopic Nissen procedures, two had herniation of the upper stomach into the chest in the early postoperative period [13]. In both cases there was evidence of breakdown of the crural repair. It was postulated that if routine crural repair had not been performed, the incidence of this complication would have been higher.

Partial Versus Total Fundoplication

The fundoplication in laparoscopic antireflux surgery can be partial or total. The "total" or Nissen fundoplication consists of a loose 360-degree fundic wrap that is 1–2 cm in length. Partial fundoplications include the Dor and Toupet procedures. The Dor procedure represents a 180-degree anterior wrap that is often used after the Heller myotomy. The Toupet fundoplication, which has been modified from its original 180 degrees to a 270-degree posterior wrap, is the most commonly performed partial wrap. The question as to which wrap provides the best symptom relief while minimizing side effects such as bloating and dysphagia has been difficult to answer because of differences in the individual techniques in reports of the

Nissen and Toupet procedures. Both procedures augment the LES high-pressure zone by restoring the stomach and sphincter into the positive pressure environment of the abdomen and narrowing the LES. Furthermore, both promote gastric emptying by diminishing receptive relaxation while augmenting postprandial LES tone. However, it appears that the Nissen fundoplication creates a higher pressure zone around the LES. The Toupet fundoplication leaves 90 degrees of the esophagus exposed and lower LES resting pressures are generated. Theoretically this lower outflow resistance allows for easier passage of the food bolus, the ability to belch and less dysphagia. This was confirmed by McKernan [14] who found that in 37 patients who underwent a Nissen fundoplication, 79% had an excellent result, 2 required esophageal dilation, and most resumed normal swallowing within 24 days. By comparison he noted excellent results in 89%, no dilations, and resumption of normal swallowing within 6 days in the Toupet fundoplication group. However, this has not always been proven in clinical trials. Hunter showed equal long-term dysphagia rates of 2% when prospectively comparing his laparoscopic Nissen and Toupet fundoplications [9] and Jobe has reported dysphagia after the Toupet fundoplication in 20% at 3 months and 9% at 9 months [15]. Regarding the efficacy against reflux, most have found the Toupet fundoplication to be less effective than the Nissen. Jobe et al. reported their Toupet patients to have a 22% symptomatic failure and 51% positive pH score at 22 months postoperatively [15]. Similarly Lund et al. found that in patients with abnormal esophageal motility treated with a laparoscopic Toupet fundoplication, 17% had a positive acid-reflux score [16]. Others, such as Laws [17], have found no difference in postoperative symptomatology regarding both bloating and recurrent reflux using Visick scores in comparing the Toupet and Nissen fundoplications at an average follow-up of 27 months. Thus it appears that the Nissen fundoplication provides better protection from reflux symptoms but sometimes at a higher cost in terms of dysphagia and bloating. There are no prospective randomized trials comparing the Toupet and Nissen fundoplications in patients with poor esophageal body motility but it is our opinion that the Toupet fundoplication should be used in this group to minimize postoperative dysphagia.

Conclusions

Laparoscopic antireflux surgery is becoming the treatment of choice for many patients with gastroesophageal reflux disease. It should be offered to young patients with a long-term need for aggressive medical therapy and to those who do not wish to continue with medical therapy. Patients with severe esophagitis, a large hiatal hernia, and pulmonary symptoms are best treated surgically. The laparoscopic antireflux procedure should involve crural closure, division of the short gastric vessels, and the avoidance of esophageal dilators during surgery. The laparoscopic "floppy" Nissen fundoplication has a low incidence of recurrent symptoms and should be performed in patients with normal esophageal motility. Patients with poor esophageal body motility or with a Heller myotomy should receive a Toupet fundoplication. The mandatory use of esophagogastroduodenoscopy and esophageal manometry with selective use of 24-h pH, barium esophagogram, and gastric emptying studies provides a reasonable work-up of patients prior to surgery.

References

1. Monnier P, Ollyo JP, Fontolliet C, Savory M (1995) Epidemiology and natural history of reflux esophagitis. Semin Laparosc Surg 2:2–9
2. Hutzel DJ, Dent J, Reed WD, et al. (1988) Healing and relapse of severe peptic esophagitis after treatment with omeprazole. Gastroenterology 95:903–912
3. Coley CM, Barry MJ, Spechler SJ, et al. (1993) Initial medical versus surgical therapy for complicated or chronic reflux disease: a cost effectiveness analysis (abstract). Gastroenterology 104:A5
4. Kahrilas PJ 1999) Laparoscopic antireflux surgery: silver bullet or the emperor's new clothes? (editorial; comment). Am J Gastroenterol 94:1721–1723
5. Klingler PJ, Hinder RA (1999) Laparoscopic antireflux surgery for the treatment of esophageal strictures refractory to medical therapy. Am J Gastroenterol 94:632–636
6. Wetscher GJ, Hinder RA, et al. (1997) Respiratory symptoms in patients with gastroesophageal reflux disease following medical therapy and following antireflux surgery. Am J Surg 174:639–643
7. Campos GM, Peters JH, DeMeester TR, et al. (1994) Multivariate analysis of factors predicting outcome after laparoscopic Nissen fundoplication. Ann Surg 3:292–300
8. Jamieson GG, Watson DI, et al. (1994) Laparoscopic Nissen fundoplication. Ann Surg 220:137–145
9. Hunter JG, Swanstrom L, Waring PJ (1996) Dysphagia after laparoscopic antireflux surgery. The impact of operative technique. Ann Surg 224:51–57
10. Laycock WS, Trus TL, Hunter JG (1996) New Technology for the division of short gastric vessels during laparoscopic Nissen fundoplication. A prospective randomized trial. Surgical Endoscopy 10:71–73
11. Lowham AS, Filipi CJ, et al. (1996) Mechanisms and avoidance of esophageal perforation by anesthesia personnel during laparoscopic foregut surgery. Surg Endosc 10:979–982
12. Schauer PR, Meyers WC, et al. (1996) Mechanisms of gastric and esophageal perforations during laparoscopic Nissen fundoplication. Ann Surg 223:43–52
13. Hinder RA, Filipi CJ, et al. (1994) Laparoscopic Nissen fundoplication is an effective treatment for gastroesophageal reflux disease. Ann Surg 220:472–483
14. McKernan JB, Champion JK (1995) Laparoscopic antireflux surgery. Am Surg 61:530–536
15. Jobe BA, Wallace J, Hansen PD, Swanstrom LL (1997) Evaluation of laparoscopic Toupet fundoplication as a primary repair for all patients with medically resistant gastroesophageal reflux. Surgical Endoscopy 11:1080–1083
16. Lund RJ, Wetcher GF, Raiser F, et al. (1997) Laparoscopic Toupet fundoplication for gastroesophageal reflux disease with poor esophageal body motility. J Gastrointest Surg 1:301–308
17. Laws HL, Clements RH, Swillie CM (1997) A randomized, prospective comparison of the Nissen fundoplication versus the Toupet fundoplication for gastroesophageal reflux disease. Ann Surg 225:647–654

Invited Comment on Laparoscopic Antireflux Surgery

Santiago Horgan · Lloyd M. Nyhus

This well-written section by Rodriguez and Hinder emphasizes some of the controversies in laparoscopic antireflux surgery.

Although we agree with the majority of what is written, we believe, as published by DeMeester et al., that on many occasions the 24-h pH test is and should be the gold standard study in the diagnosis of GERD. Not only is it important to quantify the reflux, but the pH study also plays an important role in identifying those patients with extraesophageal symptoms of gastroesophageal reflux disease. We believe, as many other authors do, that this study should always be performed.

The barium swallow is another important study that not only allows the surgeon to understand the anatomy of the esophagus (presence of epiphrenic diverticulum, paraesophageal hernia, or short esophagus), but also the motility of the esophagus and the size of the hiatal hernia. This is very important because it allows the surgeon to identify these abnormalities and plan the surgery accordingly.

We agree with the authors that the short gastric vessels should always be divided to diminish the incidence of postoperative dysphagia.

During the open fundoplication era, the use of a dilator was important to tailor the closure to help avoid the so-called tight wrap. The lack of sensorial feedback that laparoscopic surgery brought makes the use of dilator even more important to avoid tight wraps. The 0.8%-perforation rate reported in the paper is high and has not been reported in larger series. The question is what to do with patients that present with early dysphagia after a laparoscopic total fundoplication where a dilator was not used.

We agree with Rodriguez and Hinder that a total fundoplication gives the patient a better control of symptoms than fundoplication following the partial wrap

References

1. Horgan S, Pellegrini CA (1997) Nissen Fundoplication. Surg Clin North Am 77:1063–1082
2. Horvath K, et al. (1999) Laparoscopic Toupet fundoplication is an inadequate procedure for patients with severe reflux disease. J Gastroint Surg 3:583

Thoracic Surgery

Toni Hau

Introduction

Thoracoscopy was first introduced into clinical medicine by Jakobäus in 1912 [1]. During the following decades it was used extensively as a diagnostic tool especially in patients with suspected tuberculosis. Only after the introduction of laparoscopic cholecystectomy by Dubois [2] did thoracoscopy evolve rapidly from a diagnostic technique to a therapeutic modality. Thoracoscopic surgery is a safe procedure; the mortality rate is under 1% and the complication rate between 10% and 15%. The most common procedure-specific complication is a prolonged air-leak. Depending on the procedure performed the conversion rate to open thoracotomy ranges from 10% to 20% [4–6]. Table 1 gives an overview of the current indications for thoracoscopic surgery.

The term thoracoscopic surgery has recently been replaced by the term video-assisted thoracic surgery (VATS). The latter expression probably more accurately

Table 1. Indications for thoracoscopic pulmonary surgery (modified from [6])

Generally accepted
Lung biopsy
Biopsy for pleural disease
Staging of lymph nodes in the aorto-pulmonary window
Excision of pulmonary nodules
Sclerosis of the pleura space for malignant disease
Excision of benign pleural lesions
Excision of benign lung tumors
Stapling of blebs
Not generally accepted, but commonly performed
Wedge resection of T1 lung cancer in patients with poor pulmonary function
Volume reduction for pulmonary emphysema
Not generally accepted and not commonly performed
Thoracoscopic lobectomy

describes the procedure because it is frequently necessary to perform a small thoracotomy to remove the specimen. On the other hand, it is somewhat vague as to the parts of the procedure, which are actually performed by a closed as opposed to an open technique [3].

Thoracoscopic Versus Open Surgery

Thoracoscopic procedures have gained rapid acceptance not only by physicians, but especially with patients because it is felt that, compared with conventional thoracotomy, postoperative pain and impairment of pulmonary function are less, the hospital stay is shorter, the patient can return earlier to full activity, and the incidence of the postthoracotomy syndrome is decreased [6–9]. In a concurrent, not randomized study, Landreneau et al. found that patients undergoing VATS procedures had less pain, a decreased requirement for intercostal block or epidural analgesia, fewer narcotic requirements, better shoulder girdle strength, and quicker recovery of pulmonary function as compared to patients undergoing lateral thoracotomy [8].

This impression based on retrospective comparisons was confirmed by prospective studies. Förster et al. did a prospective analysis of matched pairs of patients undergoing atypical lung resection either by VATS or conventional thoracotomy and found a quicker restitution of forced expiratory volume (FEV) and a shorter hospital stay in the thoracoscopy group [10]. Santambrogio et al. in a prospective randomized trial comparing the two surgical approaches also found a shorter hospital stay and less postoperative pain in the VATS group [11]. Two prospective randomized trials compared pulmonary function after VATS with open thoracotomy. Waller et al. found that the decrease in FEV 7 hours after surgery was only 25% after VATS compared to 43% after thoracotomy [12]. Sekine et al. compared pulmonary function after surgery for spontaneous pneumothorax either by VATS or axillary thoracotomy. Patients operated upon by VATS had a continously higher pO_2, a smaller alveolar arterial oxygen gradient, less incidence of atelectasis, and a decreased use of analgesics compared with patients undergoing thoracotomy [13].

However, Kirby et al., in a prospective randomized study of patients undergoing lobectomies performed either by VATS or through a muscle sparing thoracotomy, found no difference in analgesia requirements, duration of chest tube drainage length of hospital stay, recovery time, and return to work [14]. Also, the incidence of chronic postoperative pain (postthoracotomy syndrome) does not seem to be decreased after video-assisted thoracic surgery as compared to open thoracotomy. In a retrospective study it was found that the incidence of chronic pain and the limitation in shoulder function one year after surgery were the same regardless of whether an open or video-assisted procedure was done [15].

In summary, most prospective studies comparing VATS with open thoracotomy show that the impairment of postoperative pulmonary function, postoperative pain, hospital stay, and time off work is reduced after VATS.

Pulmonary Malignancies

In view of these findings we now would like to examine the role of thoracoscopy in the management of pulmonary malignancies. There is no doubt that thoracoscopy plays a major role in the diagnosis and staging of pulmonary cancer [15, 16] and the evaluation of malignant pleural effusions [17]. An indeterminate pulmonary nodule less than 3 cm in diameter and located in the outer third of the lung parenchyma is usually considered an indication for a VATS approach [16]. Conversion to open thoracotomy is necessary in approximately 15% of all patients [18, 19]. Even though intraparenchymal hemorrhage and other artifacts are more common and extensive after VATS biopsy compared to open techniques, this does not effect the diagnostic yield [20]. Another indication for VATS is the assessment of enlarged lymph nodes not accessible by mediastinoscopy. Landreneau et al. [21], in a retrospective analysis, found a sensitivity and specificity of thoracoscopic mediastinal lymph node sampling, especially in the aorto-pulmonary window, of 100%.

Pulmonary Metastases

Thoracoscopic wedge resection in the treatment of pulmonary metastases is widely practiced. The lesions seem to be ideally suited for the VATS approach because they are located in the periphery and have been treated with a parenchyma sparing wedge resection in the part [28]. However, there are several arguments against the thoracoscopic approach. Firstly, as in laparoscopic surgery for cancer, tumor disseminations have been reported not only in primary lung cancer, but also after surgery for pulmonary metastases [23, 24]. A more important limitation, however, is the inability to bimanually palpate the lung during thoracoscopy. Because CT scans underestimate the number of metastases by 25% [25], there is a danger that metastases remain undetected. Spiral CT has an increased accuracy, but comparisons with intraoperative findings have not yet been done [25, 26, 27]. Because one cannot rely on imaging methods, the lack of good palpation during thoracoscopy may cause metastatic lesions to be missed. In a study in which pulmonary metastases were resected by VATS followed by thoracotomy, malignant lesions were missed in 10 of 18 patients during VATS surgery [28]. On the other hand, experience with open surgery shows that the frequent occurrence of occult metastases, which escape detection and resection, does not influence survival [29]. In a recent study, therefore, VATS has been recommended for the resection of pulmonary metastases in spite of the above-mentioned shortcomings [30]. Others take a more cautious view and recommend limiting the use of VATS in the treatment of pulmonary metastases to clinical trials [31].

Major Lung Resections

There is no question that lobectomies and pneumonectomies can be performed by the thoracoscopic technique [32–34]. Lymph-node sampling and complete systematic nodal dissection has also been accomplished via the VATS approach [35, 36]. However, several problems need to be resolved before VATS lobectomy can be recommended as a routine procedure. As in laparoscopic surgery for cancer, port site metastases and tumor dissemination has been described; until today, 44 cases have been reported [37, 38]. It remains unresolved whether this complication is solely due to improper tissue handling, i.e., extraction of the specimen without protection, or whether other factors play a role. The main problem is that large series which attest to the safety of the procedure are missing and that long-term follow-up is not available. If performed at all, anatomic VATS lobectomies should be reserved for peripheral stage I carcinoma without hilar lymph node enlargement or hilar fibrosis [16].

Patients who might benefit from VATS surgery are those with stage I non-small-cell carcinoma of the lung who have a very limited pulmonary reserve. One has to keep in mind that over a quarter of patients with T1 tumors have lymph node metastases (N1=9.5%, N2=16.3%) [39]. Furthermore, Ginsberg has shown that there is a threefold recurrence in patients treated with limited resection [40]. In a study of 67 patients, Miller found a 2-year survival of 80% and a 5-year survival of 31% in patients who underwent limited resection for T1 tumors [41]. Therefore, this procedure should be limited to patients whose poor pulmonary function precludes anatomic resection. Generally, this is felt to be the case if the FEV1 is less than 1 l, FEV25–75 less than 0.6 l, and the breathing capacity less than 35% of predicted capacity [41]. In addition, the lesion should be less than 3 cm in diameter, located in the outer third of the lung, and there should be no endobronchial extensions [16].

References

1. Jacobaeus HC (1912) Über laparo- und thorakoskopie. Beitr Klin Tuberk 25:185–354
2. Dubois F, Berthelot H, Levard H (1989) Cholecystectomie par coelioscopie. Presse Méd 18:980–982
3. Ginsberg JR, Rubinstein L for the Lung Cancer Study Group (1991) Patients with T1N0 non-SCLC lung cancer (abstract). Lung Cancer 7(suppl):83

4. Jaklitsch MT, DeCamp Jr MM, Liptay MJ, et al. (1998) Video-assisted thoracic surgery in the elderly. Chest 113:751–758
5. Jancovici R, Lang-Lazdunski L, Pons F, et al. (1996) Complications of video-assisted thoracic surgery: a five-year experience. Ann Thorac Surg 61:533–537
6. Kaiser LR, Shrager JB (1995) Video-assisted thoracic surgery: the current state of the art. AJR 165:1111–1117
7. Hazelrigg SR, Nunchuck SK, LoCicero III J, and the Video-Assisted Thoracic Surgery Study Group (1993) Video-assisted thoracic surgery study group data. Ann Thorac Surg 56:1039–1044
8. Landreneau RJ, Mack MJ, Hazelrigg SR, et al. (1992) Video-assisted thoracic surgery: basic technical concepts and intercostal approach strategies. Ann Thorac Surg 54:800–807
9. Landreneau RJ, Hazelrigg SR, Mack MJ, et al. (1993) Postoperative pain-related morbidity: video-assisted thoracic surgery versus thoracotomy. Ann Thorac Surg 56:1285–1289
10. Förster R, Weigel U, Geiger A, et al. (1994) Atypische Lungenresektion – Thorakoskopie versus thorakotomie. Minimal Invasive Chirurgie 2:98–102
11. Santambrogio L, Nosotti M, Bellaviti N, Mezzetti M (1995) Videothorascopy versus thoracotomy for the diagnosis of the indeterminate solitary pulmonary nodule. Ann Thorac Surg 59:868–871
12. Waller DA, Forty J, Morritt GN (1994) Video-assisted thoracic surgery versus thoracotomy for spontaneous pneumothorax. Ann Thorac Surg 58:372–377
13. Sekine Y, Miyata Y, Yamada K, et al. (1999) Video-assisted thoracic surgery does not deteriorate postoperative pulmonary gas exchange in spontaneous pneumothorax patients. Eur J Cardiothorac Surg 16:48–53
14. Kirby TJ, Mack MJ, Landreneau RJ, Rice TW (1995) Lobectomy-video-assisted thoracic surgery versus muscle-sparing thoracotomy. J Thorac Cardiovasc Surg 109:997–1002
15. Landreneau RJ, Mack MJ, Hazelrigg SR, et al. (1994) Prevalence of chronic pain after pulmonary resection by thoracotomy or video-assisted thoracic surgery. J Thorac Cardiovasc Surg 107:1079–1086
16. Landreneau RJ, Mack MJ, Dowling RD, et al. (1998) The role of thoracoscopy in lung cancer management. Chest 113:6–12
17. Austin EH, Flye MW (1978) The treatment of recurrent pleural effusion (collective review). Ann Thorac Surg 25:190–203
18. Bernard A and The Thorax Group (1996) Resection of pulmonary nodules using video-assisted thoracic surgery. Ann Thorac Surg 61:202–205
19. Landreneau RJ, Hazelrigg SR, Ferson PF, et al. (1992) Thoracoscopic resection of 85 pulmonary lesions. Ann Thorac Surg 54:415–420
20. Kadokura M, Colby TV, Myers JL, et al. (1995) Pathologic comparison of video-assisted thoracic surgical lung biopsy with traditional open lung biopsy. J Thorac Cardiovasc Surg 109:494–498
21. Landreneau RJ, Hazelrigg SR, Mack MJ et al. (1993) Thoracoscopic mediastinal lymph node sampling: useful for mediastinal lymph node stations inaccessible by cervical mediastinoscopy. J Thorac Cardiovasc Surg 106:554–548
22. Crow J, Slavin G, Kreel L (1981) Pulmonary metastases: a pathologic and radiologic study. Cancer 47:2595–2602
23. Fry WA, Siddiqui A, Pensler JM (1995) Thoracoscopic implantation of cancer with a fatal outcome. Ann Thorac Surg 55:1361–1366
24. Walsh GL, Nesbitt JC (1995) Tumor implants after thoracoscopicresection of a metastatic sarcoma. Ann Thorac Surg 59:215–216
25. McCormack, PM, Ginsberg KB, Bains MS (1993) Accuracy of Lung Imaging in Metastases with Implications for the Role of Thoracoscopy. Ann Thorac Surg 56:863–866
26. Remy-Jardin J, Remy-Jardin M, Giraud F (1993) Pulmonary nodules: detection with thick section spiral ct versus conventional CT. Radiology 187:513–520
27. Touliopoulos P, Costello P (1995) Helical (spiral) CT of the thorax. Radiol Clin North Am 33:843–861
28. McCormack PM, Bains MS, Begg CB, et al. (1996) Role of video-assisted thoracic surgery in the treatment of pulmonary metastases: results of a prospective trial. Ann Thorac Surg 62:213–217
29. Roth JA, Pass HI, Wesley MN (1986) Comparison of median sternotomy and thoracotomy for resection of pulmonary metastases in patients with adult soft tissue sarcomas. Ann Thorac Surg 42:134–138
30. Lin JC, Wiechmann RJ, Szwerc MF, et al. (1999) Diagnostic and therapeutic video-assisted thoracic surgery resection of pulmonary metastases. Surgery 126:636–642

31. Dowling RD, Landreneau RJ, Miller DL (1998) Video-assisted thoracoscopic surgery for resection of lung metastases. Chest 113:2S-5S
32. Kirby TJ, Rice TW (1993) Thoracoscopic lobectomy. Ann Thorac Surg 56:784-786
33. Roviaro G, Varoli F, Rebuffat C, et al. (1993) Major pulmonary resections: pneumonectomies and lobectomies. Ann Thorac Surg 56:779-783
34. Tovar EA (1998) Minimally invasive approach for pneumonectomy culminating in an outpatient procedure. Chest 114:1454-1458
35. McKenna Jr RJ (1994) Lobectomy by video-assisted thoracic surgery with mediastinal node sampling for lung cancer. J Thorac Cardiovasc Surg 107:879-882
36. Kondo T, Sagawa M, Tanita T, et al. (1998) Is complete systematic nodal dissection by thoracoscopic surgery possible? A prospective trial of video-assisted lobectomy for cancer of the right lung. J Thorac Cardiovasc Surg 116:651-652
37. Downey RJ, McCormack P, LoCicero J, The Video-Assisted Thoracic Surgery Study Group (1996) Dissemination of malignant tumors after video-assisted thoracic surgery: a report of twenty-one cases. J Thorac Cardiovasc Surg 111:954-960
38. Johnstone PAS, Rohde DC, Swartz SE, et al. (1996) Port site recurrences after laparoscopic and thoracoscopic procedures in malignancy. J Clin Oncol 14:1950-1956
39. Asamura H, Nakayama H, Kondo H, et al. (1996) Lymph node involvement, recurrence and prognosis in resected small, peripheral, non - small-cell lung carcinomas: Are these carcinomas candidates for video-assisted lobectomy? J Thorac Cardiovasc Surg 111:1125-1134
40. Ginsberg RJ, Rubenstein LV (1995) Randomized trial of lobectomyversus limited resection for t1n0 non - small cell lung cancer. Ann Thorac Surg 60:615-623
41. Miller JI (1993) Limited resection of bronchogenic carcinoma in the patient with impaired pulmonary function. Ann Thorac Surg 56:769-771

Invited Comment on Thoracoscopic Surgery

Malek Massad · Lloyd M. Nyhus

To VATS or Not to VATS?

The recent advances in video-assisted thoracic surgery (VATS) came as a natural sequelae to the introduction of television transmission of endoscopic views in the operating room and to the wide range of endoscopic instruments that became available due to an aggressive industry-driven technology [1, 2]. That revived the interest in the field and brought thoracoscopic surgery back to life. As a result, the classic indications for thoracoscopy [2, 3] broadened to include the diagnosis and management of a wide array of benign and malignant diseases of the chest as alluded to by Dr. Hau. The advantages of VATS are obviously numerous and include smaller incisions, less extensive dissection, less procedure-related pain, shortened hospital stay, and earlier recovery. The disadvantages of VATS are also numerous and include limited exposure, loss of tactile sensation, and inability to locate the pathology in some instances because of its size or depth. There are limitations of spacial orientation and instrument handling associated with transforming a three-dimensional structure into a two-dimensional television image. Operator dependability, the presence of a learning curve, cost of the procedural equipment, and last but not least, the relatively high conversion rate to an open thoracotomy must be considered. Hazelrigg et al. [4] reviewed 1,820 patients who underwent VATS for thoracoscopic procedures in 40 centers. Of those, 439 procedures were converted

Table 2. Video-assisted thoracic surgery: reasons for conversion to open thoracotomy (from [4])

Reason for conversion	Number of cases	Percentage of converted ($n=439$)	Percentage of total ($n=1820$)
Need for more extensive resection	219	50%	12%
Inability to find pathology	65	15%	4%
Too large a lesion or difficult location	62	14%	3%
Adhesions	58	13%	3%
Equipment failure	25	6%	1%
Bleeding	10	2%	1%
Total converted to open	439	100%	24%

to open thoracotomy (24%). The reasons for conversion to open thoracotomy are listed in Table 2.

Although generally regarded as safe, VATS carries a mortality of about 1% and a complication rate of 10–15%, primarily related to bleeding, persistent air leak, and lung injury. One of the frequent applications of VATS at present is drainage of malignant pleural effusions and pleurodesis in terminally ill or elderly patients with end-stage malignancy. Common sense must prevail in these situations when considering VATS versus bedside drainage as many of us who perform VATS have noted an operative mortality above the 1% mark mentioned by Dr. Hau in this patient population, primarily related to anesthetic complications, aspiration, mucous plugs, pneumonia, and respiratory failure.

Three areas that relate to the application of VATS in the diagnosis and management of lung malignancies remain controversial and will be the focus of our commentary:

- Use of VATS versus CT-guided needle biopsy for the indeterminate solitary lung nodule (SLN)
- Use of VATS for lung resection for primary lung cancer
- Use of VATS for pulmonary metastasectomy

VATS Versus CT-Guided Needle Biopsy for SLN

The diagnostic approach for the SLN continues to be a subject of debate. Once identified by a chest radiogram and computed tomography (CT scan), a tissue diagnosis is required, particularly in patients with a history of smoking or those who are over the age of 40 years. In view of the limitations of sputum cytology and bronchoscopy in the absence of endobronchial involvement, in diagnosing the small (< 3 cm) peripheral (located in the outer one-third of the lung) SLN, a tissue diagnosis becomes mandatory. Historically, these nodules are approached by a percutaneous transthoracic fluroscopic or CT-guided needle biopsy. Although a positive cytologic diagnosis can be obtained in approximately 80% of such lesions by CT-guided biopsy, a false-negative rate close to 60% is present among patients with nonspecific benign cytologic findings [1], a majority of whom have carcinoma. Mitruka et al. reported a 25% success rate of CT-directed biopsy in tumors

Table 3. Selection criteria for VATS lung resection (from [8])

Lesion less than 5 cm
Lesion in outer 1/3 of lung parenchyma
Absence of chest wall involvement
Absence of pleural adhesions
Complete or near complete interlobar fissures

less than 1 cm in diameter and a 48% success rate in tumors that are 2–3 cm in size. The success rate for tumors that were over 3 cm in diameter approached 78% [5], but was far from ideal. In view of these limitations, complete surgical resection of a newly identified suspicious SLN becomes mandatory. In these instances, wedge resection of the SLN by VATS and a frozen section histologic examination invariably yields the diagnosis and constitutes the definitive treatment for patients with benign pathology. In situations when the primary tumor is identified as cancerous on frozen section examination, a more definitive resection through open thoracotomy or VATS is indicated.

VATS for Resection of Primary Lung Cancer

Lessons learned from the surgical treatment of breast cancer over the past half century have shown that radical resection does not necessarily mean improved outcome. As a result, many patients who in the past would have been treated with a radical or modified radical mastectomy now undergo lesser resection without an adverse impact on survival.

Despite data in the lung cancer literature supporting the fact that patients who undergo less than an anatomic lobectomy for stage I non-small-cell lung cancer are at an increased risk of local recurrence [6], this has not been shown to have an impact on survival [7]. Therefore, segmental or wedge resection through VATS appears to be a reasonable alternative in a select group of patients who are considered at high risk for a standard lobectomy or pneumonectomy either because of their age, pulmonary reserve, or comorbid conditions. Although demonstrated to be feasible, VATS lobectomy can be technically demanding and requires careful patient selection (Table 3) [8] for it to be performed safely, as major complications relating to bleeding, air leak, or injury to the remaining lung may occur.

Iwasaki et al. investigated the validity of thoracoscopic surgery in patients with primary lung cancer undergoing lobectomy (56 standard and 14 VATS lobectomies) [9]. The number of dissected lymph nodes were similar among both groups of patients, indicating that sampling of the nodal stations and staging may be performed equally well by both approaches.

VATS for Pulmonary Metastasectomy

Pulmonary metastases discovered as the only site of disease in patients where the primary tumor has been under control are often treated by metastasectomy. The most common primary sites of these tumors are the colon and rectum, breast, skin, kidney, cervix, and testicles. The most consistent prognostic factor predicting survival in these patients has been complete resection of all metastatic foci [10]. Invariably, the decision on surgical resection of the metastatic focus or foci is based solely on computed tomography. McCormack et al. [11] retrospectively compared the CT findings with the surgical findings among 72 patients who had primary colon cancer metastatic to the lung and found that computed tomographic scans underestimated the surgical findings in 42% of the cases (30 patients). Subsequently, the Memorial Sloan-Kettering group prospectively enrolled 18 patients of a planned 50 who satisfied the criteria of having only one or two ipsilateral pulmonary metastases identified on computed tomography to undergo VATS metastasectomy followed by thoracotomy to assess for complete resection of all metastaic foci. After the 18 patients were entered, a cross-sectional analysis of the early results disclosed a 56% failure rate of CT scan and VATS to detect all lesions [10]. Although that study was abandoned early, no long-term survival data were available for analysis. In a similar study, Watanabe et al. compared the survival rate of patients with controlled colorectal cancer who underwent thoracoscopic resection of one or two pulmonary metastases to a similar group of patients who underwent resection through a standard thoracotomy and found no significant difference in the 3-year survival between the two (56% vs. 49%, NS) [12]. The limitation of that study was that it compared the survival of patients who underwent VATS metastasectomy to a historical control group of patients who underwent resection through a standard thoracotomy. In order to evaluate for the presence of synchronous contralateral disease in the group of patients with ipsilateral disease on chest tomography, other investigators adopted the median sternotomy approach and found that 45–66% of patients with identified unilateral disease on preoperative evaluation had bilateral metastasis [13, 14]. In view of these data, we recently implemented the practice of performing high-resolution spiral CT scan imaging on such patients hoping that improved imaging may decrease or eliminate the number of lesions missed with a VATS approach. Whether resection of these so-called missed lesions influences survival is subject to discussion [15, 16].

References

1. Landreneau RJ, Mack MJ, Dowling RD, Luketich JD, Keenan RJ, Ferson PF, Hazelrigg SR (1998) The role of thoracoscopy in lung cancer management. Chest 113:6S–12S
2. Braimbridge MV (1993) The history of thoracoscopic surgery. Ann Thorac Surg 56:610–614
3. Bloomberg AE (1978) Thoracoscopy in perspective. Surg Gynecol Obstet 147:433–443
4. Hazelrigg SR, Nunchuck SK, LoCicero J (1993) Video-assisted thoracic surgery study group data. Ann Thorac Surg 56:1039–1043
5. Mitruka S, Landreneau RJ, Mack MJ, et al. (1995) Diagnosing the indeterminate pulmonary nodule: percutaneous biopsy versus thoracoscopy. Surgery 118:676–684
6. Ginsberg RJ, Rubenstein LV (1995) Randomized trial of lobectomy versus limited resection for T1N0 non-small cell lung cancer. Ann Thorac Surg 60:615–623
7. Lewis RJ (1993) The role of video-assisted thoracic surgery for carcinoma of the lung: wedge resection to lobectomy by simultaneous individual stapling. Ann Thorac Surg 56:762–768
8. Yim AP, Liu HP (1997) Thoracoscopic major lung resection-indications, technique, and early results: experience from two centers in Asia. Surg Laparosc Endosc 7(3):241–244
9. Iwasaki A, Shirakusa T, Kawahara K, et al. (1997) Is video-assisted thoracoscopic surgery suitable for resection of primary lung cancer? Thorac Cardiovasc Surg 45:3–5

10. McCormack PM, Bains MS, Begg CB, et al. (1996) Role of video-assisted thoracic surgery in the treatment of pulmonary metastases: results of a prospective trial. Ann Thorac Surg 62:213–217
11. McCormack PM, Ginsberg KB, Bains MS, et al. (1993) Accuracy of lung imaging in metastases with implications for the role of thoracoscopy. Ann Thorac Surg 56:863–867
12. Watanabe M, Deguchi H, Soto M, et al. (1998) Midterm results of thoracoscopic surgery for pulmonary metastases especially from colorectal cancers. J Laparoendosc Adv Surg Tech A 8(4):195–200
13. Kern KA, Pass HI, Roth JA (1987) Treatment of metastatic cancer to lung. In: Rosenberg SA, (ed) Surgical treatment of pulmonary metastases. JB Lippincott, Philadelphia, pp 69–100
14. Johnston MR (1983) Median sternotomy for resection of lung metastases. J Thorac Cardiovasc Surg 85:516–522
15. Roth JA, Pass HI, Wesley MN, et al. (1986) Comparison of median sternotomy and thoracotomy for resection of pulmonary metastases in patients with adult soft tissue sarcomas. Ann Thorac Surg 42:134–138
16. Dowling RD, Landreneau RJ, Miller DL (1998) Video-assisted thoracoscopic surgery for resection of lung metastases. Chest 113:2S–5S

Laparoscopic Hernia Repair

Piotr J. Gorecki

Inguinal Hernia

Laparoscopic hernia repair has become an increasingly popular procedure ever since its introduction in the late 1980s [1]. In 1996, an expert panel concluded that the new operation was safe and effective, but the advantages over the conventional repair were only potential and unproven [2].

Controversies

The Procedure of Choice: TAPP Versus TEP Versus IPOM

In a prospective randomized study reported by Cohen [3], two methods of laparoscopic hernia repair were compared. Both transabdominal preperitoneal (TAPP) and totally extraperitoneal (TEP) procedures were found to give equally good results. TAPP, however, was found to be an easier procedure to learn. In the analysis of 339 patients with TAPP repair and 87 patients in whom the TEP technique was used, Kald [4] concluded that TEP might be the preferred method, since intra-abdominal injury and postoperative adhesions occurred more often in the TAPP group. The intraperitoneal onlay mesh technique (IPOM) leaves the viscera in contact with a prosthetic mesh, does not include dissection of the sac, and may yield higher recurrence rates than other techniques [5]. The review of laparoscopic herniorrhaphy techniques revealed that TAPP is the most frequently performed procedure followed by TEP and IPOM [6].

Is Laparoscopy Better? Analysis of Prospective Randomized Trials

I TAPP Versus Tension-Free Open (Lichtenstein) Repair

Meta-analysis of studies examining 607 patients [7–12], revealed increased duration of operation in the laparoscopic transabdominal preperitoneal (TAPP) group. There was no difference in postoperative pain but the recovery time was shorter in the TAPP group. There was no difference in early recurrences between the two groups. A study reported by Johansson [13] revealed shorter time to full recovery and shorter time to return to work in the laparoscopic group.

II TAPP/TEP Versus Sutured Repairs (Shouldice)

Meta-analysis involving 1,711 patients showed increased operating time in the laparoscopic group but less postoperative pain and shorter recovery time [7, 14–16]. A recent study reported by Jull et al. [17] revealed that patients in the laparoscopic group had significantly less postoperative pain and recovered more quickly. A large randomized study from Sweden [13] revealed that the laparoscopic technique resulted in both shorter time to full recovery and to return to work. There was no difference in the recurrence rate between the study groups.

III Laparoscopic Repairs Versus Mixed Open Repairs

Two randomized studies [7] comparing laparoscopic to mixed open techniques were flawed by the diversity of the open techniques and different definitions of the outcome measures.

IV All Laparoscopic Versus All Open Repairs

A meta-analysis of 14 randomized controlled trials with 2,471 patients analyzed [7] revealed longer operating time but shorter recovery time in the laparoscopic group. The advantage in terms of pain reduction was seen only in comparison to sutured, but not tension-free repairs [7]. Recent prospective randomized studies [17, 13, 18] confirm the observation that the laparoscopic repair results in less postoperative pain and quicker recovery compared to open repair (see Table 4).

Is Laparoscopic Repair a Minimally Invasive Approach?

Open hernia repair is an operation performed with minimal morbidity. Modern tension free repair offers less pain and quicker recovery to normal activity compared to sutured repairs [19–21]. Therefore, the laparoscopic technique offers fewer advantages of a minimally invasive approach compared to other laparoscopic procedures. Twenty-seven controlled randomized trials [7, 13, 17, 18] compared

Table 4. Analysis of recent prospective randomized studies

Current studies (reference)		Operation time	Less pain?	Recovery/ days off work	No. or % of early recurrence
I. Laparoscopic (TAPP) vs. shouldice repair					
Juul (1999) [17]	L=138	77 min $P<0.001$	Yes; $P<0.02$	13; $P<0.005$	2.9% NS (at 12 months)
	O=130	45 min		18	2.3%
II. 613 patients randomized to TAPP, OM, and OS repairs					
Johansson (1999) [13]	L	65 min	Yes; $P=0.02$	14.7; $P=0.05$	$n=4$ NS
	OM	38 min		17.7	$n=11$
	OS	37 min		17.9	$n=4$
III. TAPP + TEP vs. tension free-open					
MRC (1999) [19]	L=468	58 min	Yes; $P=0.018$ (at 1 year)	10; $P=0.01$	1.9% $P=0.017$
	O=460	43 min		14	0%

L, laparoscopic (TAPP); O, open repair (Shouldice repair); OM, open mesh repair; OS, open suture repair.

laparoscopic repair with open procedures. The analysis of these studies, however, is flawed because they compared different procedures and different outcome measures [7].

Stapled Versus Nonstapled Methods

A prospective study of stapled versus unstapled mesh in laparoscopic preperitoneal (TEP) inguinal hernia repair [22], revealed no recurrences and no complications in either group in a series of 100 randomized procedures with 12-month follow-up, suggesting that using staples may be unnecessary. Another large prospective randomized study from Australia [23] revealed similar results. In this report, 502 patients underwent 263 nonstapled and 273 stapled repairs. After a mean follow-up of 16 months, there was no difference in recurrence between the two techniques ($P=0.09$). Interestingly, there was also no difference in the incidence of chronic groin pain or neuralgia between the two study groups, suggesting that the injury to a nerve by the stapler may be overestimated as a cause for postoperative neuralgia.

Recurrence Rate

A large multicenter study [5] comparing recurrences associated with various laparoscopic hernia techniques (mean follow-up of 13 months studying 828 patients available for follow-up) revealed 2.2%, 0.7%, and 0.4% recurrence rates for IPOM, TAPP, and TEP respectively. Felix et al. [24] reported the results of a large multicenter study evaluating the rate and causes for recurrences in 10,053 hernias, present in 7,661 patients treated laparoscopically. In patients followed for more than 6 months, 35 repairs failed (0.4%). The causes of failure were inadequate lateral fixation of the mesh in 11 cases, inadequate medial fixation in eight cases, missed hernia in four cases, and hernia through a keyhole in the mesh in five cases. Meta-analysis of 14 prospective randomized studies showed the same recurrence rates for laparoscopic and open herniorrhaphy techniques [7]. In an analysis of 3178 laparoscopic repairs with a 6-month or longer follow-up [26], the recurrence rate was 1.92%. Another study [26] showed a significant reduction in early recurrences in 487 patients from the laparoscopic group as compared to conventional open repairs (3% vs. 6%, median follow-up of 607 days).

General Versus Local Anesthesia

Laparoscopic hernia repair is routinely performed under general anesthesia. However, the utilization of spinal [27] and local anesthesia [28] has been reported to be as effective. Thus the utilization of regional anesthesia is feasible and expected to become more popular.

Recurrent and Bilateral Hernia: Is Laparoscopic Repair Optimal?

A randomized trial of 79 patients with 93 recurrent hernias [29] compared a giant open preperitoneal mesh repair with laparoscopic transabdominal preperitoneal repair (TAPP). The results of this trial favored laparoscopic repair in terms of improved recovery and a shorter disability period. This, however, was balanced by a higher recurrence rate in the laparoscopic group (12.5% vs. 1.9%, with mean follow-up of 34 months). In another study, 81 patients underwent laparoscopic repair of 90 recurrent hernias with only one recurrence during a median 14-month follow-up [30]. In this study the average time required to resume normal activities was 1 week. Other authors [31, 32] confirmed favorable outcomes for of the laparoscopic treatment of recurrent and bilateral hernias.

Is Laparoscopic Hernia Repair More Expensive?

One of the criticisms of the laparoscopic technique is utilization of disposable instruments and increased operating time, which result in higher operative costs. In a prospective randomized study focusing on cost comparison between the laparoscopic and open Lichtenstein hernia operation, Heikkinen reported that the hospital costs were higher in the laparoscopic group [11]. The total costs for the working patients, however, were lower with the laparoscopic technique when the cost of lost workdays was factored into the overall expense.

Laparoscopic Repair: More Or Less Traumatic?

In a prospective randomized study, Shrenk et al. [33] compared the cytokine response to operation in patients undergoing laparoscopic and open Shouldice repair. No difference was found in the two groups in postoperative levels of interleukin-1 and -6, TNF-alpha, C-reactive protein, fibrinogen, transferrin, $alpha_1$-antitrypsin, and white blood cells.

Are Complications of Laparoscopic Hernia More Frequent and More Severe?

Multiple studies revealed the same complication rates in laparoscopic and open hernia repairs [17, 25]. In a large randomized study from the UK [18], the authors found fewer complications in the laparoscopic group (29.9% vs. 43.5%, $P<0.001$), but all three serious complications occurred in the group treated with laparoscopic techniques.

Advantages of the Laparoscopic Method

- Inlay rather than onlay patching of the defect has mechanical advantages
- Small incision, minimizing wound pain and infection rate
- Excellent visualization of the groin anatomy (including the contralateral side)
- Easy access to bilateral hernias
- Easy approach to recurrent hernias

Summary

Laparoscopic hernia repair is a safe and viable surgical option for the treatment of groin hernias [2]. It is more technically challenging with a substantial learning curve [34]. The optimal laparoscopic technique is still evolving [189]. Although operating room costs are slightly higher in this group, the advantage in terms of less perioperative pain and quicker recovery time seems to compensate for its disadvantages [11]. It is a particularly appealing technique in operating on bilateral and recurrent hernias [29–32]. It also provides an excellent diagnostic modality for evaluation of the contralateral groin. The design of the prospective studies, which can be subjected to a meta-analysis, is not uniform and there were more than two techniques compared: TAPP, TEP, Shouldice, McVay, Bassini, and Lichtenstein. The study outcomes are not uniformly defined and some of the significant confounding variables such as the learning curve [34] or insurance coverage [35, 36] could have been underestimated. With growing surgeon experience and refinement of laparoscopic techniques and instrumentation, laparoscopic inguinal herniorrhaphy will remain a good alternative to open repairs.

Laparoscopic Ventral Hernia Repair

Incisional hernias develop in 2–11% of patients who undergo laparotomy [37, 38]. Open ventral hernia repair can result in a 30–50% recurrence rate, particularly if prosthetic material is not used [39, 40]. Traditionally, open repair carries significant morbidity [41], prolonged hospitalization [37], and infection rates reaching 12% [42]. The first laparoscopic ventral hernia procedures were performed in the early 1990s, but they have only recently attracted the attention of laparoscopic surgeons [43].

Controversies

Is Laparoscopy Better?

To date there has been no report of a prospective randomized study comparing open and laparoscopic techniques for ventral hernia repair. In a large multicenter analysis reported by Toy et al. [44], 144 patients who underwent laparoscopic ventral hernia repair were followed for a mean period of 222 days. The observed recurrence rate was 4% and the infection rate 3%. These results compare favorably with open repairs [44, 45]. A Canadian study reported by Park [46], revealed prospectively collected data of 56 consecutive laparoscopic repairs of large incisional hernias, with a 2-year mean follow-up. In this study, laparoscopic repair took significantly longer than open repair. This, however, was compensated by significantly fewer complications and a shorter hospital stay in patients who underwent laparoscopic repair. There were six recurrences in the laparoscopic group and 17 in the open group. Because of the differences in the follow-up times, meaningful comparison of recurrences was difficult. Franklin et al. [47] analyzed 176 patients who underwent laparoscopic ventral hernia repair. The reported complication rate was 5.1% with an infection rate of 1.7% and a 1.1% recurrence rate after an average follow-up of 30 months. In a recent study reported by Ramshaw [48], laparoscopic repair compared favorably with open techniques. The hernias in the open group averaged 34 cm^2 in size and in the laparoscopic group 73 cm^2. Operative time (58 min vs. 82 min), complication rate, hospital stay, and recurrences (2.5% vs. 20.7%), were all advantageous in the laparoscopic group. Other authors [49, 50] also confirmed safety, effectiveness, and favorable outcomes of laparoscopic repair of ventral hernias.

Choice of Prosthetic Material

Among the number of biomaterials available, expanded polytetrafluoroethylene (ePTFE), polypropylene, and polyester are most commonly used [51]. It has been shown that ePTFE is less likely to adhere to the underlying viscera [51, 52] and has a lower rate of infectivity than other biomaterials [53]. Its other advantages include little adhesion formation while allowing good tissue ingrowth [54, 55]. On the other hand, there is no clear evidence in the literature supporting a preference for the clinical use of any of the three materials [51].

Advantages of Laparoscopic Ventral Hernia Repair

The advantages of laparoscopic ventral hernia repair are:

- Smaller skin incision
- Excellent visualization of the entire abdominal wall
- Less tissue dissection
- Decreased exposure of the prosthetic mesh to skin flora

- No need for dissection of the hernia sac
- No need for subcutaneous drains
- Decreased incidence of wound infection
- Improved recurrence rates
- Shorter hospitalization
- Less postoperative pain
- Quicker recovery

Summary

Laparoscopic ventral hernia repair is a safe and effective procedure [47, 49, 56]. It is a promising technique for the treatment of large ventral hernias [60]. It results in quicker recovery [44, 46, 57], shortened hospital stay [44, 46, 49, 57], decreased infection rate [58], favorable recurrence rates [48, 57], and decreased wound complications [46, 57]. No complications have been encountered as a result of not excising the hernia sac [59]. Because of favorable properties [52, 53], ePTFE is becoming the preferred biomaterial used [59]. Preliminary reports suggest that with technique improvement [60] and growing surgeon experience it may become the method of choice for treatment of ventral hernias requiring prosthetic material. Prospective randomized comparison with conventional repair and longer follow-up are needed [59].

References

1. Ger R (1991) The laparoscopic management of groin hernias. Contemp Surg 39:15–19
2. Jacoby HI, Brodie DA (1995) Laparoscopic herniorrhaphy. JAMA 275:1075–1082
3. Cohen RV, Alvarez G, Roll S, Garcia ME, Kawahara N, Schiavon CA, Shaffa TD, Pereira PR, Margarido NF, Rodrigues AJ (1998) Transabdominal or totally extraperitoneal laparoscopic hernia repair? Surg Laparosc Endosc 8:264–268
4. Kald A, Anderberg B, Smedh K, Karlsson M (1997) Transperitoneal or totally extraperitoneal approach in laparoscopic hernia repair: results of 491 consecutive herniorraphies. Surg Laparosc Endosc 7:86–89
5. Tetik C, Arregui ME, Dulucq JL, Fitzgibbons RJ, Franklin ME, McKernan JB, Rosin RD, Schultz LS, Toy FK (1994) Complications and recurrences associated with laparoscopic repair of groin hernias. A multi-institutional retrospective analysis. Surg Endosc 8:1316–1322
6. Sayad P, Hallak A, Ferzli G (1998) Laparoscopic herniorrhaphy: review of complications and recurrence. J Laparoendesc Adv Surg Tech A 8:3–10
7. Chung RS, Rowland DY (1997) Meta-analyses of randomized controlled trials of laparoscopic vs conventional inguinal hernia repairs. Surg Endosc 13:689–694
8. Payne JH, Grininger LM, Izawa MT, Podoll EF, Lindahl PJ (1994) Laparoscopic or open inguinal herniorrhaphy? Arch Surg 129:973–981
9. Stoker DL, Spiegelhalter DJ, Singh R, Wellwood JM (1994) Laparoscopic versus open inguinal hernia repair: randomized prospective trial. Lancet 343:1243–1245
10. Lawrence K, McWhinnie O, Goodwin A, Doll H, Gordon A, Gray A, Britton J, Collin J (1995) Randomized controlled trial of laparoscopic vs open repair of inguinal hernia: early results. Br J Surg 311:981–985
11. Heikkinen T, Haukipuro K, Leppala J, Hulkko A (1997) Total costs of laparoscopic and Lichtenstein inguinal hernia repairs: a randomized prospective study. Surg Laparosc Endosc 7:1–5
12. Paganini AM, Lezoche E, Carle F, Carlei F, Favretti F, Felicotti F, Gesuita R, Guerrieri M, Lomanto D, Nardovino M, Panti M, Ribichini P, Sarli L, Sottili M, Tamburini A, Taschieri A (1998) A randomized, controlled, clinical study of laparoscopic vs open tension-free inguinal hernia repair. Surg Endosc 12:979–986

13. Johansson B, Hallerback B, Glise H, Anesten B, Smedberg S, Roman J (1999) Laparoscopic mesh versus open preperitoneal mesh versus conventional technique for inguinal hernia repair: a randomized multicenter trial (SCUR Hernia Repair Study). Ann Surg 230:225–231
14. Tschudi J, Wagner M, Klaiber C, Brugger J, Frei E, Krahenbuhl L, Inderbitzi R, Husler J, Hsu Schmitz S (1996) Controlled multicenter trial of laparoscopic transabdominal preperitoneal hernioplasty vs Shouldice herniorrhaphy. Early results. Surg Endosc 10:845–847
15. Schrenk P, Woisetschlager R, Rieger R, Wayand W (1996) Prospective randomized trial comparing postoperative pain and return to physical activity after transabdominal preperitoneal, total preperitoneal or Shouldice technique for inguinal hernia repair. Br J Surg 83:1563–1566
16. Kald A, Anderberg B, Carlsson P, Park PO, Smedh K (1997) Surgical outcome and cost-minimization analyses of laparoscopic and open hernia repair: a randomized prospective trial with one-year follow-up. Eur J Surg 163:505–510
17. Juul P, Christensen K (1999) Randomized clinical trial of laparoscopic versus open inguinal hernia repair. Br J Surg 86:316–319
18. MRC Laparoscopic Groin Hernia Group (1999) Laparoscopic versus open repair of groin hernia: a randomized comparison. Lancet 354:185–190, Commentary 175–176
19. MacFayden BV Jr, Mathis CR (1994) Inguinal herniorrhaphy: complications and recurrences. Semin Laparosc Surg 1:128–140
20. Lichtenstein IL, Shulman AG (1986) Ambulatory (outpatient) hernia surgery including a new concept: introducing tension-free repair. Int Surg 11:1–4
21. Shulman AG, Amid PK, Lichtenstein IL (1992) The safety of mesh repair for primary inguinal hernias: result of 3019 operations from five diverse surgical sources. Am Surg 58:255–257
22. Ferzli GS, Frezza EE, Pecoraro, AM Jr, Ahern KD (1999); Prospective randomized study of stapled versus unstapled mesh in a laparoscopic preperitoneal inguinal hernia repair. J Am Coll Surg 188:461–465
23. Smith AI, Royston CM, Sedman PC (1999) Stapled and nonstapled laparoscopic transabdominal preperitoneal (TAPP) inguinal hernia repair. A prospective randomized trial. Surg Endosc 13:804–806
24. Felix E, Scott S, Crafton B, Geis P, Duncan T, Sewell R, McKernan B (1998) Causes of recurrence after laparoscopoic hernioplasty. A multicenter study. Surg Endosc 12:226–231
25. MacFayden BV Jr, Mathis CR (1994) Inguinal herniorrhaphy: complications and recurrences. Semin Laparosc Surg 1:128–140
26. Liem MS, van der Graaf Y, van Steensel CJ, Boelhouwer RU (1997) Comparison of conventional anterior surgery and laparoscopic surgery for inguinal hernia repair. NEJM 336:1541–1547
27. Spivak H, Nudelman I, Fuco V, Rubin M, Raz P, Peri A, Lelcuk S, Eidelman LA (1999) Laparoscopic extraperitoneal inginal hernia repair with spinal anesthesia and nitrous oxide insufflation. Surg Endosc 13:1026–1029
28. Ferzli G, Syayd P, Vasisht B (1999) The feasibility of laparoscopic extraperitoneal hernia repair under local anesthesia. Surg Endosc 13:588–590
29. Beets GL, Dirksen CD, Go PM, Geisler FE, Beaten CG, Kotstra G (1999) Open or laparoscopic preperitoneal mesh repair for recurrent inguinal hernia? A randomized controlled trial. Surg Endosc 13:323–327
30. Felix EL, Michas CA, McKnight RL (1995) Laparoscopic repair of recurrent hernias. Surg Endosc 9:135–138
31. Memon MA, Feliu X, Sallent EF, Camps J, Fitzgibbons RJ Jr (1999) Laparoscopic repair of recurrent hernias. Surg Endosc 13:807–810
32. Knook MT, Weidema WF, Stassen LP, van Steensel CJ (1999) Endoscopic total extraperitoneal repair of primary and recurrent inguinal hernias. Surg Endosc 13:507–511
33. Schrenk P, Bettelheim P, Woisetschlager R, Rieger R, Waynad WU (1996) Metabolic responses after laparoscopic or open hernia repair. Surg Endosc 10:628–632
34. Votic AJ (1998) The learning curve in laparoscopci inguinal hernia repair for the community general surgeon. Can J Surg 41:446–450
35. Salcedo-Wasicek M, Thirlby RC (1995) Postoperative course after inguinal herniorrhaphy. Arch Surg 130:29–32
36. Barkun JS, Keyser EJ, Wexler MJ, Freid GM, Hinchey EJ, Fernandez M, Meakins JL (1999) Sort-term outcomes in open vs. laparoscopic herniorrhaphy: confounding impact of worker's compensation on convalescence. Gastrointest Surg 3:575–582
37. Hesselink VJ, Luijendijk RW, de Wilt JHW, Heide R (1993) An evaluation of risk factors in incisional hernia recurrence. Surg Gynecol Obstet 176:228–234
38. Santora TA, Rosslyn JJ (1993) Incisional hernia. Surg Clin North Am 73:557–570

39. Langer S, Christiansen J (1985) Long-term results after incisional hernia repair. Acta Chir Scand 151:217–219
40. Van der Linden FT, van Vroonhoven TJ (1988) Long-term results after correction of incisional hernia. Neth J Surg 40:127–129
41. White T, Santos M, Thompson JS (1998) Factors affecting wound complications in repair of ventral hernias. Am Surg 64:276–280
42. Stoppa RE (1989) The treatment of complicated groin and incisional hernias. World J Surg 13:545–547
43. Voeller G (1999) Laparoscopy outdoes open surgery in study of ventral hernias. Gen Surg News Nov:1–14
44. Toy FK, Bailey RW, Carey S (1998) Prospective multicenter study of laparoscopic ventral hernioplasty: preliminary results. Surg Endosc 12:955–959
45. Stoppa RE (1989) The treatment of complicated groin and incisional hernias. World J Surg 13:545–554
46. Park A, Birch DW, Lovrics P (1998) Laparoscopic and open incisional hernia repair: a comparison study. Surgery 124:816–821
47. Franklin ME, Dorman JP, Glass JL, Balli JE, Gonzalez JJ (1998) Laparoscopic ventral and incisional hernia repair. Surg Laparosc Endosc 8: 294–299
48. Ramshaw BJ, Esartia P, Schwab J, Mason EM, Wilson RA, Duncan TD, Miller J, Lucas GW, Promes J (1999) Comparison of laparoscopic and open ventral herniorrhaphy. Am Surg 65:831–832
49. Holzman MD, Purut CM, Reintgen K, Eubanks S, Pappas TN (1997) Laparoscopic ventral and incisional hernioplasty. Surg Endosc 11:32–35
50. Kyzer S, Alis M, Aloni Y, Charuzi I (1999) Laparoscopic repair of postoperation ventral hernia. Early postoperation results. Surg Endosc 13: 928–931
51. Morris-Stiff GJ, Hughes LE (1998) The outcomes of nonabsorbable mesh placed within the abdominal cavity: literature review and clinical experience. J Am Coll Surg 186:352–366
52. Temudom T, Siadati M, Sarr MG (1996) Repair of complex giant or recurrent ventral hernias by using tension-free intraparietal prosthetic mesh (Stoppa technique): lessons learned from our initial experience (fifty patients). Surgery 120:738–744
53. Brown GL, Richardson JD, Malangoni MA, Tobin GR, Ackerman D, Polk HC Jr (1985) Comparison of prosthetic materials for abdominal wall reconstruction in the presence of contamination and infection. Ann Surg 210:705–711
54. Cristoforoni PM, Kim YB, Preys Z, Lay RY, Montz FJ (1996) Adhesion formation after incisional hernia repair: a randomized porcine trial. Am Surg 62:935–938
55. Murphy JL, Freeman JB, Dionne PG (1989) Comparison of Marlex and Gore-tex to repair abdominal wall defects in the rat. Can J Surg 32:244–247
56. Sanders LM, Flint LM, Ferrara JJ (1999) Initial experience with laparoscopic repair of incisional hernias. Am J Surg 177:223–231
57. Costanza MJ, Heniford BT, Arca MJ, Mayes JT, Gagner M (1998) Laparoscopic repair of recurrent ventral hernias. Am Surg 64:1121–1127
58. LeBlanc KA, Booth WV (1993) Laparoscopic repair of incisional abdominal hernias using expanded polytetraflouroethylene: preliminary findings. Surg Laparosc Endosc 3:39–41
59. Park A, Gagner M, Pomp A (1996) Laparoscopic repair of large incisional hernias. Surg Laparosc Endosc 6:123–128
60. Bickel A, Eitan A (1999) A simplified laparoscopic technique for mesh placement in ventral hernia repair. Surg Endosc 13:532–534

Invited Comment on Laparoscopic Hernia Repair

Lloyd M. Nyhus

The use of the term laparoscopic inguinal hernia repair is somewhat of a misnomer. The repair is not performed in the peritoneal cavity except by the IPOM method. Both repairs by the TAPP and TEP techniques are performed extraperitoneally. The same criticism might be leveled at the overall use of the prefix "laparo" as related to esophageal, thoracic, and vascular procedures. Thus, we have tended in

Table 5. Nyhus classification of inguinal hernias

Type	Definition
Type I	*Indirect inguinal hernias* in which the internal abdominal ring is of normal size, configuration, and structure. They usually occur in infants, children, or young adults. The boundaries are well delineated and Hesselbach's triangle is normal. An indirect hernial sac extends variably from just distal to the internal abdominal ring to the middle of the inguinal canal.
Type II	*Indirect inguinal hernias* in which the internal ring is enlarged and distorted without impinging on the posterior wall (floor in American surgical anatomy) of the inguinal canal. Hesselbach's triangle (the posterior wall of the canal) is normal when palpated through the opened peritoneal sac. The hernial sac is not in the scrotum but it may occupy the entire inguinal canal.
Type III	
Type IIIA	*Direct* inguinal hernias in which the protrusion does not herniate through the internal abdominal (inguinal) ring. The weakened transversalis fascia (posterior inguinal wall medial to the inferior epigastric vessels) bulges outward in front of the hernial mass. All direct hernias, small or large, are type IIIA.
Type IIIB	*Indirect* inguinal hernias with a large dilated ring that has expanded medially and encroaches on the posterior inguinal wall (floor) to a greater or lesser degree. The hernial sac frequently is in the scrotum. Occasionally the caecum on the right or the sigmoid colon on the left makes up a portion of the wall of the sac. These sliding hernias always destroy a portion of the posterior wall of the inguinal canal. (The internal abdominal ring may be dilated without displacement of the inferior epigastric vessels. Direct and indirect components of the hernial sac may straddle those vessels to form a pantaloon hernia.)
Type IIIC	*Femoral* hernias, a specialized form of posterior wall defect.
Type IV	*Recurrent* hernias. They can be direct (type IVA), indirect (type IVB), femoral (type IVC), or a combination of these types (type IVD). They cause intricate management problems and carry a higher morbidity than do other hernias.

our presentations to refer to an endoscopy or endoscopic methodology rather than to use the global term laparoscopic when, in our estimation, it is more appropriate.

The list of literature references furnished by Dr. Gorecki is excellent. I recommend careful review of this rapidly expanding important area of interest. The entire field of laparoscopic hernia repair remains in a state of flux. Thus, controversy is rampant. In essence, no single technique has surfaced as superior within the laparoscopic milieu, although the TEP (nonlaparoscopic, extraperitoneal method) seems to be gaining adherents. TEP is my choice because intra-abdominal catastrophic complications are avoided.

It appears that the endoscopic approach generally performs well when compared with the time-tested anterior hernia repairs, i.e., Bassini, McVay, Shouldice, and the innumerable variations of these time-honored techniques. My argument is that when a classification of hernia types is used to determine operative procedures, none of the aforementioned operations, including endoscopic methods, should be used for small inguinal hernias, Types I and II and femoral hernias, Type IIIC of our classification (see Table 5) [1]. This statement can be made as well for the so-called minimally invasive operations from the anterior approach where the use of prosthetic mesh is key, but I feel contraindicated in the type I, II, and Type IIIC femoral hernias. Our editors requested controversy in our comments: our readers certainly recognize the controversial tone of this position.

Laparoscopic techniques for the repair of groin hernias have been extensively studied for a decade. The same problems are aired today as in the early 1990s. These endoscopic techniques are not minimally invasive methods considering the gross blunt dissection of the anterior abdominal wall with the TEP technique and the same pulling and tearing of tissues in the preperitoneal space by the TAPP method prior to placement of the prosthetic mesh buttress to the posterior inguinal wall. Yes, this is one way to apply intra-abdominal pressure to the mesh for correction of the defect in the posterior inguinal wall, but is it the best overall, considering the plethora of proven operations where clean, sharp dissection is the standard. Frankly, I have some doubts.

Ventral Hernia Repair

The garden variety, epigastric, umbilical, and Spigelian ventral abdominal hernias should be approached by a standard open nonprosthetic mesh repair. The massive incisional hernias of the anterior abdominal wall in the morbidly obese patient is an unsolved problem. Re-recurrence after repair of recurrent hernia is the norm. Although still unproven, the use of double layer (visceral nonadhesion provoking inner-layer and porous mesh allowing tissue ingrowth as an outer layer) inlay prosthetic mesh inserted via the laparoscope shows promise of improving our current dismal results in these unfortunate patients.

Reference

1. Nyhus, LM (1993) Individualization of hernia repair: a new era. Surgery 114:1–2

Spleen and Adrenal Gland

Emma J. Patterson · Michel Gagner

Introduction

Since the introduction and general acceptance of laparoscopic cholecystectomy in the late 1980s and early 1990s, the realm of laparoscopic surgery has increased exponentially. Laparoscopic splenectomy and adrenalectomy have both been shown to be feasible and safe, and are currently performed by many expert laparoscopic surgeons. Splenectomy and adrenalectomy are two ideal procedures for laparoscopic surgery, as the ratio of access to procedural trauma was relatively high in the open operation [1]. This ratio, plus the fact that no anastomosis or reconstruction is required, makes splenectomy and adrenalectomy ideal procedures to perform laparoscopically.

Just a few years ago, laparoscopic splenectomy or adrenalectomy would have been considered controversial under any circumstances. Both of these procedures have now been generally accepted as the procedure of choice in ideal circumstances, even among conventional surgeons. However, there are still many controversies surrounding laparoscopic spleen and adrenal surgery: there are those that relate to spleen or adrenal surgery in general and those that are specific to laparoscopic spleen and adrenal surgery. This chapter will address only the latter.

Indications

Splenic Trauma

The spleen is injured in approximately 25% of patients with blunt abdominal trauma and 7% of patients with penetrating abdominal trauma. Diagnostic laparoscopy has recently been introduced into various trauma protocols for the management of both blunt and penetrating abdominal trauma. Acceptance of laparoscopy into trauma algorithms has evolved slowly, even though large series have demonstrated very low false-negative rates since the 1970s [2].

The pervasive conservatism by surgeons when it comes to laparoscopy in trauma may be understandable, since some surgeons have reported a low sensitivity for hollow viscus injuries in penetrating trauma, which is the main argument supporting the traditional approach of mandatory laparotomy if tract exploration shows anterior fascial penetration [3]. The lack of enthusiasm for laparoscopy in abdominal trauma may also partially be due to the fact that trauma surgeons generally perform few laparoscopies, and laparoscopic surgeons often manage few trauma patients. Therefore, many general surgeons are not adept at both trauma and laparoscopy.

Thus the use of laparoscopy in trauma is quite varied even in the few published papers on this topic. Laparoscopy in trauma may be used as a screening tool, as a diagnostic test, or as a therapeutic procedure. As a screening tool it is used to detect or exclude a positive finding (e.g., peritoneal penetration, gastrointestinal spillage, or hemoperitoneum) that requires operative exploration or repair [4]. As a diagnostic tool it is used to thoroughly explore the abdomen and identify all injuries, rather than as a screening tool to identify the first indication for a laparotomy. In a recent review of over 1,900 trauma patients, laparoscopy missed 1% of injuries as a screening tool and helped prevent 63% of patients from having a "full" laparotomy. However, laparoscopy is obviously operator-dependent, and some surgeons have reported unacceptably high rates of missed injuries (40–70%) using laparoscopy as a diagnostic tool. A basic principle of laparoscopic surgery must be adhered to, in that the same procedure should be performed laparoscopically as open. Missed injuries should be avoidable if the surgeon can confidently perform a thorough intra-abdominal exploration laparoscopically [4].

The primary advantage of laparoscopy in penetrating abdominal trauma is the potential to decrease the nontherapeutic or negative laparotomy rate significantly, from 80% to 50%. Reductions in morbidity and mortality are expected to result from this decrease in the number of laparotomies performed for penetrating trauma, but such a benefit has not yet been demonstrated.

Laparoscopy in blunt abdominal trauma is more controversial. In our opinion, laparoscopy is rarely required, since decisions to operate are usually easily made based on the patient's clinical condition and radiographic findings such as focused ultrasound or double contrast CT scan. Occasionally, hemodynamically stable patients with equivocal abdominal findings may benefit from laparoscopy, provided the surgeon is technically skilled enough to perform a thorough evaluation laparoscopically, including running the entire small bowel and mobilizing the splenic and hepatic flexures of the colon.

Recent trends in management of blunt splenic injuries have included a transition from a primarily operative to nonoperative approach. This strategy has improved splenic salvage rates and reduced the morbidity related to nontherapeutic laparotomies. However, nonoperative management has been associated with higher rates of blood transfusion and associated morbidity and mortality [5]. Thus some trauma surgeons have recommended nonoperative management of splenic injuries only if blood transfusion is not required, with early laparotomy when transfusion appears necessary [5].

An interesting alternate approach involves the use of early laparoscopy and autotransfusion in the clinical scenario of a stable patient with a blunt splenic injury, where transfusion is imminently necessary. At least two such cases have been reported, in which laparoscopy was performed to inspect the spleen, and intraperitoneal blood was collected, washed and autotransfused, preventing transfusion of banked blood products [6, 7]. Therapeutic laparoscopy for splenic trauma is uncommon, but successful laparoscopic splenorrhaphy and partial splenectomy have been reported [8, 9].

Splenomegaly

Splenomegaly was initially considered a contraindication for laparoscopic splenectomy (LS), but refinement of techniques has allowed some experienced laparoscopic surgeons to successfully remove enlarged spleens laparoscopically, albeit with longer operating times [8, 10, 11]. A recent retrospective comparison of laparoscopic to open splenectomy showed that patients with large spleens had lower morbidity, transfusion rate, and shorter hospital stay when the laparoscopic approach was used [12]. However, in this study, all five patients with massively enlarged spleens greater than 3200 g required conversion to open surgery due to insufficient working space. Spleens that surpass the costal margin generally weigh more than 750 g. Targarona et al. compared their results of LS in normal versus enlarged spleens weighing more than 1000 g and found that postoperative analgesic requirements were increased, but there were no differences in transfusion requirements, length of hospital stay, or morbidity [13].

Recommendations regarding maximum spleen size for LS vary widely and must be individualized based on surgeon experience. In general, a maximum splenic size of 20 cm in diameter is recommended, and spleens larger than 20 cm should definitely not be attempted for surgeons during the learning curve for the first 15–

20 cases [14]. Poulin found that all spleens larger than 30 cm required conversion to an open procedure, and regards size greater than 30 cm as a contraindication to laparoscopic splenectomy [11]. In a small Greek series on LS for 12 β-thalassemia major patients, only two patients were converted, and the mean spleen size was 35 cm [15].

However, a disadvantage of attempting laparoscopic removal of enlarged spleens is that these are more often malignant and are given to the pathologist intact. Since many surgeons feel that spleen morcellation is contraindicated in this situation, a large counterincision is made for specimen removal. This may negate some of the benefits of the laparoscopic approach. Another disadvantage is the greater potential for massive bleeding since there is a greater number of large vessels to divide.

The first few laparoscopic splenectomies in any surgeon's series should ideally be normal-sized spleens of patients with idiopathic thrombocytopenic purpura (ITP), since these are the most straightforward to remove. Modification of the laparoscopic technique with the hand-assisted approach has been described and may add an additional level of safety and ease of dissection for enlarged spleens [16–18]. Massive spleens that reach the anterior superior iliac spine or cross the midline of the abdomen are more likely to be converted, and may be better treated with an open approach.

Technique

Preoperative Embolization

Some surgeons routinely perform splenic artery embolization prior to laparoscopic removal of an enlarged spleen [11, 19, 20]. However, this is an invasive technique that can increase pain and morbidity, and it has not been widely adopted [21]. Embolization may not be necessary if the technique of early hilar devascularization is performed laparoscopically [22, 23]. In our own limited experience with preoperative splenic artery embolization, we found it to be beneficial in patients with portal hypertension and hypersplenism [24].

Hanging Spleen Versus Detached Spleen

Initially, laparoscopic splenectomy was performed with the patient in the anterior position, mimicking open surgery. Since then, the importance of using gravity to help expose intra-abdominal organs has been appreciated, and the lateral approach has been widely adopted [11, 24, 25]. This allows the spleen to hang by its diaphragmatic attachments, providing a natural countertraction while gravity retracts the stomach, transverse colon, and greater omentum inferiorly, and places the hilum of the spleen under tension. Some surgeons still prefer supine positioning in selected cases where concomitant procedures are performed, such as cholecystectomy in β-thalassemia major patients or abdominal staging of Hodgkin's lymphoma [15, 26].

There are two variations of the technique of laparoscopic splenectomy in the lateral position. These are known as the anterolateral hanging spleen (HS) technique described by Delaitre and the posterolateral detached spleen (DS) technique introduced in 1992 for adrenalectomy and subsequently adapted for LS [24, 27, 28]. In the HS technique, the patient is positioned in a partial right lateral decubitus position at 60° and tilted in 15 of reverse Trendelenburg. The spleen is left attached to the diaphragm until it has been completely devascularized.

The DS technique mimics the open approach and thus may be more intuitive and familiar to surgeons [29]. The patient is positioned in full right lateral decubitus and the phrenic attachments are divided first to provide medial retraction of the spleen and excellent visualization of the pancreatic tail and the splenic pedicle from the back. Differences in these two methods may affect outcome, as it has been shown that the pancreatic tail lies within 1 cm of the splenic hilum 75% of the time and touches the splenic hilum in 30% of patients [30]. Superior visualization of the tail of the pancreas via the detached spleen technique may prevent inadvertent injuries resulting in pancreatitis or pancreatic fistulas.

Proponents of the hanging spleen technique feel that the patient position is more amenable to urgent conversion to laparotomy if necessary. Other potential advantages are minimal manipulation of the spleen during dissection, which may reduce the risk of capsular tears and the potential for splenosis [31].

Localization of Accessory Spleens

Accessory spleens occur in 10% of the normal population and 15–30% of patients undergoing open splenectomy for ITP [32]. As in open surgery, a thorough search for accessory spleens must be performed at laparoscopic splenectomy. Failure to remove accessory spleens (AS) at the primary operation can result in recurrent ITP. Recent series of laparoscopic splenectomy have reported wide ranges of AS (6–40%), with conflicting data regarding the ability of surgeons to find and remove accessory spleens laparoscopically compared with open procedures [8, 13, 24, 32–36].

Most ASs occur in the left upper quadrant (LUQ) of the abdomen, which can readily be explored during LS in the lateral position [32]. A systematic search for AS should routinely be undertaken at the beginning of LS for ITP, prior to the splenectomy. The search should begin around the splenic hilum and greater curve of the stomach, followed by the gastrocolic, gastrosplenic, and splenocolic ligaments, greater omentum, and mesentery. During splenectomy, care should be taken to avoid rupturing the splenic capsule, and morcellation should be performed within a durable specimen bag to prevent splenic seeding and splenosis, which can also cause recurrent ITP.

It has been suggested that preoperative imaging, with either CT scan or radionuclide imaging with denatured red blood cell scintigraphy (DRBCS), might reduce the incidence of retained accessory spleens. However, the literature has not supported this approach, as thorough laparoscopic exploration is more sensitive at detecting AS (75%) than is CT (25%) and DRBCS (25%) alone or in combination (44%) [36]. Preoperative nuclear scans are inaccurate due to the overwhelming uptake of tracer by the liver and spleen, whereas their usefulness prior to reoperation is undisputed [32, 37]. DRBCS can also be performed intraoperatively to locate a small accessory spleen and confirm its successful laparoscopic removal [34].

Morcellation of Malignant Spleens

Laparoscopic splenectomy is sometimes indicated for patients with Hodgkin's or non-Hodgkin's lymphoma. Surgical staging of Hodgkin's became redundant when combined chemotherapy and radiation treatment protocols were offered to all patients regardless of stage. A resurgence of surgical staging is anticipated in the near future due to adoption of a more tailored approach to treatment with less aggressive chemotherapy being considered for some patients with early-stage Hodgkin's disease. Reduction in the surgical morbidity may be decreased by laparoscopic staging instead of laparotomy [38].

After laparoscopically excising the spleen, the standard extraction technique is to place the spleen in a bag within the abdomen, and crush it into pieces to facilitate removal through a port site. However, this morcellation process is controversial in the case of a malignancy involving the spleen, with some surgeons favoring making a counter incision for extraction of an intact spleen [26]. After discussing this with our pathologists, they felt spleen fragments were adequate for a diagnosis of lymphoma, and we therefore continue to morcellate these spleens, as do others [38].

Controversies in Laparoscopic Adrenal Surgery

Since its introduction in 1992, laparoscopic adrenalectomy has become the gold standard for resection of adrenal masses.

Indications

Large Masses

We still consider large masses, greater than 15 cm, a contraindication to laparoscopic adrenalectomy due to technical difficulties. There is no prospective data to answer this question, and surgeons' size limit for laparoscopic adrenalectomy will vary somewhat depending on their experience. Other authors use smaller size limits (such as 8 or 10 cm) for attempting laparoscopic adrenalectomy [39]. The largest mass that we have resected is 14 cm, but such a mass makes dissection difficult and time-consuming, and frequently large masses have numerous retroperitoneal feeding vessels which are difficult to expose and require tedious dissection [40]. Hand-assisted laparoscopic surgery is another option for large adrenal masses [41]. However, the primary concern with size should be more a debate regarding neoplastic potential and the safety of laparoscopy in cancer, rather than the technical feasibility of laparoscopic adrenalectomy.

Malignancy

Early in the experience of any laparoscopic procedure, malignancy is intuitively a contraindication. However, several series of laparoscopic adrenalectomies for cancer have recently been reported. Any surgeon with a large volume of laparoscopic adrenalectomies for incidentalomas will eventually find an incidental adrenal carcinoma or unsuspected metastasis, and this is how the first malignant adrenal masses were removed laparoscopically. Now that we have more experience with laparoscopic adrenal surgery, and laparoscopic cancer surgery in general, some surgeons will knowingly excise adrenal malignancies laparoscopically. As long as the malignancy is confined to the adrenal gland on preoperative imaging and at operation, we feel that a laparoscopic removal that does not violate the principles of open oncologic resection should be considered adequate [40, 42].

This topic is controversial, as with laparoscopy for any malignancy. Some surgeons experienced in laparoscopic adrenalectomy still feel strongly that any tumor suspected of being malignant should not be removed laparoscopically [43]. Strictly speaking, this includes any operation to remove a nonfunctioning adrenal mass due to large size or growth. They argue that the best opportunity for cure is with wide en bloc excision at the initial operation, which is optimally accomplished using open methods for adrenalectomy [39]. These tumors are often large, technically difficult to remove, and vulnerable to breakage or incomplete resection [43].

Pheochromocytomas

Pheochromocytoma was initially considered a contraindication to the laparoscopic approach to adrenalectomy. Theoretical concerns include the larger size of the tumors compared with other adrenal tumors (mean 6.3 cm vs. 3.9 cm) and the potential for hemodynamic instability due to widely fluctuating catecholamine levels, which occur intraoperatively in over 50% of patients [40]. Recent studies have demonstrated that pheochromocytomas can be safely resected laparoscopically despite blood pressure variations and most experts would no longer consider this issue a controversy [44–46]. However, pheochromocytomas with metastases to periaortic lymph nodes are considered a contraindication to this approach.

Incidentalomas

Incidental adrenal masses are discovered in 0.29–1.30% of patients imaged with CT for reasons other than suspected adrenal pathology [47]. Most of these are benign if three conditions are met: (1) no history of previous malignancy, (2) no signs or symptoms of adrenal hormone excess, and (3) normal physical examination [48]. Approximately 25% of these will be hypersecretory tumors, consisting mostly of pheochromocytomas and a mixture of functioning cortical tumors. However, approximately 5% will be adrenocortical carcinomas.

Size is the most important factor in the management of nonfunctioning adrenal incidentalomas. Traditional indications for resection have included tumors larger than 6 cm, enlarging on repeat imaging, or unfavorable appearance (suspicious for malignancy) on computed tomography (CT) or T2-weighted magnetic resonance imaging (MRI). Although much of the literature suggests that tumors larger than 6 cm can be observed, we side with those who believe that young, healthy patients with smaller tumors (3–6 cm) and indeterminate imaging studies should be resected. Albeit most of these tumors will be benign, the morbidity of laparoscopic adrenalectomy is minimal, and the patient is spared the anxiety, expense, and time lost from repeated follow-up appointments and imaging studies [48].

Technique

Approach: Transabdominal Versus Retroperitoneal

During the era of open adrenalectomy, the approach of choice evolved from anterior to posterior (retroperitoneal) for most adrenal diseases. An anterior approach was preferred when large adrenal carcinomas, pheochromocytomas, or additional intra-abdominal surgery, including bilateral adrenalectomy, was anticipated. Originally described by Young in 1936, the posterior retroperitoneal (RP) approach is considered one of the earliest examples of minimally invasive surgery [49]. Since the peritoneal cavity is not entered, the potential for bowel injury is almost nonexistent, and the ileus is minimal [39]. Compared to the open anterior approach, a smaller incision is used which is less painful, and allows patients to recover more quickly. The advantages of the posterior approach to adrenalectomy are now being challenged by the laparoscopic approach [50, 51].

However, a laparoscopic retroperitoneal approach has been advocated by a minority of laparoscopic surgeons [52, 53]. The technique of choice by most surgeons performing laparoscopic adrenalectomy is the transabdominal lateral approach, originally described by Gagner in 1992 [28, 54, 55].

A theoretical benefit of the RP approach is decreased physiologic impact on the cardiovascular and respiratory systems. Animal experiments have demonstrated greater changes in cardiac output, pulmonary artery, central venous and iliac pressures in intraperitoneal compared with RP insufflation at the same pressures [56]. Fernandez-Cruz and his group have published several studies on the physiology of the retroperitoneal approach [52, 57]. In one small study they found a greater rise in $PaCO_2$ level in transabdominal adrenalectomy compared with RP adrenalectomy [58]. However, a more recent update with twice as many patients did not support the hypothesis that the retroperitoneal approach is advantageous in avoiding the respiratory and hemodynamic effects of CO_2 pneumoperitoneum. They found no difference in partial pressure of carbon dioxide between patients undergoing peritoneal versus retroperitoneal laparoscopic adrenalectomy [52].

Another proposed benefit of the retroperitoneal approach is direct access to the adrenal gland without the need to mobilize intra-abdominal organs, which is thought to be particularly advantageous in patients who have adhesions from previous abdominal surgery. The presence of adhesions from previous surgery in the vicinity, such as nephrectomy or splenectomy, can add to the difficulty of dissection and exposure in this space; however, it is rare that conversion to the open technique is required due to adhesions [40].

Disadvantages of the retroperitoneal approach include a lack of anatomic landmarks and a restricted working space. This combination of technical difficulties renders the retroperitoneal approach unsuitable for tumors larger than 6–7 cm. A major advantage of the transperitoneal approach is that the abdominal cavity, and particularly the liver, can be explored. In patients with pheochromocytomas, the liver can be examined by inspection and ultrasound, and suspicious lesions can be biopsied. In our personal experience with the retroperitoneal approach, the exposure was inferior to that which an experienced laparoscopic surgeon can readily obtain via the transperitoneal approach to the adrenal gland.

Bilateral Adrenalectomy: Supine Versus Lateral with Repositioning

Bilateral laparoscopic adrenalectomy is infrequently required for Cushing's disease or bilateral pheochromocytoma, and rarely for bilateral adenoma or bilateral macronodular hyperplasia. Intuitively there are two options regarding patient position: either to perform both adrenalectomies via the anterior approach or to reposition in each lateral decubitus position for each adrenal gland. There are no studies comparing these alternatives, but due to the superior exposure as explained above, we prefer to position the patients laterally for left adrenalectomy, and after the trocar sites are closed, reposition for right adrenalectomy in the lateral position. We prefer to do the left side first since it is technically easier and may be less likely to be converted to an open procedure. The chances that the patient will benefit from a laparoscopic technique may therefore be better [45].

References

1. Cuschieri SA, Jakimowicz JJ (1998) Laparoscopic pancreatic resections. Semin Laparosc Surg 5:168–179
2. Gazzaniga AB, Stanton WW, Bartlett RH (1976) Laparoscopy in the diagnosis of blunt and penetrating injuries to the abdomen. Am J Surg 131:315–318
3. Ivatury RR, Simon RJ, Stahl WM (1993) A critical evaluation of laparoscopy in penetrating abdominal trauma. J Trauma 34:822–827
4. Villavicencio RT, Aucar JA (1999) Analysis of laparoscopy in trauma. J Am Coll Surg 189:11–20
5. Feliciano PD, Mullins RJ, Trunkey DD, Crass RA, Beck JR, Helfand M (1992) A decision analysis of traumatic splenic injuries. J Trauma 33:340–347
6. Collin GR, Bianchi JD (1997) Laparoscopic examination of the traumatized spleen with blood salvage for autotransfusion. Am Surg 63:478–480
7. Smith RS, Meister RK, Tsoi EK, Bohman HR (1993) Laparoscopically guided blood salvage and autotransfusion in splenic trauma: a case report. J Trauma 34:313–314
8. Poulin EC, Thibault C, DesCoteaux JG, Cote G (1995) Partial laparoscopic splenectomy for trauma: technique and case report. Surg Laparosc Endosc 5:306–310
9. Koehler RH, Smith RS, Fry WR (1994) Successful laparoscopic splenorrhaphy using absorbable mesh for grade III splenic injury: report of a case. Surg Laparosc Endosc 4:311–315
10. Schlachta CM, Poulin EC, Mamazza J (1999) Laparoscopic splenectomy for hematologic malignancies. Surg Endosc 13:865–868
11. Poulin EC, Mamazza J, Schlachta CM (1998) Splenic artery embolization before laparoscopic splenectomy. An update. Surg Endosc 12:870–875
12. Targarona EM, Espert JJ, Cerdan G, et al. (1999) Effect of spleen size on splenectomy outcome. A comparison of open and laparoscopic surgery. Surg Endosc 13:559–562
13. Targarona EM, Espert JJ, Balague C, Piulachs J, Artigas V, Trias M (1998) Splenomegaly should not be considered a contraindication for laparoscopic splenectomy. Ann Surg 228:35–39

14. Klingler PJ, Tsiotos GG, Glaser KS, Hinder RA (1999) Laparoscopic splenectomy: evolution and current status. Surg Laparosc Endosc 9:1-8
15. Laopodis V, Kritikos E, Rizzoti L, Stefanidis P, Klonaris P, Tzardis P (1998) Laparoscopic splenectomy in beta-thalassemia major patients. Advantages and disadvantages. Surg Endosc 12: 944-947
16. Gossot D, Meijer D, Bannenberg J, De Wit L, Jakimovicz J (1995) La splénectomie laparoscopique revisitée. [Laparoscopic splenectomy revisited] Ann Chir 49:487-489
17. Ballaux KE, Himpens JM, Leman G, Van den Bossche MR (1997) Hand-assisted laparoscopic splenectomy for hydatid cyst. Surg Endosc 11:942-943
18. Klingler PJ, Smith SL, Abendstein BJ, Hinder RA (1998) Hand-assisted laparoscopic splenectomy for isolated splenic metastasis from an ovarian carcinoma: a case report with review of the literature. Surg Laparosc Endosc 8:49-54
19. Phillips EH, Carroll BJ, Fallas MJ (1994) Laparoscopic splenectomy. Surg Endosc 8:931-933
20. Poulin E, Thibault C, Mamazza J, Girotti M, Cote G, Renaud A (1993) Laparoscopic splenectomy: clinical experience and the role of preoperative splenic artery embolization. Surg Laparosc Endosc 3:445-450
21. Kuriansky J, Ben Chaim M, Rosin D, et al. (1998) Posterolateral approach. An alternative strategy in laparoscopic splenectomy. Surg Endosc 12:898-900
22. Cuschieri A, Shimi S, Banting S, Vander VG (1992) Technical aspects of laparoscopic splenectomy: hilar segmental devascularization and instrumentation. J R Coll Surg Edinb 37:414-416
23. Nicholson IA, Falk GL, Mulligan SC (1998) Laparoscopically assisted massive splenectomy. A preliminary report of the technique of early hilar devascularization. Surg Endosc 12:73-75
24. Park A, Gagner M, Pomp A (1997) The lateral approach to laparoscopic splenectomy. Am J Surg 173:126-130
25. Trias M, Targarona EM, Espert JJ, Balague C (1998) Laparoscopic surgery for splenic disorders. Lessons learned from a series of 64 cases. Surg Endosc 12:66-72
26. Johna S, Lefor AT (1998) Laparoscopic evaluation of lymphoma. Semin Surg Oncol 15:176-182
27. Delaitre B (1995) Laparoscopic splenectomy. The "hanged spleen" technique. Surg Endosc 9:528-529
28. Gagner M, Lacroix A, Bolte E (1992) Laparoscopic adrenalectomy in Cushing's syndrome and pheochromocytoma [letter]. N Engl J Med 327:1033
29. Katkhouda N, Hurwitz MB, Rivera RT, et al. (1998) Laparoscopic splenectomy: outcome and efficacy in 103 consecutive patients. Ann Surg 228:568-578
30. Baronofsky ID, Walton W, Noble JF (1951) Occult injury to the pancreas following splenectomy. Surgery 29:852-856
31. Cadiere GB, Verroken R, Himpens J, Bruyns J, Efira M, De Wit S (1994) Operative strategy in laparoscopic splenectomy. J Am Coll Surg 179:668-672
32. Morris KT, Horvath KD, Jobe BA, Swanstrom LL (1999) Laparoscopic management of accessory spleens in immune thrombocytopenic purpura. Surg Endosc 13:520-522
33. Watson DI, Coventry BJ, Chin T, Gill PG, Malycha P (1997) Laparoscopic versus open splenectomy for immune thrombocytopenic purpura. Surgery 121:18-22
34. Coventry BJ, Watson DI, Tucker K, Chatterton B, Suppiah R (1998) Intraoperative scintigraphic localization and laparoscopic excision of accessory splenic tissue. Surg Endosc 12:159-161
35. Katkhouda N, Waldrep DJ, Feinstein D, et al. (1996) Unresolved issues in laparoscopic splenectomy. Am J Surg 172:585-589
36. Gigot JF, Jamar F, Ferrant A, et al. (1998) Inadequate detection of accessory spleens and splenosis with laparoscopic splenectomy. A shortcoming of the laparoscopic approach in hematologic diseases [see comments]. Surg Endosc 12:101-106
37. Diaz J, Eisenstat M, Chung RS (1996) Laparoscopic resection of accessory spleen for recurrent immune thrombocytopenic purpura 19 years after splenectomy. J Laparoendosc Surg 6:337-339
38. Walsh RM, Heniford BT (1999) Role of laparoscopy for Hodgkin's and non-Hodgkin's lymphoma. Semin Surg Oncol 16:284-292
39. Godellas CV, Prinz RA (1998) Surgical approach to adrenal neoplasms: laparoscopic versus open adrenalectomy. Surg Oncol Clin N Am 7:807-817
40. Gagner M, Pomp A, Heniford BT, Pharand D, Lacroix A (1997) Laparoscopic adrenalectomy: lessons learned from 100 consecutive procedures. Ann Surg 226:238-246
41. Duh, QY (1999) Hand-assisted laparoscopic technique for large adrenal mass. (Personal Communication)
42. Heniford BT, Arca MJ, Walsh RM, Gill IS (1999) Laparoscopic adrenalectomy for cancer. Semin Surg Oncol 16:293-306

43. Wells SA, Merke DP, Cutler GBJ, Norton JA, Lacroix A (1998) Therapeutic controversy: the role of laparoscopic surgery in adrenal disease. J Clin Endocrinol Metab 83:3041-3049
44. McClellan MW, Keiser HR, Linehan WM (1999) Pheochromocytoma: evaluation, diagnosis, and treatment. World J Urol 17:35-39
45. Gagner M, Breton G, Pharand D, Pomp A (1996) Is laparoscopic adrenalectomy indicated for pheochromocytomas? Surgery 120:1076-1079
46. Fernandez-Cruz L, Taura P, Saenz A, Benarroch G, Sabater L (1996) Laparoscopic approach to pheochromocytoma: hemodynamic changes and catecholamine secretion. World J Surg 20:762-768
47. Murai M, Baba S, Nakashima J, Tachibana M (1999) Management of incidentally discovered adrenal masses. World J Urol 17:9-14
48. Godellas CV, Staren ED, Prinz RA (1998) Adrenal incidentaloma. In: Cameron JL (ed) Current surgical therapy. St. Louis, Mosby, Inc., pp 584-587
49. Young HH (1936) A technique for simultaneous exposure and operation on the adrenals. Surg Gynecol Obstet 54:179-188
50. Linos DA, Stylopoulos N, Boukis M, Souvatzoglou A, Raptis S, Papadimitriou J (1997) Anterior, posterior, or laparoscopic approach for the management of adrenal diseases? Am J Surg 173:120-125
51. Ting AC, Lo CY, Lo CM (1998) Posterior or laparoscopic approach for adrenalectomy. Am J Surg 175:488-490
52. Fernandez-Cruz L, Saenz A, Taura P, Benarroch G, Astudillo E, Sabater L (1999) Retroperitoneal approach in laparoscopic adrenalectomy: is it advantageous? Surg Endosc 13:86-90
53. Duh QY, Siperstein AE, Clark OH, et al. (1996) Laparoscopic adrenalectomy. Comparison of the lateral and posterior approaches. Arch Surg 131:870-875
54. Gagner M, Lacroix A, Prinz RA, et al. (1993) Early experience with laparoscopic approach for adrenalectomy. Surgery 114:1120-1124
55. Gagner M, Lacroix A, Bolte E, Pomp A (1994) Laparoscopic adrenalectomy. The importance of a flank approach in the lateral decubitus position. Surg Endosc 8:135-138
56. Giebler RM, Kabatnik M, Stegen BH, Scherer RU, Thomas M, Peters J (1997) Retroperitoneal and intraperitoneal CO_2 insufflation have markedly different cardiovascular effects. J Surg Res 68:153-160
57. Fernandez-Cruz L, Saenz A, Taura P, Sabater L, Astudillo E, Fontanals J (1998) Helium and carbon dioxide pneumoperitoneum in patients with pheochromocytoma undergoing laparoscopic adrenalectomy. World J Surg 22:1250-1255
58. Fernandez-Cruz L, Saenz A, Benarroch G, Astudillo E, Taura P, Sabater L (1996) Laparoscopic unilateral and bilateral adrenalectomy for Cushing's syndrome. Transperitoneal and retroperitoneal approaches. Ann Surg 224:727-734

Invited Comment on Advanced Laparoscopic Surgery: Spleen and Adrenal Gland

Santiago Horgan · Lloyd M. Nyhus

This section emphasizes the ups and downs of laparoscopic splenectomy and adrenalectomy. The authors address the controversial issues in a very balanced way.

Laparoscopic treatment of splenic trauma is still a very controversial issue since most trauma patients are handled today either through a conservative approach (no surgery) or on the other hand a decision is made to rush the patient to the OR. To perform a laparoscopic splenectomy, advanced laparoscopic skills are needed. To perform the same operation in an emergency setting, with the abdomen full of blood and a hypotensive patient, a surgical team is needed with experience in advanced laparoscopic surgery. This becomes difficult to achieve in many trauma centers.

Splenomegaly is another controversial issue. Laparoscopic surgery is performed after creating an artificial intra-abdominal space (to allow visualization) either through the use of CO_2 or through the use of mechanical abdominal wall lift devices. Splenomegaly creates a problem when the size of the spleen limits the view of vital structures. The lack of view translates into lack of control in the case of an intraoperative emergency. Laparoscopic surgeons with experience in advanced laparoscopic surgery can still get around these limitations, but the majority of surgeons cannot. The data published today regarding laparoscopic treatment of splenomegaly are still limited and the procedure is only performed in centers with large experience in standard laparoscopic splenectomy.

Michel Gagner, the co-author of this paper, is one of the surgeons with the largest experience in the treatment of adrenal diseases through the laparoscopic approach. He emphasizes very well the indications and limitations of the technique. The referral of patients with adrenal diseases is limited and only few centers are able to capture this pool of patients. As with any other operation, the ability to perform it correctly is dependent upon the number of cases performed. Here is where the problem starts, because it becomes very difficult for the average surgeon to achieve the complete learning curve. The right-sided adrenalectomy can be a very challenging operation if the adrenal tumor is big or is too close to the inferior vena cava. The risk of injury to this vessel can become a life-threatening situation especially when laparoscopic techniques are used. On the left side the most common complication is disorientation with the anatomy which leads the surgeon to improperly dissect in the region of the pancreatic tail.

Laparoscopic adrenalectomy as published by Gagner and others is a great operation if performed in centers with a large referral base so that the learning curve can be completely achieved.

References

1. Gagner M, Pomp A, Haniford BT, et al. (1997) Laparoscopic Adrenalectomy: lessons learned from 100 consecutive procedures. Ann Surg 226:238–246
2. Horgan S, Sinanan M, Helton S, Pellegrini C (1997) Use of laparoscopic technique improves outcome from adrenalectomy. Am J Surg 173:371–374

Bile Ducts

Eli Mavor · Namir Katkhouda

Complete laparoscopic management of biliary tract problems, mainly choledocholithiasis, but also palliative treatment for malignant distal biliary obstruction, is feasible today with the recent advances in surgical techniques and instrumentation. The recently introduced imaging modality of magnetic resonance cholangiopancreatography (MRCP) [1] allows for a noninvasive, preoperative evaluation of biliary tract anatomy and pathology, and it may obviate the need for preoperative diagnostic endoscopic retrograde cholangiography (ERC), which, even in the presence of strong clinical predictors of common bile duct (CBD) stones, will be normal in over 50% of patients [2, 3].

Laparoscopic Management of Choledocholithiasis

About 10% of patients undergoing laparoscopic cholecystectomy (LC) will require extraction of stones from their biliary tract, detected either preoperatively or by the routine performance of intraoperative cholangiogram (IOC). The ideal management of choledocholithiasis would have been complete clearing of the biliary tree during the same setting of the laparoscopic cholecystectomy; however, the algorithm for management of detected CBD stones is not yet decided because an experienced and skilled laparoscopic surgeon who can perform laparoscopic CBD procedures is not available in all hospitals at all times.

Current controversies in the treatment of CBD stones center on the issues of a staged versus a single-stage approach to the problem of choledocholithiasis: what is the preferred method of intraoperative imaging for detecting choledocholithiasis during LC, IOC, or laparoscopic ultrasound, and what is the preferred laparoscopic approach to common duct exploration, either by the transcystic approach or via direct choledochotomy?

In most institutions, whenever CBD stones are detected, they are treated endoscopically by ERC and endoscopic sphincterotomy (ES), either before or after LC. This staged approach, however, is associated with unnecessary preoperative ERCs performed in over 50% of patients [4, 5]. Endoscopic sphincterotomy is associated with a significant morbidity of up to 32%, and mortality of 0.5–2.2% that may reach 8–10% in patients over 70 years of age [6, 7]. On the other hand, the strategy of postoperative ERC and ES for CBD stones detected during LC has the advantage of reducing the number of unnecessary ERC examinations, but is running the risk of a 7%- to 14%-failure rate, requiring a further procedure to clear the duct [5, 8]. An alternative approach of ES performed during LC, though having the potential advantage of managing CBD and gallbladder stones at the same procedure, is cumbersome and associated with prolonged OR time and logistic problems.

Laparoscopic exploration of the common bile duct has the major advantage of dealing with CBD stones during LC, thus avoiding the problems associated with ERC and ES. Though technically more demanding, it has been shown in numerous studies to carry success rates of over 95% [9–12]. The European Association of Endoscopic Surgery (EAES) ductal stone study, prospectively compared a single-stage laparoscopic management of patients with ductal calculi and gallstone disease to a two-stage management consisting of a preoperative endoscopic stone extraction followed by LC. It demonstrated equivalent success rates and patient morbidity between the two management options, but a shorter hospital stay with the single-stage laparoscopic treatment [13]. The conclusion of the study was that single-stage laparoscopic treatment is the better option and the role of endoscopic stone extraction should change to selective use in those patients in whom laparoscopic ductal stone extraction has failed.

Another issue of controversy is the preferred method of intraoperative evaluation of the biliary tract [14–16]. Both methods currently used, fluorocholangiography and laparoscopic ultrasound, have similar sensitivity and specificity rates of over 95% [14, 15]. The IOC has the advantages of clear definition of the anatomy and superior evaluation of the cystic duct. It is associated, however, with a high failure rate during LC, a false-positive rate of up to 16% leading to unnecessary CBD explorations, exposure to x-ray radiation and contrast material, and can be performed only once after dissection of the cystic duct [15]. The major advantage of laparoscopic ultrasound is the possibility to perform it repeatedly, starting before dissection, allowing assessment of not only the CBD but of neighboring structures and blood vessels. It is the method of choice for detection of intrahepatic biliary stones. However, it does not give a full picture of the anatomy, does not demonstrate flow into the duodenum, and most important, requires a lot of experience for accurate interpretation [14].

Transcystic Duct CBD Exploration

The transcystic approach is usually accepted as the initial method of managing CBD stones [17]. This is a difficult maneuver that has not, in the authors' experience, had the 95% success rate that some authors have reported and requires training [9, 10]. This approach is indicated for small and a limited number of stones, and in cases where a relatively large cystic duct is implanted to the lateral edge of the CBD. It is contraindicated in cases where CBD stones are located proximal to the entrance of the cystic duct, for large stones, and for stones impacted in the distal CBD [18].

The first step of this technique is to dilate the cystic duct. This is achieved either by inserting Kelly forceps into the duct, or by using a dilating kit with an inflatable balloon, a biliary Fogarty, or even stents of different calibers. The next step is the insertion of a Dormia wire basket to retrieve the stones. This may be attempted without fluoroscopic guidance because IOC will already have located the stones. However, when retrieval of the stones proves difficult, fluoroscopic guidance can be called upon, before resorting to a choledochoscope. If a choledochoscope is needed to locate the stones, they can be removed using a wire basket introduced through its operating channel. If all these techniques combined with flushing of the CBD are not successful, it will be necessary to convert to a laparoscopic choledochotomy. Intraductal laser or shockwave electrolithotripsy to crunch the stones is dangerous, as small fragments can be pushed into the papilla, leading to biliary pancreatitis.

The transcystic approach is applicable in over 85% of the cases, and has an overall reported success rate between 54% and 95% [2, 9–11, 18]. Its major advantages are lower postoperative morbidity and shorter hospital stay because no T-tube is required.

CBD Exploration via Choledochotomy

Direct approach to the CBD is indicated when the transcystic approach has failed or is not possible, or when there are more than three to four CBD stones larger than 8 mm in diameter [17]. It has a reported success rate of over 96% with a 2–3.2% incidence of residual stones [10, 11].

The first step is dissection of the CBD, as in open surgery. The peritoneal adhesions are peeled from the CBD. It is not necessary to peel the entire CBD, as there is a real risk of devascularizing the duct; only an area appropriate for the choledochotomy is dissected out. A choledochotomy is performed longitudinally using sharp microscissors. The size of the choledocotomy should be appropriate for the size of the CBD, and should also match the size of the stones. The same technique as in open surgery then applies, with the introduction of a choledochoscope with a 2.8 French channel, through the midclavicular port, to locate the stones. Introduction of the wire basket, either directly into the choledochotomy or via the operating channel of the choledochoscope, will usually allow extraction of the stones from the CBD under direct vision. If a flexible choledochoscope is unavailable or stone removal by this method proves difficult, a traditional rigid choledochoscope can be introduced into the subxyphoid incision after removal of the 10 mm trocar. A suture can be tightened around the choledochoscope to keep the abdomen airtight. This can also be done directly through a separate skin incision.

When the CBD has been cleared of all stones, it should be closed around a T-tube which is introduced through a separate small skin incision. Either interrupted or continuous 4-0 PDS sutures, depending on the size of the CBD, are used to close the choledochotomy. Interrupted sutures tied intracorporeally are best for thin CBDs, while continuous sutures can be used on larger, dilated CBDs. Extracorporeal knot-tying is not useful in this setting. The T-tube is then tested for leaks by injecting some saline, before being properly fixed to the skin. A completion cholangiogram is performed. A drain is always inserted adjacent to the choledochotomy to monitor bile leaks.

Primary closure of the choledochotomy without T-tube may be considered if complete clearance of the CBD stones has been achieved, if there is no distal edema or obstruction, and if there is good tissue quality [18].

Laparoscopic Management of Malignant Distal Biliary Obstruction

Whenever palliative treatment is indicated for malignant stenoses of the biliary tract, because of the very poor prognosis, the management of these lesions should alleviate the symptoms safely with a more comfortable and short hospital stay, allowing the patient to spend the rest of his life as independently as possible. Endoscopic or transhepatic stents have a low initial morbidity, but they require frequent readmissions to treat stent obstructions, whereas surgery has a better long-term result [19]. The laparoscopic palliation of malignant biliary obstruction may be an alternative for patients with an intact gallbladder and an obstruction below the level of the cystic duct. The palliation can be performed as a cholecystoduodenostomy or choledochoduodenostomy.

Laparoscopic Cholecystoduodenostomy

Cholecystoduodenostomy is performed after a Kocher maneuver which will allow the duodenum to be mobilized and approximated to the gallbladder. The duodenum is carefully incised at the ideal location, as is the gallbladder, and both are anastomosed using a continuous running suture of 4-0 PDS using intracorporeal suture and blocking the knots additionally with the laparotie (Ethicon Endosurgery Inc., Cincinnati, OH).

Laparoscopic Choledochoduodenostomy

A more radical way of performing a duodenal biliary anastomosis is the performance of choledochoduodenostomy. This procedure may also be used in cases of recurrent choledocholithiasis and biliary obstruction due to benign biliary strictures [20]. The procedure is similar to open surgery except that the choledochotomy should be performed transversely. The duodenum is then approximated and incised. Interrupted sutures are applied and knotted intracorporeally to avoid the tension that might occur were they to be knotted extracorporeally. Running sutures are possible if the CBD is very dilated.

The ideal suture is 3-0 PDS and square knots are tied using standard techniques. The key to success is proper mobilization of the duodenum. This can be achieved easily by a partial Kocher maneuver of the duodenum. A drain should be left in place.

Laparoscopic Hepaticojejunostomy

Biliary bypass procedures using the gallbladder for the anastomosis have an initial failure to relieve jaundice in approximately 10% of patients and recurrent jaundice or cholangitis occurs in up to 64% [21, 22]. Newer evaluations of bilioenteric bypass procedures clearly favor the Roux-en-Y hepatico- or choledochojejunostomy, approaching a failure rate of near zero [23]. However, laparoscopic hepaticojejunostomy is a very difficult operation that should be attempted only by highly skilled laparoscopic surgeons.

Six ports are used. The operation starts with dissection of the CBD and separation from the structures of the porta hepatis, passing an umbilical tape around it to allow retraction of the duct. The CBD is then transected. The distal part is ligated using an Endoloop with 2-0 PDS. The proximal end of the CBD is trimmed conservatively, care being taken to avoid devascularization. One then proceeds to prepare the Roux-en-Y loop. The angle of Treitz is first identified. Following the small bowel, the second jejunal loop is picked up and windows are created in the jejunal mesentery. Ligation of primary and secondary vascular arcades is done using clips, and finally a transsection of the loop is performed using an Endo-linear Cutter-60 (Ethicon Endosurgery). The distal closed part of the jejunum is then brought up and approximated to the end of the CBD. An enterotomy is performed, followed by creation of an anastomosis using a continuous suture on the posterior aspect of the jejunal wall. An interrupted 3-0 PDS is used on the anterior jejunal wall, making sure to avoid a stricture of the bile duct. Finally, a reconstruction is performed by approximating the proximal part of the jejunum to the side of the Roux-en-Y loop. A stapler is introduced into the two enterotomies and fired, and the enterotomies are closed using either an extra stapler or, better still, intracorporeal suturing to avoid potential narrowing of the enterotomies.

References

1. Lomanto D, Pavone P, Laghi A, Panebianco V, Mazzocchi P, Fiocca F, Lezoche E, Passariello R, Speranza V (1997) Magnetic resonance cholangiopancreatography in the diagnosis of biliopancreatic diseases. Am J Surg 174:33–38
2. Liberman MA, Phillips EH, Carroll BJ, Fallas MJ, Rosenthal R, Hiatt J (1996) Cost-effective management of complicated choledocholithiasis: laparoscopic transcystic duct exploration or endoscopoic sphincterotomy. J Am Coll Surg 182:488–494
3. Liu CL, Lai ECS, Lo CM, Chu KM, Fan ST, Wong J (1996) Combined laparoscopic and endoscopic approach in patients with cholelithiasis and choledocholithiasis. Surgery 119:534–537
4. Millat B, Fingerhut A, Deleuze A, Briandet H, Marrel E, de Seguin C, Soulier P (1995) Prospective evaluation in 121 consecutive unselected patients undergoing laparoscopic treatment of choledocholithiasis. Br J Surg 82:1266–1269
5. Lorimer JW, Lauzon J, Fairfull-Smith RJ, Yelle JD (1997) Management of choledocholithiasis in the time of laparoscopic cholecystectomy. Am J Surg 174:68–71
6. Perissat J, Huibregtse K, Keane FBV, Russell RCG, Neoptolemos JP (1994) Management of bile duct stones in the era of laparoscopic cholecystectomy. Br J Surg 81:799–810
7. Phillips EH, Liberman M, Carroll BJ, Fallas MJ, Rosenthal RJ, Hiatt JR (1995) Bile duct stones in the laparoscopic era. I preoperative sphincterotomy necessary? Arch Surg 130:880–886
8. Cox MR, Wilson TG, Toouli J (1995) Peroperative endoscopic sphincterotomy during laparoscopic cholecystectomy for choledocholithiasis. Br J Surg 82:257–259
9. Petelin JB (1993) Laparoscopic approach to common duct pathology. Am J Surg 165:487–491
10. Berthou JC, Drouard F, Charbonneau P, Moussalier K (1998) Evaluation of laparoscopic management of common bile duct stones in 220 patients. Surg Endosc 12:16–22
11. Dorman JP, Franklin ME, Jr, Glass JL (1998) Laparoscopic common duct exploration by choledochotomy. Surg Endosc 12:926–928
12. Paganini AM, Lezoche E (1998) Follow-up of 161 unselected consecutive patients treated laparoscopically for common bile duct stones. Surg Endosc 12:23–29
13. Cuschieri A, Croce E, Faggioni A, Jakimowicz J, Lacy A, Lezoche E, Morino M, Ribeiro VM, Toouli J, Visa J, Wayand W (1996) EAES ductal stone study. Preliminary findings of multi-center prospective randomized trial comparing two-stage vs single-stage management. Surg Endosc 10:1130–1135
14. Thompson DM, Arregui ME, Tetik C, Madden MT, Wegener M (1998) A comparison of laparoscopic ultrasound with digital fluorocholangiography for detecting choledocholithiasis during laparoscopic cholecystectomy. Surg Endosc 12:929–932
15. Birth M, Ehlers KU, Delinikolas K, Weiser HF (1998) Prospective randomized comparison of laparoscopic ultrasonography using a flexible-tip ultrasound probe and intraoperative dynamic cholangiography during laparoscopic cholecystectomy. Surg Endosc 12:30–36
16. Falcone RA, Fegelman EJ, Nussbaum MS, Brown DL, Bebbe TM, Merhar GL, Johannigman JA, Luchette FA, Davis K, Jr, Hurst JM (1999) A prospective comparison of laparoscopic ultrasound vs intraoperative cholangiogram during laparoscopic cholecystectomy. Surg Endosc 13:784–788
17. Katkhouda N, Heimbucher J, Mills S, Mouiel J (1994) Management of problems in laparoscopic surgery of the biliary tract. Ann Chir Gynaecol 83:93–99
18. SSAT/SAGES (1998) Minimally invasive surgery: advanced laparoscopic hepatobiliary surgery (symposium). Surg Endosc 12:361–373
19. Bornmann PC, Harries-Jones EP, Tobias R, Van Stiegmann G, Terblanche J (1986) Prospective controlled trial of transhepatic biliary endoprothesis versus bypass surgery for incurable carcinoma of the head of pancreas. Lancet 1:69–71
20. Gurbuz AT, Watson D, Fenoglio ME (1999) Laparoscopic choledochoduodenostomy. Am Surg 65:212–214

21. De Rooij PD, Rogatko A, Brennan MF (1991) Evaluation of palliative surgical procedures in unresectable pancreatic cancer. Br J Surg 78:1053–1058
22. Tarnasky PR, England RE, Lail LM, Pappas TN, Cotton PB (1995) Cystic duct patency in malignant obstructive jaundice. An ERCP-based study relevant to the role of laparoscopic cholecystojejunostomy. Ann Surg 221:265–271
23. Schöb OM, Schmid RA, Morimoto AK, Largiadère F, Zucker KA (1997) Laparoscopic Roux-en-Y choledochojejunostomy. Am J Surg 173:312–319

Invited Comment on Laparoscopic Management of Choledocholithiasis

Santiago Horgan · Lloyd M. Nyhus

Management of common bile duct stones during the open surgery era changed dramatically when endoscopic retrograde cholangiopancreatography (ERCP) became a gold standard in the preoperative approach to this disease. When laparoscopic cholecystectomy became available it was almost standard care to study patients who where suspected of having stones present in the biliary tree with a preoperative ERCP. The experience with the laparoscopic techniques and the development of new tools have allowed surgeons to perform retrievals of the stones either transcystically or through a choledochotomy using laparoscopic techniques. One of the limitations is the necessity for extra equipment in the OR: if the choledocoscope is needed, two cameras, two light sources, an extra monitor, and a mixer are needed, equipment that is not always available in every institution. Others have shown, as did Mavor and Katkhouda in this paper, that if performed by experienced surgeons, the use of laparoscopic techniques to retrieve stones is very effective.

Some questions remain unanswered:

- Should ERCP be performed preoperatively or postoperatively?
- Should laparoscopic common bile duct exploration be performed as the first option in patients who are suspected of having common bile duct stones?
- Should we use intraoperative ERCP once the surgeon fails to retrieve the stones laparoscopically so that a single stage is used to clear the biliary tree?

Time and only time will answer these important questions.

Reference

1. Cotton et al. (1991) Consensus. Gastrointest Endosc 37:383–393

Laparoscopic Vascular Surgery

Yves-Marie Dion · Carlos Gracia · Hassen Ben El Kadi

Introduction

It is with doubt and skepticism that the vascular surgery community contemplated the change in practice that has occurred in general surgery since the development of laparoscopy. For a time, vascular surgeons, without denying the potential benefits of this technique, were convinced that laparoscopic vascular surgery was a utopia. Several reasons put forward, such as basic requirements of vascular surgery (i.e., good exposure, safe control of the blood vessels, and meticulous completion of the anastomoses), proved at first difficult under laparoscopy. Furthermore, the pathophysiologic effects of the pneumoperitoneum, and the risk of CO_2 embolization appeared to disqualify a laparoscopic approach in vascular surgery.

During the same period, the wide enthusiasm provided by the development of endovascular procedures appeared to end the debate: vascular surgery seemed to have its own minimally invasive procedure. The laparoscopic approach was considered by some a useless and hazardous technique for vascular surgery.

However, in the early 1990s, surgeons made the first step toward a laparoscopic access to aortoiliac vessels. Animal studies were first performed to establish the feasibility and the safety of this procedure. Clinical studies were later started [1–3]. The laparoscopy-assisted approach was first described, which allowed the surgeon to become familiar with dissection around the aortoiliac vessels. After this stage, and after further laboratory work, totally laparoscopic aortoiliac surgery could be done [3]. As with any new technique, controversies remain. What is the best laparoscopic approach to aortoiliac vessels? Where should laparoscopic vascular surgery stand among endovascular and open techniques?

Different Approaches to Aortoiliac Vessels

Trans- Versus Retroperitoneal Approach

Transperitoneal access [2, 4, 5], even if used commonly in open surgery, was found to be difficult. Indeed, the main problem was the exposure of the aorta without the intrusion of intraperitoneal organs in the operative field (Figs. 1–3). Several methods were used to retract the small bowel and to keep it away from the aorta. Among these methods, fan and fish retractors and the use of the Trendelenburg position did not win overall approval. As a result, other approaches have been developed. The lateral retroperitoneal approach [3, 6, 7], keeping the abdominal organs off the aorta, seemed attractive. However, several problems arose: the retroperitoneal cavity is not easy to create and to maintain, the lateral positioning of the patient does not facilitate right femoral access, the tunnelization of the graft is not easy, and the surgeon is unable to inspect the abdominal cavity, particularly the left colon. The anterior retroperitoneal approach developed by Shumacker et al. [8]

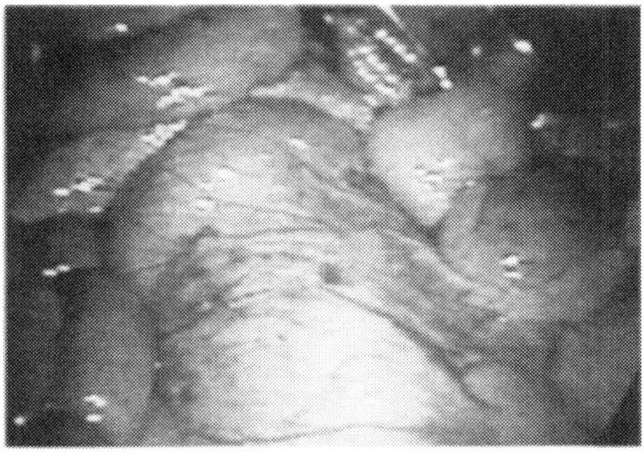

Fig. 1. The intraperitoneal approach. Despite the presence of two fan-shaped retractors, and the Trendelenburg position, the small bowel is seen to surround the retroperitoneum overlying the aorta

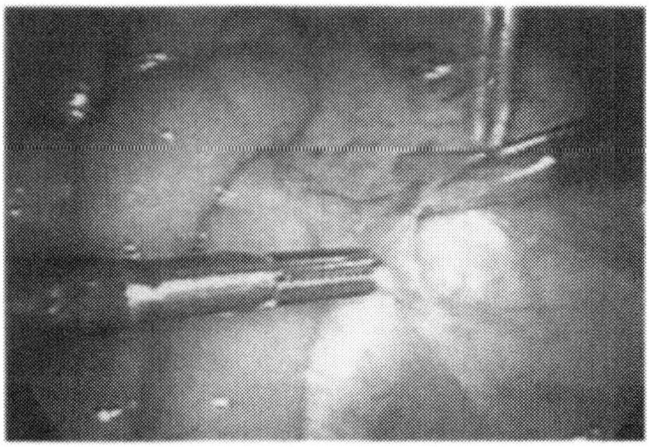

Fig. 2. The intraperitoneal approach. The retroperitoneum overlying the aortic bifurcation is being incised. Note the proximity of the small bowel which could lead to a dangerous situation

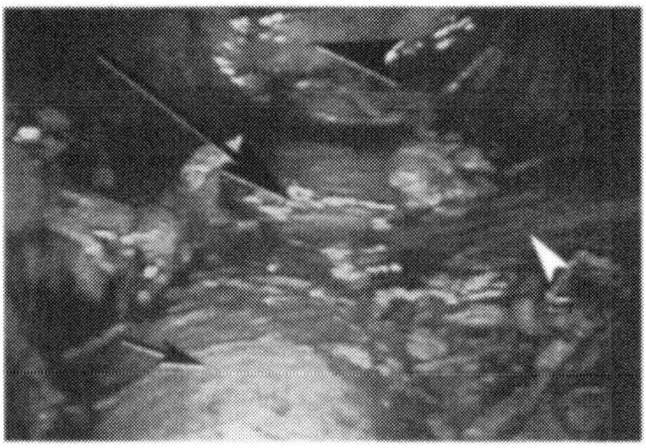

Fig. 3. The intraperitoneal approach to the aorta (*short arrow*) up to the renal vein (*long arrow*) is made difficult by the presence of the small bowel (*large arrowhead*) which inevitably falls over the operative site. The tip of a suction device (*small arrowhead*) is seen to push against the inferior aspect of the renal vein

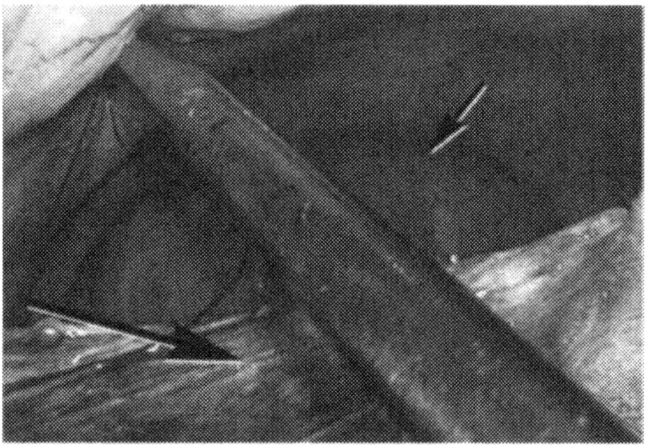

Fig. 4. The left parietal peritoneum along with the retroperitoneum have been dissected from the abdominal wall and will be used to create an "apron" (*long arrow*) which will separate the peritoneal content (*short arrow*) from the retroperitoneal working field. The caecum is visible behind the peritoneal apron. A 0 nylon suture is being inserted in the anterior portion of the peritoneal apron and when it will be pulled to the right, the content of the peritoneal cavity will disappear from view

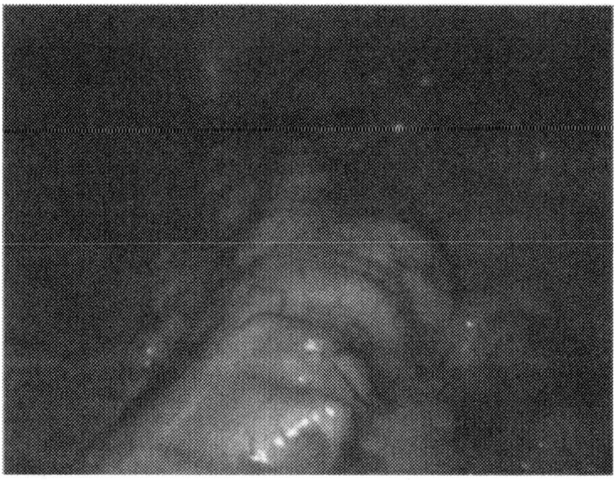

Fig. 5. The sigmoid colon can be inspected using the apron technique

was applied to laparoscopy to facilitate the tunnelization of the graft and the femoral dissection, but it was also not judged totally satisfactory [9].

Controversy remains concerning the best approach to the aortoiliac vessels. We devised a new technique that in our opinion could offer a valuable alternative to these approaches [10]. The "apron" technique involves the creation of a flap of retroperitoneum that is used to separate the intraperitoneal organs from the content of the retroperitoneal cavity (Fig. 4). We found many advantages to this technique: an easier retraction of intraperitoneal structures, a larger retroperitoneal cavity, the ability to inspect the left colon at any moment (Fig. 5), and a peritoneal coverage of the entire graft at the end of the procedure, which is presently very difficult to obtain using the transabdominal approach.

The Gasless Technique

Under CO_2 pneumoperitoneum, fear of CO_2 embolism, of leaks at the trocars sites, and of an eventual collapse of the working cavity after prolonged suctioning led to the use of a gasless technique to maintain sufficient space. Berens [4] summarized the potential advantages of working in a gasless environment: it is possible to use standard vascular instruments, to use vigorous suction if needed, and to eliminate potential CO_2 complications. However, he noted how difficult it was to work in a pyramid-shaped rather than in a dome-shaped cavity (Fig. 6) and emphasized that it was impossible to maintain good exposure without the use of classical bowel packing with laparotomy pads inserted through a 4-cm incision. In the author's experience [3, 9], the gasless technique was abandoned because many judged it to be of little help. Indeed, since dedicated instrumentation has become available, including laparoscopic vascular clamps and appropriate trocars, the need for standard instrumentation and the possibility of leaks and collapse of the cavity appear to be remote. However, the potential risk of gas embolism (0.2–0.002% in most series) [11] must not be forgotten. In an experimental study evaluating the risk of pulmonary embolization following major venous laceration occurring during laparoscopic surgery, it was suggested that gas embolism occurred in 18% of the cases after 1-cm venotomies were performed in the inferior vena cava [12]. However, in these cases, small and clinically insignificant quantities of CO_2 were traced in the right heart cavities with transoesophageal ultrasound (Figs. 7, 8).

Even if caution is suggested when laparoscopic surgery is performed in the vicinity of large veins, we found that the large dome-cavity and the better visualiza-

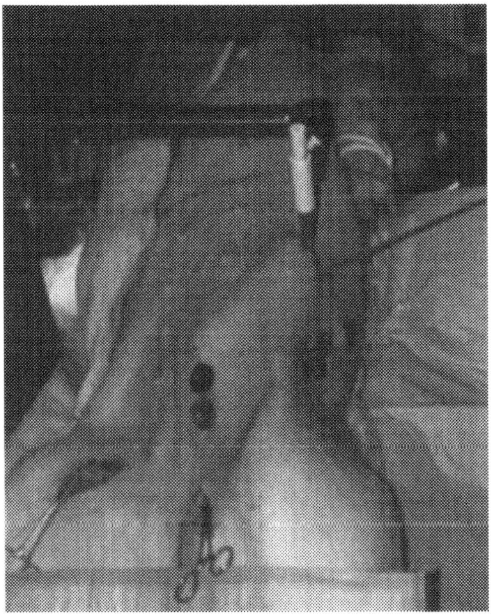

Fig. 6. This animal model demonstrates how an abdominal wall lift creates a pyramid-shaped cavity since there is no lateral force expanding the cavity medially and laterally, unlike the pneumoperitoneum

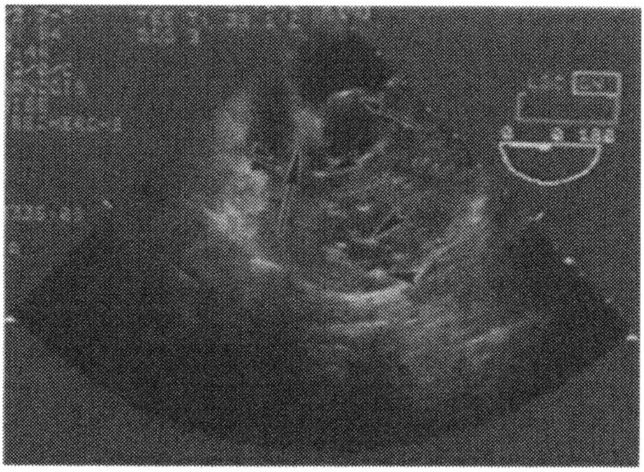

Fig. 7. Transoesophageal echocardiography after a 1-cm venotomy was created on the anterior wall of the inferior vena cava under a 15 mmHg pneumoperitoneum. Only a few CO_2 bubbles can be seen in the right atrium and left ventricle (*arrowheads*) in 18% of the cases. *Long arrows* point to the tricuspid and mitral valves

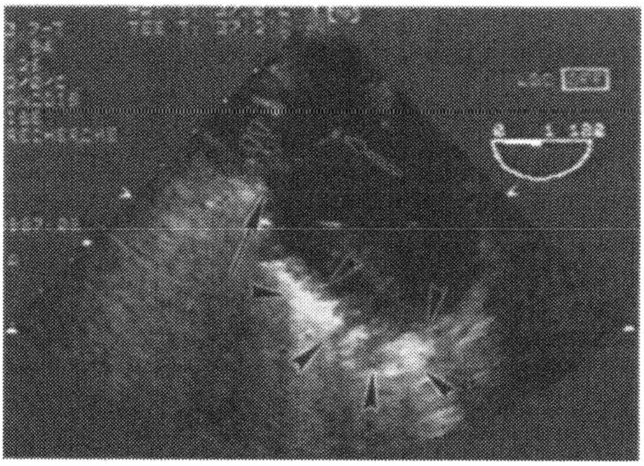

Fig. 8. 15 cc of CO_2 has been bolused through the right internal jugular vein. *Arrowheads* point to a definitely larger quantity of CO_2 in the left cardiac cavities; *arrows* represent the previously mentioned valves

tion provided by the pneumoperitoneum make it the method of choice to maintain a sufficient and stable working cavity.

The Place of Laparoscopy in Vascular Surgery

The management of many surgical conditions has been revolutionized by endovascular techniques. Endovascular procedures have proven their safety and effectiveness. Concerning aortoiliac disease (i.e., occlusive and aneurysmal disease), one may wonder where laparoscopy will stand in the future between the standard open repair and endovascular surgery.

Aortoiliac Occlusive Disease

In aortoiliac occlusive disease, the gold standard treatment is the open aortobifemoral bypass. The major reasons of this primary role lie in its well-documented long-term patency rate (90% at 5 years and 75% at 10 years) [13], its excellent functional results, and its applicability to most patterns of disease.

The other alternative more recently developed aortoiliac occlusive disease treatment is percutaneus transluminal angioplasty (PTA). The potential advantages that it provides (i.e., reduced risk, reduced hospital stay, quicker recovery, and cost effectiveness) explain its major impact on the management of aortoiliac occlusive disease. Furthermore, studies reported a 5-year patency of 70% for a stenosis of the lower aorta [14] and 72% for iliac stenoses [15]. However, only few randomized prospective data exist. Comparing patients with diseases suitable for treatment by each modality, Wilson [16] found that the cumulative long-term success rate favored surgery (81% vs. 62% success rate at 3 years). Another prospective study of 667 iliac PTA procedures confirmed a 3-year success rate of 60% in the most favorable circumstance (i.e., localized common iliac stenosis in patients with claudication alone and good runoff) [17]. Concerning iliac occlusion, the role of PTA appears to be more limited. Johnston [17] reported a 3-year success rate of only 48% and 17% in patients with long-segment occlusions and multiple stenoses.

These studies demonstrated that the chance of long-term success depends on the following major variables: indication, site and severity of the lesion, and runoff quality. PTA does not appear to be applicable to patients with extensive patterns of disease. Thus, this approach has an important role to play in the management of only selected patients with aortoiliac occlusive disease.

The fact that laparoscopy differs from the conventional method only by the approach used represents a great advantage. Long-term results are not available but they are expected to be similar to those reported for the open technique. Among the variety of approaches used, several points have to be emphasized. Laparoscopic surgery for occlusive disease has proven feasible. Operative time has decreased from 8 h to 4 h, dissection of the aortoiliac vessels can be done safely and anastomosis can be now performed in 18–30 min. Laparoscopic surgery also appears reproducible. We have now operated on 40 patients. Barbera [18] showed positive results after studying 31 patients. End-to-side anastomosis and reimplantation of the inferior mesenteric artery are also feasible under laparoscopy [19, 20].

It has been suggested that the laparoscopic approach could decrease the ICU stay and the hospital stay. It could cause less disabling pain and allow for a quicker recovery [21, 22]. Furthermore, a recent prospective study comparing the interleukin level between standard open, laparoscopic-assisted, and retroperitoneal repair revealed that laparoscopy reduces surgical trauma [23].

In summary, the feasibility and reliability of the laparoscopic technique, the ability to perform a standard aortobifemoral bypass (Fig. 9), its wide applicability among different patterns of occlusive disease, and the fact that it should provide the same advantages as those demonstrated in general surgery make the laparoscopic approach appear as a serious contender for the treatment of occlusive aortoiliac disease.

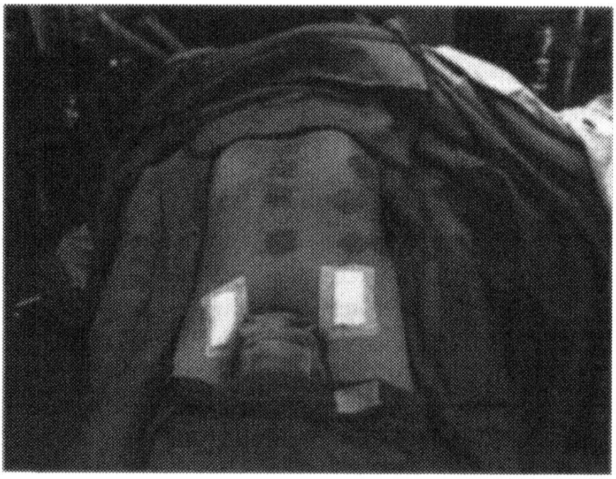

Fig. 9. A patient who just underwent a totally laparoscopic aortobifemoral bypass

Abdominal Aortic Aneurysm Repair

The first laparoscopy-assisted abdominal aortic aneurysm (AAA) repairs were performed by Chen and al. [1]. They observed decreased postoperative ileus, less hypothermia, lower fluid requirements, and less postoperative pain compared to open surgery [5, 24]. The minilaparotomy associated with the laparoscopy-assisted technique allowed for a standard endoaneurysmorraphy popularized by Creech in 1966 [25].

Edoga [7, 26] and Jobe [27] performed laparoscopic AAA repairs using the exclusion technique. They clipped the lumbar arteries from outside and performed aortobifemoral or aortoiliac bypass. The authors emphasized the technical difficulty of this procedure and the long learning curve required, but they noticed a quicker recovery and less disabling pain than in their previous open repair. In our opinion, the gold standard endoaneurysmorrhaphy should not be altered (i.e., employing the exclusion technique) to allow the performance of laparoscopic repair. Indeed, it appears that the long-term fate of the exclusion technique has not been determined and concern exists that the excluded blood-filled aneurysm may not thrombose or may be the source of late sepsis [28].

We have performed totally laparoscopic aneurysmorrhaphy (Figs. 10–12). We believe that the most significant difficulties in AAA repair (i.e., occlusion of the lumbar arteries, safe dissection of the aneurysmal neck, and removal of the intraluminal thrombus) will soon be resolved by appropriate instrumentation.

Endovascular AAA repair is also another field where the laparoscopic approach could be helpful. Indeed, the anatomic requirements that make an AAA suitable for endovascular repair seem to be more and more stringent. A recent study revealed that based on currently available technology, 80% of the patients were not candidates for an endovascular AAA repair because of proximal calcification, short aortic or distal cuff, coexisting distal iliac aneurysm, and stenotic iliac disease [29]. Furthermore, even after the learning curve and the correction of device-related problems, this evolving field seems to carry a significant number of compli-

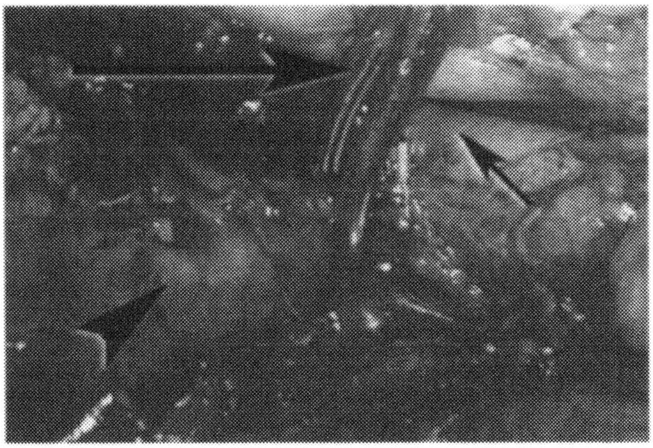

Fig. 10. The aortic clamp (*long arrow*) has been placed at the level of the aneurysm neck just distal to the left renal vein (*short arrow*). The proximal portion of the aneurysm mass can be seen to the left of the picture (*arrowhead*)

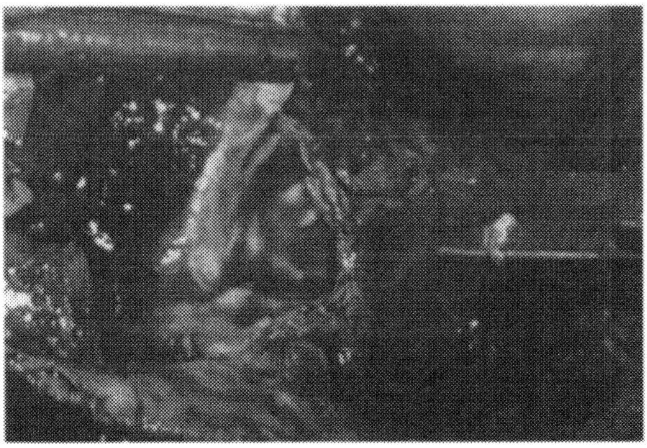

Fig. 11. The aneurysm neck as is often seen in open surgery

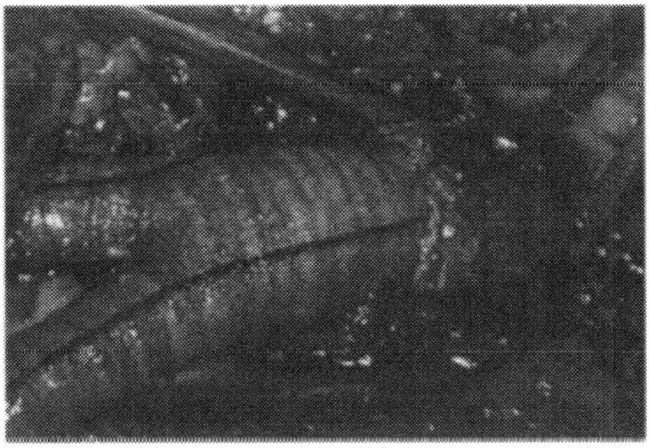

Fig. 12. The aortic anastomosis has been unclamped. The aneurysm wall can be seen pushed aside by the suction device

cations, mainly endoleaks [30, 31]. One could easily emphasize the added value of laparoscopy in such cases. The laparoscopic approach to aortoiliac vessels could help prevent or manage such endoleaks. Kolvenbach and al. described an original approach to treat iatrogenic pseudoaneurysm with combined endovascular and laparoscopic techniques [32].

At the present time, the development of the laparoscopic technique for AAA repair depends on the availability of dedicated instrumentation which will soon be available. A realistic animal model [9, 33] has to be developed for teaching purposes.

Conclusion

Laparoscopy in vascular surgery is in development. Obesity, high-risk patients, and the hostile abdomen are the present contraindications to this type of surgery, which presently requires technical expertise. However, this technique is very attractive. It differs from standard surgery only by the approach used, and does not carry much incertitude on its outcome. Randomized studies should prove that laparoscopy will provide the same benefits for vascular patients as it did for general surgery patients.

References

1. Chen MH, Murphy EA, Halpern V, Faust GR, Cosgrove JM, Cohen JR (1995) Laparoscopic-assisted abdominal aortic aneurysm repair. Surg Endosc 9:905–907
2. Dion YM, Katkhouda N, Rouleau C, Aucoin A (1993) Laparoscopy-assisted aortobifemoral bypass. Surg Laparosc Endosc 3:425–429
3. Dion YM, Chin AK, Thompson TA (1995) Experimental laparoscopic aortobifemoral bypass. Surg Endosc 9:894–897
4. Berens ES, Herde JR (1995) Laparoscopic vascular surgery: four case reports [see comments]. J Vasc Surg 22:73–79
5. Kline RG, AJ DA, Chen MH, Halpern VJ, Cohen JR (1998) Laparoscopically assisted abdominal aortic aneurysm repair: first 20 cases. J Vasc Surg 27:81–88
6. Edoga J, James K, Resnikoff M, Asgarian K, Singh D, Romanelli J (1998) Laparoscopic aortic aneurysm resection. J Endovasc Surg 5:335–344
7. Edoga JK, Asgarian K, Singh D, et al. (1998) Laparoscopic surgery for abdominal aortic aneurysms. Technical elements of the procedure and a preliminary report of the first 22 patients. Surg Endosc 12:1064–1072
8. Shumacker HB, Jr (1972) Midline extraperitoneal exposure of the abdominal aorta and iliac arteries. Surg Gynecol Obstet 135:791–792
9. Dion YM, Gracia C (1996) Experimental laparoscopic aortic aneurysm resection and aortobifemoral bypass. Surg Laparosc Endosc 6:184–190
10. Dion YM, Gracia CR (1997) A new technique for laparoscopic aortobifemoral grafting in occlusive aortoiliac disease. J Vasc Surg 26:685–692
11. Wolf JS, Jr, Stoller ML (1994) The physiology of laparoscopy: basic principles, complications and other considerations. J Urol 152:294–302
12. Dion YM, Levesque C, Doillon CJ (1995) Experimental carbon dioxide pulmonary embolization after vena cava laceration under pneumoperitoneum. Surg Endosc 9:1065–1069
13. Brewster DC (1997) Current controversies in the management of aortoiliac occlusive disease. J Vasc Surg 25:365–379
14. Charlebois N, Saint Georges G, Hudon G (1986) Percutaneous transluminal angioplasty of the lower abdominal aorta. AJR Am J Roentgenol 146:369–371
15. Becker GJ, Katzen BT, Dake MD (1989) Noncoronary angioplasty. Radiology 170:921–940

16. Wilson SE, Wolf GL, Cross AP (1989) Percutaneous transluminal angioplasty versus operation for peripheral arteriosclerosis. Report of a prospective randomized trial in a selected group of patients. J Vasc Surg 9:1–9
17. Johnston KW (1993) Iliac arteries: reanalysis of results of balloon angioplasty. Radiology 186:207–212
18. Barbera L, Kemen M, Mumme A, Zumtobel V (1998) Results of 31 laparoscopic interventions of the aorto-iliac vessels for arterial occlusive disease. Langenbecks Arch Chir Suppl Kongressbd 115:528–531
19. Dion Y, Hartung O, Gracia C, Doillon C (1999) Experimental laparoscopic aortobifemoral bypass with end-to-side aortic anastomosis. Surg Laparosc Endosc 9:35–38
20. Dion Y, Hartung O, Gracia C, Doillon C (1999) Laparoscopic end-to-end aortobifemoral bypass with reimplantation of the inferior mesenteric artery:an experimental study. Surg Edosc 13:449–451
21. Ahn SS, Hiyama DT, Rudkin GH, Fuchs GJ, Ro KM, Concepcion B (1997) Laparoscopic aortobifemoral bypass. J Vasc Surg 26:128–132
22. Barbera L, Mumme A, Metin S, Zumtobel V, Kemen M (1998) Operative results and outcome of twenty-four totally laparoscopic vascular procedures for aortoiliac occlusive disease. J Vasc Surg 28:136–142
23. Kolvenbach R, Deling O, Schwierz E, Landers B (1998) Reducing the operative trauma in aortoiliac reconstructions: a prospective study to evaluate the role of video-assisted vascular surgery. Eur J Vasc Endovasc Surg 15:483–488
24. Chen MHM, AJ DA, Murphy EA, Cohen JR (1996) Laparoscopically assisted abdominal aortic aneurysm repair. A report of 10 cases. Surg Endosc 10:1136–1139
25. Creech O, Jr (1966) Endo-aneurysmorrhaphy and treatment of aortic aneurysm. Ann Surg 164:935–946
26. Edoga JK, James KV, Resnikoff M, Asgarian K, Singh D, Romanelli J (1998) Laparoscopic aortic aneurysm resection. J Endovasc Surg 5:335–344
27. Jobe BA, Duncan W, Swanstrom LL (1999) Totally laparoscopic abdominal aortic aneurysm repair. Surg Endosc 13:77–79
28. Shah DM, Chang BB, Paty PS, Kaufman JL, Koslow AR, Leather RP (1991) Treatment of abdominal aortic aneurysm by exclusion and bypass: an analysis of outcome [see comments]. J Vasc Surg 13:15–22
29. Treiman GS, Lawrence PF, Edwards WH, Jr, Galt SW, Kraiss LW, Bhirangi K 1999) An assessment of the current applicability of the EVT endovascular graft for treatment of patients with an infrarenal abdominal aortic aneurysm. J Vasc Surg 30:68–75
30. Schurink GW, Aarts NJ, van Bockel JH (1999) Endoleak after stent-graft treatment of abdominal aortic aneurysm: a meta-analysis of clinical studies. Br J Surg 86:581–587
31. Schurink GW, Aarts NJ, van Baalen JM, Chuter TA, Schultze Kool LJ, van Bocke JH (1999) Late endoleak after endovascular therapy for abdominal aortic aneurysm. Eur J Vasc Endovasc Surg 17:448–450
32. Kolvenbach R, Schwierz E (1998) Combined endovascular/laparoscopic approach to aortic pseudoaneurysm repair (letter). J Endovasc Surg 5191–193
33. Dion YM, Cardon A, Gracia CR, Doillon C (1999) A model for laparoscopic aortic aneurysm resection. Surg Endosc 13:654–657

Invited Comment on Endoscopic Vascular Surgery

David S. Landau · Lloyd M. Nyhus

The application of endoscopic techniques to vascular surgery has lagged in comparison to other surgical disciplines, for reasons mentioned by the authors. While endoscopy has gained favor in the area of perforator ligation surgery and saphenous vein harvesting, it has not in regards to abdominal vascular procedures. With the alternatives to conventional vascular procedures already available, namely extra-anatomic bypass grafting, angioplasty with and without stenting, endoluminal techniques for aneurysmal and occlusive disease, and retroperitoneal exposures, the question is not whether abdominal or retroperitoneal endoscopic vascular surgery can be performed, but rather should it be performed, and if so, when? In regard to aortoiliac procedures, the authors have justifiably stated that since endoscopic methods of repair utilize grafting techniques similar to traditional approaches, the patency rates should also be similar. However, in order to gain acceptance within the vascular community, such procedures will need to be simple to perform while offering something new, such as reduced risk and fewer complications. Edoga et al. have commented, in their preliminary report of 22 aneurysmal patients treated endoscopically, that the procedure does not alter the outcome in high-risk patients, with the risk of death being largely determined by associated comorbid conditions [1]. Presently, it would appear that endovascular repair of abdominal aortic aneurysms (AAA) would be a better alternative for high-risk patients if future trials yield results similar to Edoga's and if endovascular methods of repair prove durable. Disqualifications for endovascular repair of aortic aneurysms, such as suprarenal aneurysms, short necks, heavy calcification, associated distal iliac aneurysms, and aberrant visceral anatomy, will likely make endoscopic repair difficult, if not impossible. Barbera et al. consider severe obesity, pulmonary disease, and prior aortoiliac surgery as contraindications to endoscopy [2], while Dion et al. excluded patients with concomitant aberrant renal arteries, large inferior mesenteric arteries, and external iliac artery occlusions from endoscopic treatment of occlusive disease [3]. It would appear that the patient best suited for endoscopic surgery is the low-risk patient with ideal anatomy, namely, the same patient suitable for straightforward open repair. Due to the inherent difficulties encountered during endoscopic aortoiliac surgery, it is unlikely that surgeons would prefer this approach to standard methods of repair for lower-risk patients. One must, however, consider the reported benefits of endoscopic approaches such as earlier resumption of bowel activity, decreased overall hospital stay, earlier return to functional status, and others [3, 4]. It is ironic however that Cerveira et al. have found that by repairing AAAs via open but smaller 8–10-cm transabdominal incisions, the same as those utilized during their endoscopically assisted AAA repairs, many of the same benefits of the endoscopic approach are still observed, while maintaining the durability of conventional repair [5].

When then might endoscopy play a role in the vascular surgeon's armamentarium? A Type-2 endoleak is defined as persistent flow within an aneurysm sac following endograft placement caused by patent side branches arising from that segment of aorta or iliac arteries. Endoscopic clipping of patent lumbar and inferior mesenteric arteries has already been used to eliminate such endoleaks, and will probably be the method of choice for controlling these leaks should embolization techniques fail [6]. Continued expansion of aneurysms despite successful endograft placement and no demonstrable endoleaks has been observed. The changing morphology of the native aorta can lead to endograft migration and at times rupture. Long-term data may reveal that aneurysm sacs themselves may require some sort of treatment. Endoscopy may prove to be a technique by which the sac can be either pressure transduced, injected with pro-thrombotic or sealing devices, and even opened should the need arise. For very-high-risk patients with infrarenal aneurysms not suitable for endografting, endoscopic AAA exclusion with extra-anatomic grafting, as described by Edoga et al., may be a safer alternative than conventional open repair [1]. Finally, it is almost inevitable that the next frontier of surgical technology, namely endoscopic-robotic assistance, will find a niche in vascular surgery - perhaps as an adjunct to endovascular procedures.

As has been noted time and time again, with anticipated technological improvements, increasing use of vascular endoscopy will undoubtedly occur. Dion's group and all other investigators involved in the advancement of endoscopic vascular techniques should be congratulated on their efforts, perseverance, and contributions thus far.

References

1. Edoga JK, Asgarian K, Singh D et al. (1998) Laparoscopic surgery for abdominal aortic aneurysm. Technical elements of the procedure and a preliminary report of the first 22 patients. Surg Endosc 12:1064–1072
2. Barbera L, Mumme A, Metin S, Zumtobel V, Kemen M (1998) Operative results and outcome of twenty-four totally laparoscopic vascular procedures for aortoiliac occlusive disease. J Vasc Surg 28:136–142
3. Dion YM, Gracia CR (1977) A new technique for laparoscopic aortibifemoral grafting in occlusive aortoiliac disease. J Vasc Surg 26:685–692
4. Kline RG, Aj DA, Chen MH, Halpern VJ, Cohen JR (1998) Laparoscopically assisted abdominal aortic aneurysm repair: first 20 cases. J Vasc Surg 27:81–88
5. Cerveira JJ, Halpern VJ, Faust G, Cohen JR (1999) Minimal incision abdominal aortic aneurysm repair. J Vasc Surg 30:977–984
6. Wisselink W, Cuesta M, Berends F (2000) Retroperitoneal endoscopic ligation of lumbar and inferior mesenteric arteries as a treatment of persistent endoleak after endoluminal aortic aneurysm repair. J Vasc Surg 31:1240–1244

Dr. Dion and colleagues requested to rebut the invited comment by Drs. Landau and Nyhus. We allowed them 600 words.

The Editors

Invited Rebuttal

Yves-Marie Dion · Carlos Gracia · Hassen Ben El Kadi

Landau and Nyhus refer to standard surgery as an ideal means of treating "low-risk" patients. However, over the past 20 years, there has been no significant change in the deaths associated with repair of either elective or ruptured abdominal aortic aneurysms (AAAs) despite improvements in the preoperative evaluation and perioperative care [1].

We agree with Cerveira that laparoscopy is not necessary when a 10-cm anterior incision is made. However, having used it 8 years ago, we found the limitations imposed by working through a short incision are such that surgeons will inevitably abandon this technique.

A laparoscopic aortobifemoral bypass can be performed in about 3 h. Until January 2001, there were no vascular clamps for the distal aorta and the iliacs. They are now available as deployable clamps for AAA resection. A newly developed needle driver allows suturing even when the needle faces the surgeon. We have now operated on patients with severe aortic calcifications, with bilateral external iliac occlusions, and in whom the inferior mesenteric artery (IMA) needed to be preserved.

There is no question about the durability of the laparoscopic repair. We, like many vascular surgeons, insert endovascular grafts. Patient selection is mandatory. This means that between 40% and 60% of the patients with AAA are not candidates. Should we then consider a laparotomy or a laparoscopic approach? Between 30% and 40% of endograft patients need secondary procedures, and 8%–10% require conversion within a 3-year period [2]. These patients have to be followed up rigorously for the rest of their lives. Persistent leaks may be expected in nearly one of four endograft patients [3]. Several costly embolization sessions may be required. Complete aneurysm exclusion as defined by absence of an endoleak does not indicate an event-free postoperative course [4]. The response of an AAA to endovascular grafting is unpredictable [5]. Guidant/EVT reports that only 68.5% of patients had shrinking aneurysms at 2 years. Patients may continue to have pressurized AAA sacs despite endovascular AAA repair. Endoleaks transmit pulsatile pressure into the aneurysm sac regardless of type, and in most cases this pressure is systemic. It is possible to have systemic sac pressures without evidence of endoleaks on CT or angiography [5]. There are potential solutions which could make endografts more secure in the long term and allow for a more general use. The cost of these grafts is another issue. Moreover, most teams are composed of at least one interventional radiologist and one surgeon. Endovascular grafting is still under investigation and a considerable learning curve is anticipated before the average vascular surgeon feels comfortable inserting such a graft without assistance.

Laparoscopic aortoiliac surgery for aneurysmal disease is just beginning. The vascular surgeon can easily learn how to approach the vessels. Courses are now available where he can perform arterial clamping and anastomoses, and learn to occlude the IMA and the lumbar arteries.

The next decade should witness improved patient benefits with these less invasive endovascular and laparoscopic technologies.

References

1. Heller JA, Weinberg A, Arons R et al. (2000) Two decades of abdominal aortic aneurysm repair: have we made any progress? J Vasc Surg 32:1091–1098
2. Fry PD, Martin M, Machan L (2000) Endoleaks and the need for a paradigm shift (letter to the editor). J Endovasc Ther 7:521–522
3. Ermis C, Kramer S, Tomczak R et al. (2000) J Endovasc Ther 7:441–445
4. Lee AW, Wolf YG, Fogarty TJ, Zarins CK (2000) Does complete aneurysm exclusion ensure long-term success after endovascular repair? J Endovasc Ther 7:494–500
5. Baum RA, Carpenter JP, Cope C et al. (2001) Aneurysm sac pressure measurements after endovascular repair of abdominal aortic aneurysms. J Vasc Surg 33:32–40

Editorial Comment

Bob Condon once said that "everything in surgery is complicated until one learns to do it well; then it is easy." The laparoscopic maestros who kindly provided us with the above sections are certainly masters in their field; for them, advanced and ultra-advanced laparoscopic surgery appear "simple."

Since Llyod Nyhus and his associates from Chicago provide us with balancing comments to these chapters, we will limit ourselves to a few general observations. We wish to emphasize the comment made by Drs. Patterson and Gagner that laparoscopic procedures are mostly beneficial in situations in which the *access trauma/procedure trauma ratio* is high. In other words, when the operative access is "simple" (e.g., appendectomy) and/or the procedural trauma is extensive (e.g., Whipple), the benefits of laparoscopic procedure are marginal, if any.

Typically, "leading experts" from centers of excellence report excellent results of advanced laparoscopic procedures. But the rosy picture tends to change when results of multi-institutional experience, or prospective randomized trials, are published. Thus, for example, a recent randomized trial from The Netherlands, comparing laparoscopic to conventional Nissen fundoplication for gastroesophageal reflux, concluded that "although laparoscopic Nissen fundoplication was as effective as the open procedure in controlling reflux, the significantly higher risk of reaching a primary endpoint in the laparoscopic group led us to stop the study" [1]. A review of 5,502 antireflux operations performed in Finland concluded that "laparoscopic fundoplication was associated with more life-threatening complications than open fundoplication. This may compromise the advantages of the laparoscopic technique" [2]. The predictably automatic response of the "leading experts" to such reports is that "they do not know how to do it as safely as we do." This of course may be true and brings us back to the universal and endless dilemma of who should be doing what.

As advanced laparoscopic procedures are becoming fancier, even less invasive alternatives are being invented by our radiological or gastroenterological competitors. Thus, sooner or later we will see antigastroesophageal reflux procedures performed through the endoscope [3, 4]. In the scene of vascular surgery, as stated by Drs. Landau and Nyhus, endoluminal procedures hamper the introducton and acceptance of laparoscopic vascular procedures.

The section on laparoscopic bile duct operations by Drs. Mavor and Katkouda, followed by comments by Drs. Horan and Nyhus, is pertinent to this whole section in that today, as more and more therapeutic alternatives are available, we should stress the importance of proper tailoring of the (best) procedure to the individual patient and local facilities. What is the purpose of laparoscopic acrobatics such as a Roux-en-Y jejunohepaticostomy when simple endoscopic stenting is available?

References

1. Bais JE, Bartelsman JF, Bonjer HJ, Cuesta MA, Go PM, Klinkenberg-Knol EC, van Lanschot JJ, Nadorp JH, Smout AJ, van der Graaf Y, Gooszen HG (2000) Laparoscopic or conventional Nissen fundoplication for gastro-oesophageal reflux disease: randomised clinical trial. The Netherlands Antireflux Surgery Study Group. Lancet 355:170–174

2. Rantanen TK, Salo JA, Sipponen JT (1999) Fatal and life-threatening complications in antireflux surgery: analysis of 5,502 operations. Br J Surg 86:1573–1577
3. Kadirkamanathan SS, Evans DF, Gong F, Yazaki E, Scott M, Swain CP (1996) Gastrointest Endosc 44:133–143
4. Mason RJ, Filipi CJ, DeMeester TR, Peters JH, Lund RJ, Flake AW, Hinder RA, Smyrk TC, Bremner CG, Thompson S (1997) A new intraluminal antigastroesophageal reflux procedure in baboons. Gastrointest Endosc 45:283–290

CHAPTER 12

Vascular Trauma

Evaluation and Nonoperative Management

JAMES W. DENNIS

Introduction

Experience over the past four decades has clearly shown which penetrating injuries to the extremities and neck require immediate surgical repair. No one disputes the need to operate on patients presenting with hard signs of arterial injury which include: (1) active hemorrhage, (2) expanding hematoma, (3) distal pulse deficit, (4) bruit or thrill over the injury, or (5) distal ischemia (manifested in the neck as a central neurologic deficit). Several specific types of injuries, however, have sparked intense controversy in the surgical literature in the past 10 years and will be discussed in this chapter. These debates have centered around questions concerning the proper management of penetrating injuries in proximity to the major arteries of the extremities and neck without any evidence of hard signs (clinically occult). Secondly, there are questions concerning which abnormalities identified on arteriograms need to be surgically repaired and which ones are "minimal" and will heal without surgical intervention. Thirdly, whether these treatment principles can be applied in the management of posterior knee dislocations is also still being debated.

Management of Penetrating Proximity Injuries to the Extremities

Treatment of penetrating arterial injuries to the extremities beyond simple ligation was first demonstrated during the 1950s, first in the Korean War [1, 2] and then in the civilian sector [3]. Papers appeared showing that physical examination (PE) alone could miss some injuries to arteries that were later detected on surgical exploration [4]. The devastating consequences of missing a significant arterial injury and lack of any readily available diagnostic imaging led to the practice of routine exploration of all penetrating injuries in proximity to the major arteries of the arms or legs [5, 6]. This policy was followed until the late 1970s and early 1980s when diagnostic arteriography (AG) became widely available in most trauma centers. The diagnostic accuracy of these examinations was shown to be 98%–99%

[7, 8] and they had the appeal of allowing surgeons to avoid unnecessary operations in the majority of patients with proximity injuries and no hard signs of vascular injury. Studies consistently showed a 10%–20% incidence of abnormalities on AGs obtained for proximity alone [9, 10]. The downside to routine AG was the tremendous expense in personnel and equipment required to do these examinations. Occasional complications such as contrast allergies and puncture site bleeding or thrombosis could also occur [11, 12]. What remained poorly defined for years was an accurate description of the types of injuries identified, which types were actually limb-threatening and which were benign with a natural history of healing spontaneously.

In the late 1980s, Frykberg and colleagues first published articles that critically examined these issues [13, 14]. He found that nearly 90% of clinically occult arterial injuries identified by AG alone would not deteriorate into large pseudoaneurysms or occlusions that required operative repair. Repeated AG showed that smooth segmental narrowings almost never worsen, most intimal injuries resolve and their morphology is not helpful in predicting which few would eventually deteriorate. Also, the small subset that did worsen usually deteriorated within a few days and could be treated at that time with no additional morbidity or limb loss. In addition, the huge expense required in routine AG could be eliminated by doing repeated, simple, close physical examinations. Thus, the diagnostic accuracy of PE alone in identifying arterial injuries *that required surgical repair* (1%–2% overall) was similar to that of AG.

This paradigm shift in the management of penetrating proximity injuries initially brought a hailstorm of criticism from the surgical community. Studies from other trauma centers during the 1990s, however, have supported the use of PE alone in managing these injuries [15, 19] (Table 1). Some resistance still exists as indicated by the number of articles from centers unwilling to rely on PE alone and advocating ultrasound (US) as the best means whereby arterial injuries can be identified [20–23]. These reports show that a good duplex study of the artery at risk from a penetrating proximity injury can be determined with 96%–98% diagnostic accuracy by US. These examinations, however, are highly operator-dependent, incur significant additional expense to the patient, and may have low specificity in some nonocclusive injuries [24].

Perhaps this controversy concerning the best management approach to penetrating proximity injuries is starting to resolve. Most major trauma centers have

Table 1. Prospective studies of asymptomatic penetrating injuries in proximity to extremity arteries

Author	No. of proximity wounds	No. of occult vascular injuries (%)	No. of occult vascular injuries requiring surgery (%)
Dennis [14]	254	25 (10)	2 (0.8)
Francis [16]	160	17 (11)	7 (4.4)
Kauffman [19]	92	22 (24)	0
Trooskin [18]	153	7 (5)	2 (1.3)
Weaver [17]	157	17 (11)	1 (0.6)
Total	816	88 (9.3)	12 (1.5)

adopted the use of PE alone in handling these injuries. AG is rarely utilized routinely, although the use of US as an adjunct to PE continues to be argued. Recent long-term data indicate the use of physical examination alone to be safe and accurate with up to 10 years follow-up in patients followed with minimal injuries [25]. In addition, over 5 years follow-up in patients managed by PE alone has not demonstrated any delayed complications not seen within the first 3 months after injury. Exceptional situations may occasionally exist when some form of imaging may still be helpful in determining the existence and location of an arterial injury even in the presence of hard signs. These include shotgun blasts, elderly patients with chronic vascular disease, and missile tracts that parallel the course of a major artery.

Management of Penetrating Injuries to Zone 2 of the Neck

In many ways, the management of penetrating Zone 2 neck injuries has paralleled the trends seen for penetrating extremity injuries; however, these changes have been delayed several years and not as widely accepted. Like in the extremities, the initial management of penetrating Zone 2 neck injuries during the two World Wars was ligation of actively bleeding vessels and observation of all other wounds [26, 27]. The risk of this procedure was that approximately 30% of patients would suffer a permanent neurologic deficit or stroke. Initial experience in Korea and later in Vietnam showed that vascular repair resulted in a much lower incidence of stroke (<10%) with no additional risk to the patient [28, 29]. This approach was carried into the civilian sector in the late 1950s when Fogelman and his colleagues demonstrated a significant advantage to exploring all penetrating wounds to Zone 2 of the neck and open vascular repair if at all possible [30]. They also demonstrated that outcome success was directly related to the time required to get the patient to the operating room. Routine exploration of all wounds penetrating the platysma became the standard of care for years. In the middle 1960s, Freeark and Saletta described the three zones of the neck and recommended routine exploration of Zone 2 and AG for Zones 1 and 3 [31]. This approach continued until the 1980s when several reports indicated that selective management of Zone 2 injuries based on AG had similar results and avoided the high rate of negative neck explorations [32–34].

Selective management based on AG remains the most common approach used by trauma centers today. Duplex US has also been shown to be highly accurate in identifying vascular injuries in Zone 2 [35]. A third line of management has also appeared in the past 8 years. Following the data obtained for extremities, the Jacksonville group reviewed their experience with using AG and physical examination in managing these injuries. The first retrospective review found the rate of finding significant injuries by AG not manifested by physical findings was less than 1% [36], and this was later confirmed in a prospective study [37]. This accuracy was similar to that found with AG, but again saved the enormous cost in time and resources. Other centers have subsequently published similar findings [38–40], yet there seems to be a resistance to adopting this approach in the neck, even more so than the extremities (Table 2). This continues despite prospective studies confirm-

Table 2. Studies evaluating the use of physical examination in the management of Zone 2 penetrating neck injuries

Author	Total no. wounds	No. undergoing surgery	No. observed with no injury	Missed injuries No. (%)	No. with AG -AG	No. with AG +AG	No with +AG requiring surgery (%)
Menawat [36]	110	23	42	0	27	18	1 (3.7)
Biffl [38][a]	143	15	128	1 (0.7)	0	0	0
Byers [39]	106	62	24	0	19	1	0
Atteberry [37][a]	36	2	28	0	6	0	0
Rivers [40]	65	0	3	0	57	6	1 (1.7)
Total	460	102	225	1 (0.4)	109	25	2 (1.8)

[a] Prospective.
No, number; -AG, negative angiogram; +AG, positive angiogram.

ing the earlier retrospective findings that using physical examination alone in managing these injuries is as accurate and safe as AG or US [1 out of 156 injuries missed (0.64%) when prospectively managed with PE exam alone].

Similar questions concerning the natural history of minimal injuries in cervical arteries have also arisen and the possible risk of stroke if these lesions are treated nonoperatively. Although the number of such lesions is smaller than that reported in the extremities, the same benign pattern has been demonstrated, particularly the smooth narrowings and intimal irregularities [41]. Long-term safety for this approach has yet to be demonstrated and thus the controversy remains.

Of note, when dealing with the other zones of the neck, most Zone 1 penetrating injuries are actually within the thorax or torso and must be dealt with either operatively (if unstable) or by AG. Zone 3, however, represents a unique challenge. Although less amenable to physical examination, it is also very difficult to access technically. With the evolvement of advanced endovascular techniques, the role of AG is changing from one of primarily diagnosis to that of treatment. Further studies continually need to be done as new devices and techniques become available.

Posterior Knee Dislocations and Vascular Injuries

Posterior knee dislocations can result in popliteal artery injuries up to 32% of the time [42]. Data from DeBakey's World War II experience also demonstrated the popliteal artery to be the major artery most likely (over 70% chance) to lead to amputation if acutely occluded [43]. These reports led to the policy in most institutions that all patients with posterior knee dislocations need AG to rule out arterial injury, no matter what physical findings are present. This policy is still the routine approach to diagnosing vascular injuries in many trauma centers today and is still supported in much of the orthopedic literature [44, 45].

Following publication concerning the benign history of most clinically occult arterial injuries in penetrating extremity trauma, reports have also appeared which show that the same pattern holds true for minimal popliteal artery injuries caused

Table 3. Studies demonstrating the accuracy of physical examination in identifying arterial injuries requiring surgery following knee dislocations

Author	No. dislo-cations	+AG with hard signs	+AG with hard signs requiring surgery	-AG with no hard signs	+AG with no hard signs	No. AG with no hard signs	No. hard signs needing surgery
Dennis [46]	38	2 (5.0)	2 (5.3)	10 (44.7)	7[a] (18.4)	19	0
Kendall [48]	37	6 (16.2)	6 (16.2)	15 (40.5)	1[b] (2.7)	15	0
Treiman [47]	115	29 (25.2)	23 (20.0)	77 (66.9)	9[c] (7.8)	0	0
Total	190	36 (19.4)	31 (16.3)	102 (53.7)	17 (8.9)	34 (17.9)	0

[a] Narrowing in 4, intimal defect in 3, no complications.
[b] Focal intimal injury resolved.
[c] Spasm in 5, intimal flap in 4, no complications.

by knee dislocations (Table 3) [46–48]. These reports indicate that occult arterial injuries are detected by AG less than 10% of the time. These defects are usually smooth narrowings, spasm, or intimal flaps that on follow-up usually do not deteriorate into occlusions or large pseudoaneurysms which require repair. In the absence of any hard signs, no intervention is warranted. Serial examinations must be performed in these situations both before and after orthopedic manipulation. Arguments have been made that this area of trauma is one of high litigation (thus indicating AG); however, in almost all instances the physicians have ignored hard signs on PE and treated the patient conservatively with disastrous consequences. It should be emphasized that, like in penetrating extremity injuries, the presence of a Doppler signal in the pedal arteries in no way excludes the possibility of a significant popliteal injury and should have no role in the management of these injuries. More prospective studies are needed in this controversial area of vascular trauma.

References

1. Spencer FC, Grewe RF (1955) The management of arterial injuries in battle casualties. Ann Surg 141:304–313
2. Hughes CW (1958) Arterial repair during the Korean War. Ann Surg 147:555–561
3. Ferguson IA, Byrd WM, McAfee DK (1961) Experiences in the management of arterial injuries. Ann Surg 153:980–986
4. Saletta JD, Freeark RJ (1968) The partially severed artery. Arch Surg 97:198–205
5. Spencer AD (1962) The reliability of signs of peripheral vascular injury. Surg Gynecol Obstet 114:490–494
6. Fomon FJ, Warren D (1965) Late complications of peripheral arterial injuries. Arch Surg 91:610–616
7. Snyder WH, Thal ER, Bridges RA, et al. (1978) The validity of normal arteriography in penetrating trauma. Arch Surg 113:424–428
8. O'Gorman RB, Feliciano DV, Bitondo CG, et al. (1984) Emergency center arteriography in the evaluation of suspected peripheral vascular injuries. Arch Surg 119:568–573
9. McCorkell SJ, Harley JD, Morishima MS, et al. (1985) Indications for angiography in extremity trauma. AJR 145:1245–1247
10. Menzoian JO, Doyle JE, Cantelmo NL, et al. (1985) A comprehensive approach to extremity vascular trauma. Arch Surg 120:801–805
11. Rose SC, Moore EE (1988) Trauma arteriography: the use of clinical findings to improve patient selection and case preparation. J Trauma 28:240–245

12. Sclafani SJA, Cooper R, Shaftan GW, et al. (1986) Arterial trauma: diagnostic and therapeutic angiography. Radiology 161:165–172
13. Frykberg ER, Crump JM, Vines FS, et al. (1989) A Reassessment of the role of arteriography in penetrating proximity extremity trauma. J Trauma 29:1041–1046
14. Dennis JW, Frykberg ER, Crump JM, et al. (1990) New perspectives on the management of penetrating trauma in proximity to major limb arteries. J Vasc Surg 11:84–95
15. Itani KMF, Burch JM, Spjut-Patrinely V, et al. (1992) Emergency center arteriography. J Trauma 32:302–308
16. Francis H, Thal ER, Weigelt JA, et al. (1991) Vascular proximity: is it a valid indication for arteriography in symptomatic patients? J Trauma 31:512–520
17. Weaver FA, Yellin AE, Bauer M, et al. (1990) Is arterial proximity a valid indication for arteriography in penetrating extremity trauma? A prospective analysis. Arch Surg 125:1256–1261
18. Trooskin SZ, Sclafani S, Winfield J, et al. (1993) The management of vascular injuries of the extremity associated with civilian firearms. Surg Gynecol Obstet 176:350–354
19. Kauffman JA, Parker JE, Gillespie DL, et al. (1991) Arteriography for proximity of injury in penetrating extremity trauma. J Vasc Intervent Radiol 42:527–535
20. Fry WR, Smith S, Sayers DV, et al. (1993) The success of duplex ultrasonographic scanning in diagnosis of extremity penetrating extremity trauma. Arch Surg 128:1368–1375
21. Bynoe RP, Miles WS, Bell RM, et al. (1991) Noninvasive diagnosis of vascular trauma by duplex ultrasonography. J Vasc Surg 14:346–354
22. Johansen K, Lynch K, Paun M, et al. (1991) Noninvasive vascular tests reliably exclude occult arterial trauma in injured extremities. J Trauma 31:515–522
23. Knudson MM, Lewis FR, Atkinson K, et al. (1993) The role of duplex US arterial imaging in patients with penetrating extremity trauma. Arch Surg 128:1033–1040
24. Berstein JM, Blair J-F, Edwards J, et al. (1992) Pitfalls in the use of color-flow duplex ultrasound for screening of suspected arterial injuries in penetrated extremities. J Trauma 33:395–403
25. Dennis JW, Frykberg ER, Veldenz HC, et al. (1998) Validation of nonoperative management of occult vascular injuries and accuracy of physical examination alone in penetrating extremity trauma: 5- to 10-year follow-up. J Trauma 44:243–253
26. Makin GH (1922) Injuries to the blood vessels. In: Official History of the Great War Medical Services: Surgery of the War, Vol. 2. His Majesty's Stationery Office, London, England, pp 170–296
27. Lawrence KB, Shefts LM, McDaniel JR (1948) Wounds of common carotid arteries: report of seventeen cases from World War II. Am J Surg 124:46–59
28. Hughes CW (1958) Arterial repair during the Korean War. Ann Surg 147:555–561
29. Spencer FC, Grewe RF (1955) The management of arterial injuries in battle casualties. Ann Surg 141:304–313
30. Fogelman MJ, Stewart RD (1956) Penetrating wounds of the neck. Am J Surg 91:581–596
31. Monson DO, Saletta JD, Freeark RJ (1969) Carotid vertebral trauma. J Trauma 9:987–999
32. Hiatt JR, Busuttil RW, Wilson SE (1984) Impact of routine arteriography on management of penetrating neck injuries. J Vasc Surg 1:860–866
33. Mansour MA, Moore EE, Moore FA, et al. (1991) Validating the selective management of penetrating neck wounds. Am J Surg 162:517–521
34. Gertst PH, Sharma SK, Sharma PK (1990) Selective management of penetrating neck trauma. Am Surg 56:553–555
35. Ginzburg E, Montalvo B, LeBlang S, et al. (1996) The use of duplex ultrasonography in penetrating neck trauma. Arch Surg 131:691–693
36. Menawat SS, Dennis JW, Laneve L, et al. (1992) Are arteriograms necessary in penetrating Zone 2 neck injuries? J Vasc Surg 16:397–401
37. Atteberry LR, Dennis JW, Menawat SS, et al. (1994) Physical examination alone is safe and accurate for evaluation of vascular injuries in penetrating Zone 2 neck trauma. J Am Col Surg 179:657–662
38. Biffl WL, Moore EE, Rehse BA, et al. (1997) Selective management of penetrating neck trauma based on cervical level of injury. Am J Surg 174:678–682
39. Byers PM, Kopelman T, Fine E, et al. (1990) Penetrating cervical trauma: Is routine angiography indicated? Panam J Trauma 2:1–5
40. Rivers SP, Patel Y, Delany HM, et al. (1988) Limited role of arteriography in penetrating neck trauma. J Vasc Surg 2:112–116
41. Frykberg ER, Vines FS, Alexander RH (1989) The natural history of clinically occult arterial injures: a prospective evaluation. J Trauma 29:577–583

42. Green NE, Allen BL (1979) Vascular injuries associated with dislocation of the knee. J Bone Jt Surg Am 59:236–239
43. DeBakey ME, Simeone FA (1946) Battle injuries of the arteries in World War II: an analysis of 2471 cases. Ann Surg 123:534–579
44. Varnell RM, Coldwell DM, Sangeorzan BJ, et al. (1989) Arterial injury complicating knee disruption. Am Surg 55:699–675
45. Bryan T, Nerritt P, Hack B (1991) Popliteal arterial injuries associated with fractures or dislocations about the knee as a result of blunt trauma. Ortho Rev 20:525–530
46. Dennis JW, Jagger C, Butcher L, et al. (1993) Reassessing the role of arteriograms in the management of posterior knee dislocations. J Trauma 35:692–697
47. Treiman GS, Yellin AE, Weaver FA, et al. (1992) Examination of the patient with a knee dislocation: the case for selective anteriography. Arch Surg 127:1056–1063
48. Kendall RW, Taylor DC, Salvain AJ, et al. (1993) The role of arteriography in assessing vascular injuries associated with dislocations of the knee. J Trauma 35:875–878

Operative Management

David A. Spain · Eddy H. Carrillo · J. David Richardson

Introduction

There are numerous areas in the management of vascular trauma that remain controversial. Issues such as optimal methods of establishing the diagnosis and management of minimal vascular injuries are being widely debated. These nonoperative issues are extremely important, but are outside the scope of this chapter. Intraoperative decision-making in vascular trauma is challenging and equally controversial. Some of the difficulties are due simply to the nature of the injuries and the circumstances under which they occur. These are generally young and previously healthy individuals without underlying vascular disease who sustain life- or limb-threatening injuries. Preoperative decisions must be made rapidly and often with only incomplete information. Additional injuries are common and often complicate decision-making. Most intra-abdominal vascular injuries are due to penetrating trauma and usually have associated intestinal injuries, making choice of conduit and sequencing of repair difficult. Injuries in the lower extremities may be due to blunt trauma with bone, soft tissue, and nerve injury. The vascular injury usually has both arterial and venous components. Staging repair of these injuries requires consideration of numerous factors, including severity of the various injury components, ischemia time, and associated injuries. Although there are several areas of controversy, we will focus on four topics of operative management that remain controversial. These are: (1) the role of preoperative, intraoperative and completion angiography; (2) management of associated venous injuries occurring with arterial trauma; (3) intraoperative decision-making in iliac vascular trauma; and (4) sequencing of vascular and orthopedic repair in complex lower extremity fractures with vascular injury.

The Role of Angiography in Vascular Injuries

At first consideration it would seem that issues regarding angiography could scarcely be considered controversial. However, there is considerable debate over the role of preoperative angiography versus an intraoperative arteriogram in patients with suspected arterial injuries or in patients with known injuries but in whom the exact location of the wound is unclear [1, 2]. Surgeons whose experience is primarily in elective vascular surgery would likely favor a standard preoperative angiogram as they would obtain in their routine practice. However, several authors, most notably Feliciano and associates, have questioned this practice [3]. These authors note that preoperative angiography is not necessary and may place the patient's life and limb in jeopardy. While patients who are stable and have an intimal injury, as opposed to major hemorrhage, may safely have a standard angiogram, many patients are not hemodynamically stable and face major delays in obtaining contrast studies. Given the nocturnal occurrence of the majority of these wounds, it is often difficult to obtain angiography promptly.

Depending on the location and nature of the wound, angiography may not be indicated at all and certainly not preoperatively [3]. Wounds in the extremities may often be explored and the arterial injury controlled without the necessity of an angiogram. Wounds of the arm and thigh are particularly amenable to exploration alone as the most expeditious diagnostic and therapeutic approach. On-table angiography is a very useful technique that probably has not been used widely enough in the evaluation of arterial injury. On-table angiography is particularly useful in those potential injuries where the surgeon can obtain proximal control and then place a needle or catheter in the artery and inject contrast distally to obtain an angiogram.

There are several instances when standard angiography appears to be superior provided the patient is stable enough to travel to the radiology suite. Visualization of potential carotid injuries, particularly in neck Zones 1 and 3, are best accomplished by formal techniques, although some injuries can be evaluated by an on-table study if needed. Injuries of arteries that have rich collaterals are best evaluated with standard angiography. The dye required and timing of the injection to demonstrate multiple collateral vessels is difficult to accomplish with an on-table study. Therefore, potential injuries around the shoulder and pelvic girdle are best evaluated by preoperative studies in the radiology suite.

The other facet of angiographic evaluation in arterial trauma that remains controversial is the performance of completion angiography after a repair of an injured vessel. There is precious little literature on this subject, and the inference that angiography is needed comes from the fact that such a practice is often common after elective vascular operations. If the patient is stable, one could argue that the performance of a completion angiogram is a safe practice that should be followed even if data demonstrating its necessity are lacking. If the patient is unstable, cold, or coagulopathic and has palpable pulses, one can logically argue that the time required to complete an angiogram makes it unnecessary. Popliteal injuries are frequently mentioned when recommendations about completion angiogram are made. Since popliteal injuries are fraught with problems that may result in limb loss with attendant medicolegal consequences, we generally perform completion angiograms with this injury.

Management of Associated Venous Injuries Occurring with Arterial Trauma

One of the issues that remains controversial is the management of venous injuries that occur in conjunction with arterial trauma. There are several scenarios in which virtually all surgeons will agree on management: if there is an injury of a major vein that can be repaired in a stable patient, then it should ideally be repaired [4, 5]. There are also several anatomic areas in which repair is highly desirable and others in which repair is less critical. Injuries to the jugular vein can be ligated with relative impunity if they are unilateral and are not amenable to repair. On the other hand, in the unusual case of bilateral injuries, repair of at least one vessel should be undertaken. Ligation of both internal jugular veins may result in cerebral edema and/or cavernous sinus thrombosis.

Upper extremity venous injuries can usually be ligated without undue consequences if a major venous injury is present. There is usually a rich collateral network that will maintain outflow from the arm. On the other hand, ligation of a major vein in the leg is likely to cause problems with swelling and long-term venous insufficiency. There are several studies which have shown that ligation of the popliteal vein with popliteal artery injuries is associated with a higher rate of limb loss when compared to vein injuries that are repaired. The most notable example of the effect of popliteal vein repair comes from the Vietnam vascular registry where 18 of 82 amputations for combined arterial and venous injuries were thought to be due to venous gangrene [6, 7].

Every reasonable effort should be made to maintain flow in the popliteal vein. If the vein is destroyed such that no primary repair is feasible, the use of a venous conduit is indicated. Even though the long-term patency rate may be low, temporary patency improves limb salvage. The type of venous conduit used for repair may vary. With smaller veins, the saphenous vein may be used as a replacement. A spiral or panel graft may be constructed for use in large veins. It is clear that the fate of these repairs is not good. Whether they warrant the time and risk in the hopes of even short-term patency is unclear. The fate of venous repairs is known to be less than ideal, with many failing either short- or long-term. Hobson noted that three-quarters of repairs were patent on early follow-up [8]. Limb edema was three times more likely in the ligated vein group compared to those who had venous repair. Borman noted that 75% of veins repaired by venorrhaphy were patent, whereas only 45% of complex repairs were patent [9].

When the veins are injured, there are several adjuncts to management that are clearly helpful. Elevation and fasciotomy will decrease the edema and may improve limb salvage itself. The role of anticoagulant therapy is uncertain, but its use is often precluded by associated injuries.

Iliac Vascular Injuries

Injuries to the iliac vessels present a challenge for trauma surgeons. Patients are often in hypovolemic shock with multiple associated injuries and occasionally require complex reconstructions [10–14]. Mortality rates remain 25%–40% and usually are a reflection of the significant hemorrhage associated with these injuries, the difficult exposure of the iliac vessels, and the need to repair multiple associated injuries [12]. Common controversies surrounding the management of these injuries include:

- Ideal type of repair
- Use of vascular prostheses in presence of intestinal contamination
- Role of abbreviated laparotomy with planned reoperation and timing of extra-anatomic reconstructions
- Value of temporary intraluminal shunts
- Routine use of fasciotomies after venous ligation
- Need for prophylaxis against leg swelling and deep venous thrombosis after ligation

Segmental resection with end-to-end anastomosis or insertion of an interposition graft is used in 38%–43%, while lateral arteriorrhaphy is sufficient in 25%–40%. Ligation with or without crossover femoral-femoral bypass is necessary in 17%–24% and arterial transposition or autograft in 1%–2% [13, 14]. This indicates that most injuries to the iliac vessels are managed by resection with interposition grafts to avoid narrowing and expedite the vascular repair. Intraluminal shunts and arterial transposition is described in some textbooks; however, in clinical practice are very seldom, if ever, used [14]. Reported experience from our institution and others has also shown that the use of interposition grafts in the presence of intestinal contamination and acute iliac artery repairs does not increase the incidence of graft infection [13–15]. However, in the presence of massive contamination or established infection, proximal ligation of the injured artery with the suture line covered with healthy tissue, omentum, bowel mesentery, or even a rotational flap of rectus muscle may be required to ensure this separation. Abbreviated laparotomy and planned reoperation was used in 36% of patients with iliac vascular injuries, according to a report by this institution [13].

In the presence of massive contamination or exsanguinating hemorrhage, arterial ligation followed by an ipsilateral below-knee four-compartment fasciotomy may be a reasonable alternative [13, 14, 16, 17]. If signs of ischemia develop during the resuscitation period, immediate extra-anatomic reconstruction should be entertained, ideally with a femoral-femoral crossover graft. In general, repair of iliac arterial injuries, rather than ligation, should be performed [14].

Vascular exposure and hemorrhage control can be extremely challenging in these patients. In the presence of active hemorrhage, initial vascular control should be obtained with manual compression before exposing the vessel. The technique of total pelvic vascular isolation, with proximal cross-clamping of the abdominal aorta and inferior vena cava above their bifurcations and distal cross-clamping of both external iliac artery and vein with one vascular clamp on each side of the pelvis, can be used for bilateral iliac injuries [18]. For patients with more distal injuries, vascular control can be obtained by a separate vertical incision over the inguinal ligament, extending to the common femoral vessels to facilitate exposure and repair [12, 13].

Temporary intraluminal shunts have been described to maintain distal perfusion while these patients undergo correction of their physiologic abnormalities.

Even though it is a very appealing alternative, there are no controlled reports to validate its effectiveness [13, 19], but it may be helpful in selected cases.

Another area of controversy is the management of blunt common and external iliac artery injuries. Even though these are very uncommon injuries, the clinician should be aware of their presence. Every effort should be made to document an associated iliac artery injury in patients with complex pelvic fractures and an abnormal femoral pulse or ischemic lower extremity. If the diagnosis of an iliac vascular injury is confirmed, an extra-anatomical approach and the use of vascular prostheses should be considered as the initial treatment of choice [20]. Endovascular approaches may also be useful depending on the location of the injury, ischemia time, and availability of expertise.

Significant limb swelling is frequently present in patients who undergo external iliac vein ligation and in 50%–60% of those undergoing ligation of the common iliac vein. When some type of venous repair is performed, however, significantly less postoperative swelling is observed. This observation has been supported by reports that indicate that repair is more effective than ligation [13, 21]. When ligation is used, or in patients with luminal narrowing greater than 50%, early prophylaxis against complications of extremity swelling and deep venous thrombosis should be used [13].

Combined Orthopedic and Vascular Injury of the Lower Extremity: Who Goes First?

When patients present with combined orthopedic and vascular injury, there is some controversy over who should proceed first: the orthopedic surgeon or the vascular surgeon. There are several advantages to obtaining orthopedic stabilization initially. First, the extremity is brought to length, which allows adequate estimation of conduit length. Second, it provides a stable framework and prevents further soft-tissue injury by "flopping" of the leg during operative manipulation. Third, it avoids subsequent manipulation of the lower extremity and possible damage to the graft. With the development of new external fixators, most of these can be rapidly applied, but it still takes up to 1 h and adds to ischemia time, a clear disadvantage. Additionally, the fixator may be in the trauma or vascular surgeon's way, although this can usually be avoided if it is placed more laterally. If the external fixator must cross the knee, it will make the leg stiff and hinder exposure of the popliteal artery.

Some advocate proceeding with vascular repair first. This approach minimizes ischemic time, which may be especially important in patients with long prehospital times. Many of these patients will have ongoing, significant hemorrhage from arterial or venous injuries at the fracture site that will require operative repair. Proceeding with orthopedic stabilization may increase blood loss and further compound lower-extremity ischemia. The main disadvantage to this approach is the subsequent manipulation of the lower extremity during orthopedic stabilization.

Our preference is to proceed with orthopedic stabilization first, especially if there is significant instability or shortening of the lower extremity [22]. If there is significant hemorrhage from the fracture site, we will explore this first, obtain hemostasis, and then proceed with stabilization. If the patient has complete ischemia or had prolonged prehospital transport with partial ischemia time (>2 h), then we will revascularize the lower extremity first.

Another option is to place a temporary intravascular shunt to restore perfusion. Bone stabilization of the extremity can then be performed with subsequent vascular repair. This approach can be very valuable and is probably underutilized. These shunts can usually be placed within 30 min and can be used for several hours prior to definitive vascular repair [23]. Temporary shunts may stay patent for extended periods and have even been used to facilitate the transfer of patients from rural areas and minimize ischemia time [24].

Recently, several groups have used temporary shunting in highly selected cases as a means of extending the "damage control" concept to a new group of patients [25, 26]. Damage control was initially described in patients with penetrating abdominal injuries and exsanguinating hemorrhage [25, 27]. The initial goals are rapid control of hemorrhage and contamination with subsequent definitive repair after resuscitation and correction of coagulopathy, hypothermia, acidosis, etc. This approach may be useful in some patients with injuries outside the abdomen, such as patients with massive exsanguination from penetrating injuries [26]. It may also be helpful in blunt trauma patients with an otherwise salvageable extremity but severe associated injuries that preclude prolonged attempts at revascularization initially.

References

1. Modrall JG, Weaver FA, Yellin AE (1993) Vascular consideration in extreme trauma. Ortho Clin North Amer 24;557–563
2. Geuder JW, Hobson RW II, Padberg FT Jr, Lynch TG, Lee BC, Jamil Z (1985) The role of contrast arteriography in suspected arterial injuries of the extremities. Am Surg 51:89–93
3. Feliciano DV, Herskowitz K, O'Gorman RB, Cruse PA, Brandt ML, Burch JM, Mattox KL (1988) Management of vascular injuries in the lower extremity. J Trauma 28:319–328
4. Agarwal N, Shah PM, Clauss RH, Reynolds BM, Stahl WM (1982) Experience with 115 civilian venous injuries. J Trauma 22:827–832
5. Yelon JA, Scalea TM (1992) Venous injuries of the lower extremities and pelvis: repair versus ligation. J Trauma 33:352–356
6. Rich NM, Hobson RW II, Wright CB, Fedde CW (1974) Repair of lower extremity venous trauma: a more aggressive approach required. J Trauma 14:639–652
7. Sullivan WG, Thornton FH, Baker LH, LaPlante ES, Cohen A (1971) Early influence of popliteal vein repair in the treatment of popliteal vessel injuries. Am J Surg 22:528–531
8. Hobson RW II (1990) Discussion. The early fate of venous repair after civilian vascular trauma. Ann Surg 206:463.
9. Borman KR, Jones GH, Snyder WH III (1987) A decade of lower extremity venous trauma: potency and outcome. Am J Surg 154:608–612
10. Burch JM, Richardson RJ, Martin RR, Mattox KL (1990) Penetrating iliac vascular injuries: recent experience with 233 consecutive patients. J Trauma 30:1450–1459
11. Ryan W, Snyder W, Bell T, Hunt J (1982) Penetrating injuries to the iliac vessels: early recognition and management. Am J Surg 44:642–645
12. Carrillo EH, Bergamini TB, Miller FB, Richardson JD (1997) Abdominal vascular injuries. J Trauma 43:164–171
13. Carrillo EH, Spain DA, Wilson MA, Miller FB, Richardson JD (1998) Alternatives in the management of penetrating injuries to the iliac vessels. J Trauma 44:1024–1030
14. Feliciano DV (1996) Abdominal vessels. In: Ivatury RR, Cayten CG (eds) The textbook of penetrating trauma. Williams & Wilkins, Media, PA, pp 702–715
15. Feliciano DV, Mattox KL, Graham JM, Bitondo CG (1985) Five-year experience with PTFE grafts in vascular wounds. J Trauma 25:71–75

16. Degiannis E, Velmahos GC, Levy RD, Wouters S, Badicel TV, Saadia R (1996) Penetrating injuries to the iliac arteries: a South African experience. Surgery 119:146–150
17. Cushman JG, Feliciano DV, Renz BM, Ingram WL, Ansley JD, Clark WS, Rozycki GS (1997) Iliac vessel injury: operative physiology related to outcome. J Trauma 42:1033–1040
18. Feliciano DV, Burch JM, Graham JM (2000) Abdominal vascular injury. In: Mattox KL, Feliciano DV, Moore EE (eds) Trauma, 4th ed. McGraw Hill, NY, pp 783–805
19. Bender JS (1996) Shotgun wounds. In: Ivatury RR, Cayten CG (eds) The textbook of penetrating trauma. Williams & Wilkins, Media, PA, pp 121–127
20. Carrillo EH, Wohltmann CD, Spain DA, Schmieg Jr, RE, Miller FB, Richardson JD (1999) Common and external iliac artery injuries associated with pelvic fractures. J Orth Trauma 13:351–355
21. Martin LC, McKenney MG, Sosa JL, Ginzburg E, Puente I, Sleeman D, Zeppa R (1994) Management of lower extremity arterial trauma. J Trauma 37:591–599
22. Harrell DJ, Spain DA, Bergamini TM, Miller FB, Richardson JD (1997) Blunt popliteal artery trauma: a challenging injury. Am Surg 63:228–232
23. Reber PU, Patel AG, Sapio NL, Ris HB, Beck M, Kneimeyer HW (1999) Selective use of temporary intravascular shunts in coincident vascular and orthopedic upper and lower limb trauma. J Trauma 47:72–76
24. Johansen K, Hedges G (1989) Successful limb reperfusion by temporary arterial shunt during a 950-mile air transfer: case report. J Trauma 29:1289–1291
25. Reilly PM, Rotondo MF, Carpenter JP, Sherr SA, Schwab CW (1995) Temporary vascular continuity during damage control: intraluminal shunting for proximal superior mesenteric artery injury. J Trauma 39:757–760
26. Porter JM, Ivatury RR, Nassoura ZE (1997) Extending the horizons of "damage control" in unstable trauma patients beyond the abdomen and gastrointestinal tract. J Trauma 42:559–561
27. Rotondo MF, Schwab CW, McGonigal MD, Phillips GR III, Fruchterman TM, Kauder DR, Latenser BA, Angood PA (1993) 'Damage control': an approach for improved survival in exsanguinating penetrating abdominal injury. J Trauma 35:375–382

Invited Comment

Asher Hirshberg · Martin A. Schreiber

Major vascular injuries present the trauma surgeon with a wide array of problems in diagnosis, decision-making, operative technique and postoperative care. While the approach to vascular trauma is based on the same principles and logic that guide the management of nontraumatic vascular disease, the context of multiorgan trauma introduces a fundamental difference. For many patients, the vascular injury is only one element of a multiorgan trauma complex, and other injuries often take priority or radically modify the timing and technical options of the vascular repair.

Evaluation of Peripheral Vascular Injuries

Dr. Dennis nicely describes the evolution in diagnosis of peripheral vascular injuries toward reliance on physical examination as a screening modality. He states that the presence of a Doppler signal in a pedal artery in no way excludes the possibility of a significant injury and that Doppler should play no role in the evaluation. Dr. Dennis does not comment on the use of the ankle pressure index as a screening modality. In the study he quoted by Johansen et al. [1], the ankle-pressure index was found to have a sensitivity of 94%. There were no major vascular injuries missed. The ankle pressure index is a useful adjunct to the physical examination in selecting patients for arteriography or operative management.

"Minimal" Vascular Injuries

Dr. Dennis discusses the concept of "minimal" vascular injuries in a systematic and thorough fashion. We agree that the concept is valid for penetrating peripheral vascular injuries, where long-term prospective follow-up data are available. However, the extension of this concept to major truncal arteries and particularly in blunt trauma is still highly controversial and should be studied with care. For example, it may well be that minimal blunt aortic injury presenting only with an intimal irregularity, a small flap, or even a small pseudoaneurysm can safely be managed nonoperatively, but the natural history of these lesions is still largely unknown. Pseudoaneurysms and other minimal injuries resulting from blunt carotid injury, previously thought to have a benign course, have recently been shown to progress and require a subsequent intervention [2]. Another difficulty with minimal vascular injuries is the lack of precise quantitative definitions as to what exactly constitutes a "nonthreatening" arterial injury. An objective and reliable angiographic grading system, supported by outcome studies, is therefore required to make further progress in the management of minimal vascular trauma.

Endovascular Options

The use of endovascular techniques and particularly stent-grafts is rapidly gaining in popularity as an alternative to operative repair in selected patients [3]. Deployment of an endovascular graft across a nonbleeding arterial defect such as a pseudoaneurysm or an arteriovenous fistula is a simple solution to a problem that may otherwise require operative repair. The endovascular option is particularly attractive for areas where operative access may not be straightforward, such as the thoracic inlet or within the pelvis. The use of this new technology for limb arteries remains controversial because of concerns over long-term patency rates.

Preoperative Angiography

Drs. Spain, Carrillo, and Richardson emphasize the limited role of angiography in the management of vascular trauma. We tend towards a more liberal use of formal angiography in hemodynamically stable patients, especially in those with a blunt trauma mechanism. In our view, preoperative angiography of the limb arteries provides an important road map that enables the surgeon to limit the extent of exploratory dissection when the location of the arterial injury is uncertain, such as in blunt trauma or multiple penetrations in the same extremity. In some instances, interventional angiographic techniques may offer an alternative to operative intervention. Embolization of a bleeding branch of the deep femoral artery or of a lacerated artery below the knee are two examples. These options do not exist with intraoperative angiography.

Synthetic Versus Vein Graft

The ideal vascular graft for peripheral arterial reconstruction has been the subject of controversy for many years. The traditional view that autogenous vein grafts fare better in a contaminated field has been countered by evidence that PTFE grafts, being resistant to bacterial collagenase, are less likely to result in sudden exsanguinating hemorrhage in a contaminated exposed position and are therefore preferable when soft tissue coverage is lost. Since the small diameter of the arteries in the arm and below the knee mandates the use of autologous vein, the debate focuses on the femoral artery. Currently it is becoming clear that graft protection by well-vascularized soft tissue coverage is probably more important than the choice of graft material in a hostile operative field.

Vascular "Damage Control"

Drs. Spain, Carrillo, and Richardson correctly point out that temporary shunt insertion is a "damage control" technique that is probably underutilized. The concept of damage control has revolutionized the operative management of critically injured patients, but is much more reluctantly used in the field of vascular trauma. In our view there is a distinct dividing line between "simple" vascular repair techniques (ligation, shunt insertion and lateral repair) and "complex" repairs (end-to-end anastomosis and interposition graft insertion) [4]. The former are rapid and straightforward and can be used in a hypothermic coagulopathic patient, while the latter are more time-consuming and often a bad choice in an extreme situation. In the exsanguinating trauma patient with a major vascular injury, not all that is technically feasible is in the patient's best interest. A simpler or staged technical solution, for which a temporary shunt is a good example, may be a safer option for the patient than an elegant complex arterial reconstruction.

Conclusion

Vascular trauma continues to be a highly controversial and rapidly evolving field. As with other types of trauma, the lack of long-term follow-up limits the quality of prospective studies and the ability to make straightforward conclusions regarding alternative management strategies. Current areas of development in the field include clarification of which lesions can be safely managed nonoperatively, the use of endovascular stenting, and increasing use of temporary shunts in damage control scenarios.

References

1. Johansen K, Lynch K, Paun M, et al. (1991) Noninvasive vascular tests reliably exclude occult arterial trauma in injured extremities. J Trauma 31:515–522
2. Biffl WL, Moore EE, Offner PJ, et al. (1999) Blunt carotid arterial injuries: implications of a new grading scale. J Trauma 47:845–853
3. Ohki T, Veith FJ, Marin ML, et al. (1997) Endovascular approaches for traumatic arterial lesions. Semin Vasc Surg 10:272–285
4. Aucar JA, Hirshberg A (1997) Damage control for vascular injuries. Surg Clin North Am 77:853–862

Editorial Comment

In this chapter, Dr. Dennis, Drs. Spain, Carrillo, and Richardson and Drs. Hirshberg and Schreiber indicate again that the surgeon's role in vascular trauma is not simply to repair or replace an injured vessel. Instead, it involves complex judgment processes as to whether an operation is necessary at all and, if yes, which procedure should be done, as eloquently discussed by our contributors.

Dr. Dennis, who champions a selective, clinically based, approach to vascular trauma, does not mention early non-US studies that demonstrated that selective conservatism is safe and feasible. When, in the early 1980s in South Africa, we read US-based studies, we were amazed by recommendations to explore any neck wound that penetrated the platysma. It sounded similarly ridiculous to us to perform routine angiography for proximity injuries. Already then we were guided by local evidence supporting a selective, conservative clinically based approach [1, 2]. What followed then in the United States was kind of a reinvention of the wheel and it seems that even today the wheel is still being reinvented.

References

1. Campbell FC, Robbs JV (1980) Penetrating injuries of the neck: a prospective study of 108 patients. Br J Surg 67:582–586
2. Demetriades D, Stewart M (1985) Penetrating injuries of the neck. Ann R Coll Surg Engl 67:71–74

CHAPTER 13

Lower Gastrointestinal Bleeding

Investigations and Nonoperative Treatment

I. MICHAEL LEITMAN · STEPHEN E. BURPEE

Introduction

Lower gastrointestinal (GI) bleeding may be a vexing and difficult problem to evaluate and treat. Unlike upper GI hemorrhage, where the location of the bleeding site is within the reach of the endoscope, lower GI hemorrhage challenges the clinician with a long luminal surface to inspect. There are additional difficulties with endoscopic visualization secondary to patient preparation, admixture with enteric contents, and the fact that the blood is proceeding toward the endoscope. One must keep in mind that the majority of patients with lower GI hemorrhage will stop bleeding during resuscitation, but in 10–25% of patients, some therapeutic intervention will eventually be required [1, 2]. Once the bleeding has stopped, investigation of the source of the bleed usually proceeds with routine endoscopic and radiological studies, followed by elective segmental resection, if indicated. However, on occasions, it may be impossible to determine the precise location and etiology and this forces both physician and patient to await the next bleeding episode. Difficulties in utilizing the literature to develop a diagnosis and treatment strategy are related to difficulties with comparing studies that define lower GI bleeding differently, and the variation by which some perform their diagnostic studies and therapeutic interventions.

Controversies

The controversies regarding lower GI hemorrhage revolve around:

- The proper diagnostic algorithm for identification of the bleeding site
- The patient care setting
- Whether nonoperative treatments should be employed once the site of the bleeding is determined
- What to do if the evaluation is unable to indicate the precise site of bleeding

The precise location of the source of bleeding is necessary because segmental resections result in good outcomes while *blind* colonic resection or total colectomy may result in unacceptable morbidity, mortality, and rebleeding from a small intestinal source [1, 3–5] although some advocate blind total abdominal colectomy [6].

ICU Versus Regular Ward

Patients who present with lower GI bleeding are usually adults older than 50 years. The most common etiologies of lower GI bleeding include diverticulosis, vascular ectasia, ischemic colitis, inflammatory bowel disease, and neoplasm, but several other causes have been reported [7]. Whether or not to admit these patients to an intensive care unit or a regular hospital ward has been an area of controversy. Kollef recently addressed this issue. Patients classified as high-risk based upon low blood pressure, on-going bleeding, abnormal coagulation profile, erratic mental status, or unstable comorbid illness should be admitted to an intensive care unit because of a greater risk of in-hospital complications, organ system dysfunction, and the requirement for more units of packed red-blood-cell transfusion [8].

Diagnostic Evaluation

The majority of lower GI bleeding episodes are occult or do not cause hemodynamic instability. When transfusion is, however, urgently required, a diagnostic strategy is necessary to provide an efficient and safe evaluation and treatment. Diagnostic options include colonoscopy, traditional imaging techniques (CT scan or contrast studies), nuclear scintigraphy, or mesenteric angiography.

Colonoscopy

Colonoscopy is generally considered the diagnostic procedure of choice when the bleeding has stopped or slowed down considerably. The controversy arises in cases where there is still continued severe hematochezia. Some authors feel that colonoscopy is extremely difficult in the face of large amounts of blood and in the absence of a mechanical bowel preparation, leading to a high incidence of nondiagnostic examinations. Others advocate its use even with severe hematochezia, reporting rates of successful identification of the bleeding site of 83–88%, after excluding an upper GI source [9, 10]. However, there is also controversy over the need for bowel preparation. Chaudhry [10] and Rossin [11] advocate immediate colonoscopy arguing that the cathartic effect of the blood is adequate cleansing. Others feel mechanical preparation with polyethylene glycol or a sulfate purge is required. Obviously, results will vary depending on the skill and persistence of the endoscopist, and the hemodynamic stability of the patient. Colonoscopy should be aborted if the patient becomes unstable or if the bleeding is so massive that identification of a precise origin is not possible.

Colonoscopy also has the added benefit of being potentially therapeutic as well. Endoscopic coagulation is currently the treatment of choice for bleeding vascular ectasia. Colonoscopic therapy is more difficult with diverticular hemorrhage due to the severity of the bleeding and the location of the bleeding site within the diverticulum. Colonic perforation has been reported after endoscopic coagulation in approximately 2% of patients [12].

Nuclear Scintigraphy

Nuclear scintigraphy with Tc-labeled red blood cells (Tc-RBC) is a very sensitive method to detect hemorrhage as slow as 0.1 ml/min. It has the advantage of being able to find intermittent bleeding as it can be detected on delayed scans up to 24 h after injection. It is also noninvasive and therefore relatively safe. However, it is only capable of regionalizing rather than precise localization, and it has no therapeutic benefit. False-negatives and false-positives can occur with reports of false localization ranging from 2% to 48% according to a recent review by Suzman et al. [13]. In the same review they found the detection rate to be 48% and the percentage of incorrect surgeries to be 10%. Unfortunately, the results from these various studies are difficult to interpret due to variable exclusion criteria, differing criteria for successful localization and the large number of patients in whom no source of bleeding was found.

This variable accuracy in the literature has created considerable controversy as to the optimal indications for scintigraphy. There are reports of considerable success substantiating claims for widespread use as the primary diagnostic tool [13, 14], while some report very poor results concluding that bleeding scans are of minimal value [15, 16]. Suzman argues that poor results are likely secondary to inadequate follow-up scanning. In their study, images were acquired at 5-min intervals for the first hour and at 15-min intervals for up to 4 h, and stored in dynamic mode. If needed the patient was imaged every 90 min thereafter up to 24 h. They report an overall localization rate of 42.9%, but a preoperative localization rate of 96%. However, the greatest consensus would seem to indicate that scintigraphy should be used in selected situations to increase the yield of mesenteric angiography [3, 16–20]. Ng found that bleeding scans with an immediate "blush" would predict a positive angiogram in 60.6% of patients but only 7.1% in patients with a delayed blush [18]. Others have concluded that bleeding scans do not increase the rate of positive angiograms [22]. Despite these controversies, it is the authors' opinion that bleeding scans deserve early consideration in the evaluation of lower GI hemorrhage if the patient is hemodynamically stable and colonoscopy is not feasible or visualization is poor. Positive bleeding scans can be followed by mesenteric angiography to further characterize the source and to provide a route for selective vasopressin or embolization.

Mesenteric Angiography

Selective mesenteric angiography can detect hemorrhage at a rate of 0.5–1 ml/min and it can be both diagnostic and therapeutic. It is, however, an invasive procedure with a complication rate of approximately 2% [12]. This includes dye-induced renal failure, artery dissection and occlusion, bowel infarction as well as complications related to the femoral artery puncture.

As with the literature on scintigraphy, there is a wide variation of reported success rates ranging from 40% to greater than 80% [12]. Again, the data are difficult to assess due to the differing selection and exclusion criteria. It would appear that the greatest benefit would be in patients with fairly active bleeding, especially if an immediate response had been detected on the bleeding scan. Gunderman et al. showed that scintigraphic screening more than doubled the diagnostic yield of angiography [17].

Angiography is superior to scintigraphy in precisely localizing and characterizing the source of bleeding because of its higher spatial resolution and superior depiction of vascular anatomy [17]. As a result it provides more accurate information should the need arise for surgical intervention. This must be carefully balanced against the greater sensitivity of the bleeding scan given the frequently intermittent nature of lower GI hemorrhage. This is the diagnostic study of choice for the unstable patient, especially if they are considered to be a poor surgical candidate.

Therapeutic Interventions

The next step after the bleeding site has been characterized and localized may be even more controversial as new developments have provided additional therapeutic options. Deciding to utilize these options as primary therapy, as opposed to traditional operative segmental resection, must be based upon individual patient characteristics. Colonoscopy and mesenteric angiography both offer the means for potentially controlling the hemorrhage, whereas scintigraphy does not. As previously mentioned, colonoscopy can provide the means to treat bleeding lesions through electrocautery, epinephrine injection, or sclerotherapy. Angiography can provide access for vasopressin infusion or embolization.

Vasopressin causes reliable arteriolar vasoconstriction and bowel-wall contraction when infused into a mesenteric artery resulting in reduction of blood flow. A recent review of the literature indicated a success rate of 36–100% in controlling the bleeding [12]. However, all studies were performed with small numbers of patients and rebleeding occurred in 22–71%. Complications include myocardial ischemia, peripheral ischemia, hypertension, arrythmias, fluid overload, hyponatremia, mesenteric thrombosis, intestinal infarction, and death [3].

Selective embolization is another angiographic option for controlling hemorrhage. Early success rates of 70–90% have been reported in small series [23–25]. Postembolic colonic infarction has been reported although the numbers studied are insufficient to establish a precise risk [3, 26]. The rebleeding rate is also much lower than for vasopressin, in the range of 0–23% [12]. Despite this apparent efficacy, the technique is cumbersome and can be quite time-consuming, possibly delaying appropriate surgical therapy.

The Patient with Negative Localizing Studies

The management patients with negative localizing studies may be even more complex. These patients probably have stopped bleeding at the moment. If colonoscopy and traditional CT and barium studies are negative, expectant management until the next bleeding episode is appropriate. Patients with diverticular bleeding have a 25% chance of rebleeding at 4 years [7]. If rebleeding occurs, it may be necessary to repeat these studies until the site can be localized. The unstable patient without a determined site of bleeding represents the most challenging dilemma, as blind total abdominal colectomy is associated with potential rebleeding from the small intestine and significant morbidity and mortality. If angiography does not indicate a site of bleeding, it may be most prudent to persist with resuscitation while additional diagnostic studies are completed.

References

1. Colacchio TA, Forde KA, Patsos TJ, Nunez D (1982) Impact of modern diagnostic methods on the management of rectal bleeding. Am J Surg 143:607–610
2. Zuckerman DA, Bocchini TP, Birnbaum EH (1993) Massive hemorrhage in the lower gastrointestinal tract in adults: diagnostic imaging and intervention. Am J Roentgenol 161:703–711
3. Leitman IM, Paull DE, Shires III GT (1989) Evaluation and management of lower gastrointestinal hemorrhage. Ann Surg 209:175–180
4. Britt LG, Warren L, Moore OF (1983) Selective management of lower gastrointestinal bleeding. Am Surg 49:121–125
5. Setya A, Singe JA, Minken SL (1992) Subtotal colectomy as a last resort for unrelenting, unlocalized, lower gastrointestinal hemorrhage: experience with 12 cases. Am Surg 58:295–299
6. Baker R, Senagore A (1994) Abdominal colectomy offers safe management for massive lower GI bleed. Am Surg 60:578–582
7. Longstreth GF (1997) Epidemiology and outcome of patients hospitalized with acute lower gastrointestinal hemorrhage: a population-based study. Am J Gastroenterol 92:419–424
8. Kollef MH, O'Brien JD, Zuckerman GR, Shannon W (1997) BLEED: a classification tool to predict outcomes in patients with acute upper and lower gastrointestinal hemorrhage. Crit Care Med 25:1125–1132
9. Jensen DM, Machicado GA (1997) Colonoscopy for diagnosis and treatment of severe lower gastrointestinal bleeding. Routine outcomes and cost analysis. Gastrointest Endosc Clin N Am 7:477–498
10. Chaudhry V, et al. (1998) Colonoscopy: the initial test for acute lower gastrointestinal bleeding. Am Surg 64:723–728
11. Rossini FP, et al. (1989) Emergency colonoscopy. World J Surg 13:190–192
12. Vernava AM, 3rd, et al. (1997) Lower gastrointestinal bleeding. Dis Colon Rectum 40:846–858
13. Suzman MS, et al. (1996) Accurate localization and surgical management of active lower gastrointestinal hemorrhage with technetium-labeled erythrocyte scintigraphy (see comments). Ann Surg 224:29–36
14. Emslie JT (1996) Technetium-99m-labeled red blood cell scans in the investigation of gastrointestinal bleeding. Dis Colon Rectum 39:750–754
15. Garofalo TE, Abdu RA (1997) Accuracy and efficacy of nuclear scintigraphy for the detection of gastrointestinal bleeding (see comments). Arch Surg 132:196–199
16. Voeller GR, Bunch G, Britt LG (1991) Use of technetium-labeled red blood cell scintigraphy in the detection and management of gastrointestinal hemorrhage. Surgery 110:799–804

17. Gunderman R, et al. (1998) Scintigraphic screening prior to visceral arteriography in acute lower gastrointestinal bleeding. J Nucl Med 39:1081–1083
18. Ng DA, et al. (1997) Predictive value of technetium Tc 99m-labeled red blood cell scintigraphy for positive angiogram in massive lower gastrointestinal hemorrhage. Dis Colon Rectum 40:471–477
19. Kouraklis G, et al. (1995) Diagnostic approach and management of active lower gastrointestinal hemorrhage. Int Surg 80:138–140
20. Gutierrez C, Mariano M, Vander Laan T, Wang A, Faddis DM, Stain SC (1998) The use of technetium-labeled erythrocyte scintigraphy in the evaluation and treatment of lower gastrointestinal hemorrhage. Am Surg 64:989–992
21. Richter JM (1995) Effectiveness of current technology in the diagnosis and management of lower gastrointestinal hemorrhage (see comments). Gastrointest Endosc 41: 93–98
22. Pennoyer WP, Vignati PV, Cohen JL (1997) Mesenteric angiography for lower gastrointestinal hemorrhage: are there predictors for a positive study? Dis Colon Rectum 40:1014–1018
23. Gordon RL, et al. (1997) Selective arterial embolization for the control of lower gastrointestinal bleeding. Am J Surg 174:24–28
24. Guy GE, et al. (1992) Acute lower gastrointestinal hemorrhage: treatment by superselective embolization with polyvinyl alcohol particles. Am J Roentgenol 159:521–526
25. Peck DJ, McLoughlin RF, Hughson MN, Rankin RN (1998) Percutaneous embolotherapy of lower gastrointestinal therapy. J Vasc Interv Radiol 9:747–751
26. Rosenkrantz H (1982) Postembolic colonic infarction. Radiology 142:47–51

Operative Treatment

Jonathan E. Efron · Steven D. Wexner

Introduction

Lower gastrointestinal (GI) bleeding is defined as any hemorrhage occurring in the GI tract distal to the ligament of Treitz. The surgical management of lower GI bleeding is primarily dependent on the location of the hemorrhage, with the optimal surgical intervention being a segmental resection in a hemodynamically stable patient. Ultimately, successful surgical management of lower GI bleeding depends on accurate localization of the bleeding site. The current controversy involving the operative treatment of lower GI hemorrhage focuses on when to operate, and what to resect in a patient who is persistently bleeding from an unknown location.

Etiology and Diagnosis

There are many causes of lower GI bleeding (Table 1). From a recent review of over 17,900 patients, Vernava et al. determined that diverticular disease is the most common cause of significant lower GI hemorrhage in adults, accounting for 40% of all hemorrhages [1]. The remaining colonic causes identified in descending order were inflammatory bowel disease (21%), neoplasia (14%), coagulopathy (12%), benign anorectal diseases (11%), and finally, arteriovenous malformations which were identified in only 2% of all bleeds. This list contradicted prior studies which listed diverticular disease or arteriovenous malformation as the two most common causes of lower GI bleeding; however, recent literature has confirmed diverticulosis

Table 1. Etiology of lower gastrointestinal hemorrhage

- Systemic
  - Coagulopathy
  - Drugs:
    - Anticoagulants
    - Enteric coated potassium
    - Nonsteroidal anti-inflammatory agents
  - Henoch-Schonlein purpura
  - Hereditary hemorrhagic telangiectasia
- Localized
  - Angiodysplasia
  - Aortoenteric/Aortocolic fistula
  - Colonic duplications
  - Diverticulosis
  - Endometriosis
  - Fissures
  - Hemangioma
  - Hemorrhoids
  - Ischemia - enteritis or colitis
  - Idiopathic ulcers
  - Intussusception
  - Inflammatory bowel disease
  - Infection:
    - Tuberculosis
    - Typhoid + Paratyphoid
    - HIV-related infections
    - Amoebiasis
  - Meckel's diverticulum
  - Nonspecific proctitis
  - Polyps and polypectomy
  - Radiation enteritis
  - Solitary rectal ulcer
  - Tumors:
    - Carcinoma
    - Leiomyoma
    - Lipoma
    - Carcinoid
    - Lymphoma
  - Varices

as the leading cause of significant lower GI bleeding (Table 2). Hemorrhage from the small intestine accounts for 3–5% of lower GI bleeding [8–10].

Effective surgical management of lower GI hemorrhage requires that every effort be made to identify the location of the bleeding *prior to* operative intervention, as long as the patient is hemodynamically stable. An algorithm for the management of acute lower GI bleeding was outlined by Vernava et al. [11]. The algorithm calls for aggressive resuscitation followed by determining whether the bleeding is originating from the upper or lower GI tract. An upper GI source must be excluded by placing a nasogastric tube and obtaining bile from the aspirate, or performing an upper endoscopy to show that the bleeding is not originating proximal to the ligament of Trietz. The algorithm also calls for anoscopy and proctoscopy to be performed during the initial assessment of the patient to confirm that the bleeding is not from an anal or rectal source. These examinations ensure that if a patient becomes unstable a colectomy is not performed for bleeding from an

Table 2. Studies identifying locations of lower gastrointestinal hemorrhages

Study	Year	Patient Number	Diverticular disease	Arteriovenous malformation	Carcino-mas and polyps	Ischemia and IBD
Caos et al. [2]	1986	35	23%	20%	17%	9%
Jensen and Machincado [3]	1988	80	16%	30%	14%	9%
Leitman et al. [4]	1989	68	27%	24%	9%	10%
Rossini et al. [5]	1989	409	15%	15%	33%	18%
Vernava et al. [1]	1996	17,941	40%	2%	14%	21%
Peura et al. [6]	1997	125	30%	10%	18%	14%
Wilcox and Clark [7]	1999	165	56%	5%	7%	10%

IBD, inflammatory bowel disease.

anorectal source. In addition, the embarrassing situation of the radiologist identifying a bleeding hemorrhoidal vessel by arteriography can be obviated. Colonoscopy, technetium-tagged red blood cell scan, or angiography are then employed to ascertain the location of the bleeding intestine (Fig. 1).

Indications for Operation

Of those patients who present with lower GI bleeding, 10–25% will require emergent surgery. Hemodynamic instability that does not respond to fluid and blood resuscitation is an absolute indication for surgical intervention. Likewise, if the source of bleeding is reliably identified from the colon or small intestine, segmental resection should be performed [4, 12–20]. A primary acute GI bleeding that spontaneously resolves may not require surgical intervention, as less than 25% of those patients who stop bleeding will bleed again [21]. Vernava et al. [11] established four criteria defining those patients with acute GI bleed who require surgery:

- Patients who require transfusion of more than 1.5 l of blood at the initial resuscitation with continued bleeding
- Patients who require transfusion of 2 l of blood over 24 h to maintain hemodynamic stability
- Patients who continue to bleed for more than 72 h
- Patients who rebleed within 1 week of cessation of a significant bleed

Justification for these criteria comes from numerous studies. Bender et al. [22] examined 49 total abdominal colectomies performed for massive lower GI hemorrhage. The total operative mortality rate was 27%, but when they stratified the patients into their preoperative transfusion requirements, they discovered that those patients who required ten or more units of blood prior to surgery had a 45% mortality rate, while those individuals who required nine units or less had a 9% mortality. Setya et al. [23] found that those patients operated on within 24 h of admission for massive lower GI bleeding required a mean of 4.2 units of blood, while those patients operated on between 36 h and 9 days required a mean of 6.2 units of blood.

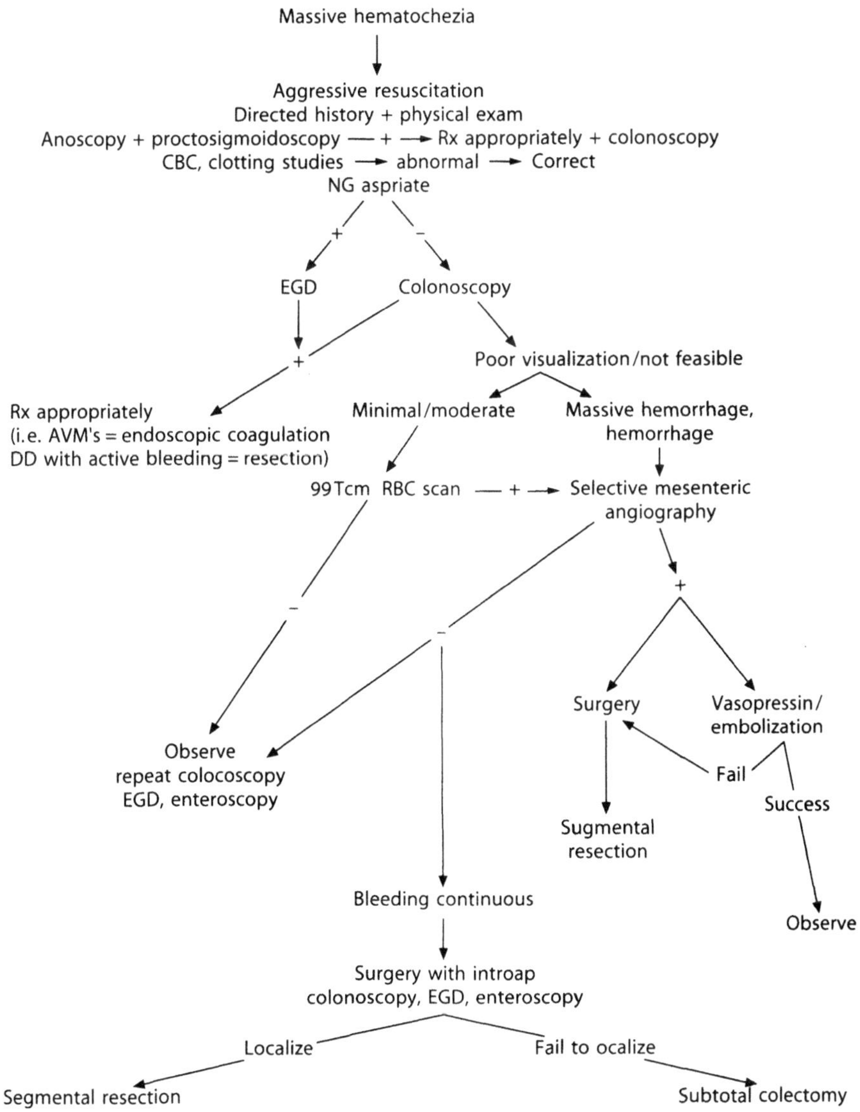

Fig. 1. Algorithm for management of lower gastrointestinal hemorrhage. *Rx*, treatment; *CBC*, complete blood count; *NG*, nasogastric tube; *EGD*, esophagogastroduodenoscopy; *AVM*, arteriovenous malformations; *DD*, diverticular disease; *99Tcm RBC*, technetium 99m red blood cell scan. (Reprinted with permission from Vernava AmIII, Moore BA, Longo WE, Johnson FE. Lower gastrointestinal bleeding. Dis Colon Rectum 1997; 40:846–858)

Additional Localizing Maneuvers

Once the decision to operate has been made, it is very important to identify the location of the bleed. If the bleeding point has been isolated by mesenteric angiography prior to surgery in an area of small intestine that is not obvious, the catheter may be left in place. The surgeon may then use the angiocatheter to identify which area of the small intestine is bleeding, allowing for a more localized resection. The catheter is usually easily palpated within the mesentery. Intraoperative injection of methylene blue may further help to define the bleeding source by forming a blue stain on the mesenteric margin. Small titanium embolization coils are also useful, provided that a resection can be performed soon thereafter before full-thickness bowel-wall necrosis and perforation ensue. When injected into the distal mesentery of the bleeding intestine, they may slow down the rate of bleeding, and can be seen and palpated within the mesentery, thereby facilitating a localized resection.

Intraoperative Colonoscopy

All patients who undergo surgery for acute GI hemorrhage should be placed in the modified lithotomy position, especially if the location of the bleeding has not been identified, as this position allows intraoperative colonoscopy to be performed. When performing colonoscopy for GI hemorrhage, it is important to use a large double-channel instrument to allow for simultaneous irrigation and suctioning. If excessive blood remains within the colon preventing adequate visualization of the mucosa, then intraoperative colonic lavage can be performed. After gentle placement of a noncrushing bowel clamp at the ileocecal junction, an appendicostomy is made to allow for placement of irrigation tubing into the cecum. The colon is irrigated with warm normal saline until clean. The irrigant and blood is drained through the rectum via a large anesthesia tubing which is placed through the anus with the aid of an anal retractor [24] (Fig. 2).

Intraoperative Enteroscopy

If the location of bleeding is not found within the colon, then complete evaluation of the small intestine is recommended. An upper endoscopy performed with a colonoscope or enteroscope will exclude bleeding proximal to the ligament of Treitz and will allow for enteroscopy. The colonoscope should be passed to the distal duodenum or proximal jejunum. The operating surgeon may then telescope the small intestine over the colonoscope, allowing direct visualization of the small-bowel mucosa. The operating room lights should be dimmed during this portion of the procedure to allow for transillumination of the small-intestine wall. Utilizing this technique, any small telangectasias that were invisible to the endoscopist can be seen by the operating surgeon. Enteroscopy will effectively diagnose the location of bleeding in 25% of cases but should only be performed in a hemodynamically stable patient [25, 26].

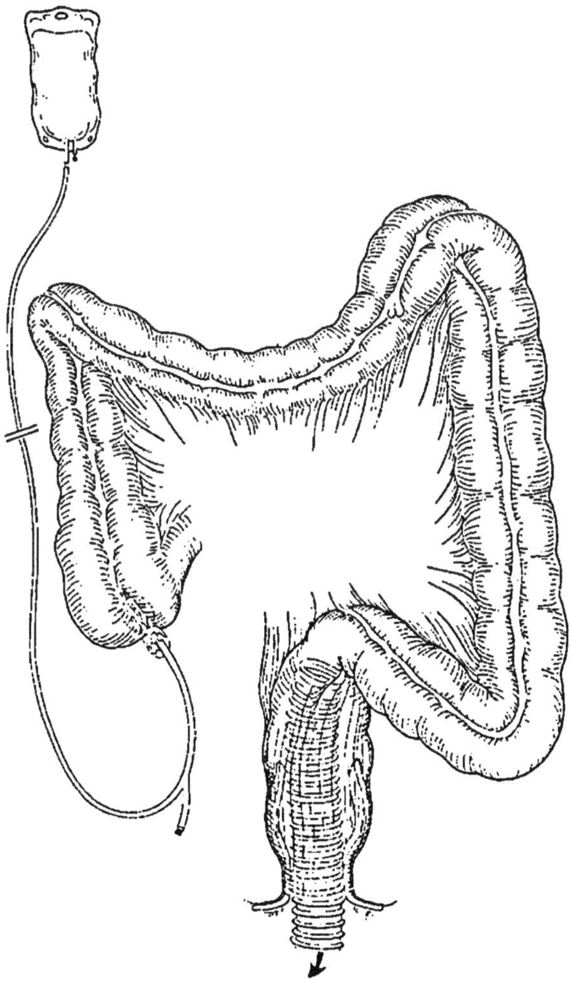

Fig. 2. Technique of on-table colonic lavage using anesthetic scavenger tubing passed into the rectum through an intra-anal retractor. (Reprinted with permission from Keighley MRB, Williams NS (eds) Surgery of the Arnus, Rectum and Colon. Vol 2. WB Saunders, London 1998, pp 2245–2287)

Extent of Resection

Historically, patients without preoperative localization of the colonic bleeding site and evidence of diverticular disease underwent left-sided resection for presumed bleeding from the diverticular disease. This practice often leads to high rebleeding rates with subsequent high mortalities. Drapanas et al. [27] demonstrated that presumptive partial colectomy led to a rebleeding rate of 50% with an overall mortality of 19%. Comparatively, total abdominal colectomy with ileorectal anastomosis had a 0% rebleeding rate and 9% mortality rate. Other series have confirmed these high rebleeding and mortality rates with presumptive segmental colonic resection [28, 29]. Directed segmental resections, however, result in rebleeding rates from 0% to 15% and mortality rates from 0% to 22% with an average mortality of 10% [4, 12–20]. Studies which have examined subtotal colectomy for massive hemorrhage have generally documented rebleeding rates ranging from 0% to 8% and mortality rates from 0% to 40%, with an average of 19% [4, 12, 17, 19, 29, 30]. An exception to these incidences was quoted in a study of ten patients by Gianfrancisco and Abcarian who documented rates of 60% and 40%, respectively [31].

Baker and Senagore [32] examined 61 patients who were admitted for massive lower GI hemorrhage. Forty-one patients had preoperative localization of the bleeding site and underwent segmental resection, while 14 underwent total abdominal colectomy. There was no difference in preoperative blood transfusion requirements or APACHE II scores; however, the time elapsed prior to surgery was significantly higher in the localized resection group. The differences in mortality rates did not reach statistical significance between the two groups - 15% for the segmental resection and 6% for the total abdominal colectomy patients. Baker and Senagore also claimed that neither group suffered from intractable diarrhea after resection. Given the slightly higher mortality associated with total abdominal colectomy when compared to directed segmental resection, a concerted effort should be made to localize the bleeding preoperatively. However, this effort should not place a hemodynamically unstable patient at risk of recurrent hypotensive episodes, or should it dramatically prolong the time before surgery, because such delay invariably results in increased transfusions. Total abdominal colectomy may be performed with low mortality and morbidity, and without significant postoperative sequelae.

To Anastomose or Not?

After resection, the decision regarding an anastomosis must be made. Patients who are hypotensive and unstable during the surgical procedure should not undergo anastomosis. After resection of the bleeding intestine, the unstable patient should undergo formation of a stoma. However, the decision in a hemodynamically stable patient is not as easy. Several studies have examined the risk of anastomotic disruption in patients who required blood transfusions prior to resection. Shrock et al. [33] examined 1,703 colonic anastomoses with a documented leak rate of 4.5%, and a subsequent mortality rate of 33% when disruption occurred. Massive hemorrhage, defined as bleeding requiring transfusion of at least four units of blood preoperatively, increased the risk of anastomotic leak. Similarly, Golub et al. [34], in a review of 764 patients, listed intraoperative transfusion of two or more units of packed red blood cells as an independent risk factor for anastomotic leak. Other factors shown to increase the rate of anastomotic leak are poor nutrition [34, 35], smoking and alcohol abuse [36], and obesity [37, 38]. Tadros et al. [39, 40] examined the effect of transfusions on colonic anastomosis in rats. They found that rats that received blood transfusions demonstrated impaired colonic healing.

The trauma literature has provided much of the data on the safety of bowel anastomosis for patients requiring preoperative and intraoperative blood transfusions. Gonzalez et al. [41] and Sasaki et al. [42] both performed randomized prospective trials which compared primary anastomosis to repair and diversion. They both found no difference in the mortality or septic complication rates between the two groups of patients who had colonic trauma. Recently, however, Corwell et al.

[43] performed a prospective study examining all patients with a full thickness colonic injury and either a penetrating abdominal index score of 25 or greater, transfusion requirement of six or more units of packed red blood cells, or 6 h between injury and surgical intervention. They found that these patients had an anastomotic leak rate of 6% and a 66% mortality rate directly related to the anastomotic disruption.

Given these findings, stable patients who have required transfusion of six or more units of blood, or have concomitant conditions associated with an increased anastomotic leak rate, should undergo primary anastomosis with proximal diversion. An exception might be if a right colectomy is performed for a localized bleed. While proximal diversion does not decrease that rate of anastomotic leak [33, 35], it does decrease the mortality and septic complications which occur in patients who do leak [37]. Our preference for diversion is the loop ileostomy which is easier to manage than loop colostomy. The diverting stoma usually is closed approximately 3 months after the initial resection. Closure of a loop ileostomy has a lower morbidity than does closure of a loop colostomy [44, 45]. Prior to closure, a water soluble contrast enema is obtained to document any leak or stricture.

Conclusions

Regardless of the etiology of a massive lower GI hemorrhage, the surgical management remains the same: resection. When the location of the hemorrhage is identified prior to surgical intervention, a limited resection should be performed. If a patient with an unrecognized bleeding location is stable in the operating room, every effort should be made to identify the source of the bleeding with intraoperative colonoscopy, upper endoscopy, and even enteroscopy. If the bleeding is believed to be coming from the colon, but the exact location within the colon is unknown, then total abdominal colectomy with or without primary anastomosis should be performed. In practice, these guidelines should allow for the management of lower GI hemorrhage with low rebleeding and mortality rates.

References

1. Vernava AM, Longo WE, Vigo KS, Johnson FE (1996) A nationwide study of the incidence and etiology of lower gastrointestinal bleeding. Surg Res Commun 18:113–120
2. Caos A, Brenner KD, Maier J, et al. (1986) Colonoscopy after Golytely preparation in acute rectal bleeding. J Clin Gastroenterol 8:46–49
3. Jensen DM, Machincado GA (1988) Diagnosis and treatment of severe hematochezia: The role of urgent colonoscopy after purge. Gastroenterology 95:15690–15694
4. Leitman IM, Paul DE, Shires GT (1989) Evaluation and management of massive lower gastrointestinal hemorrhage. Ann Surg 209:175–180
5. Rossini FP, Ferrari A, Spandre M, et al. (1989) Emergency colonoscopy. World J Surg 13:190–192
6. Peura DA, Lanza FL, Gastout CJ, Foutch PG (1997) The American College of Gastroenterology Bleeding Registry: Preliminary Findings. Am J Gastroenterol 2:924–928
7. Wilcox CM, Clark WS (1999) Causes and outcome of upper and lower gastrointestinal bleeding: the Grady Hospital experience. South Med J 92:44–50

8. Netterville R, Hardy J, Martin R (1968) Small bowel hemorrhage. Ann Surg 167:949–957
9. Gilmore PR (1988) Angiodysplasia of the upper gastrointestinal tract. J Clin Gastroenterol 10:386–394
10. Lewis B, Wayne JD (1992) Bleeding from the small intestine. In: Sugawa C, Schuman BM, Lucas CE (eds) Gastrointestinal Bleeding. Igaku-Shoin, New York, pp 178–188
11. Vernava AM, Moore BA, Longo WE, Johnson FE (1997) Lower gastrointestinal bleeding. Dis Colon Rectum 40:846–858
12. Colacchio TA, Forde KA, Patsos TJ, Nunez D (1982) Impact of modern diagnostic methods on the management of rectal bleeding. Am J Surg 143:607–610
13. Boyley SJ, Dibiase A, Brandt LJ, Sammartano R (1979) Lower intestinal bleeding in the elderly. Am J Surg 137:57–64
14. Casarella WJ, Galloway SJ, Taxin RN, et al. (1974) Lower gastrointestinal tract hemorrhage: new concepts based on arteriography. Am J Roentgenol 121:357–368
15. Nath RL, Sequeira JC, Weitzman AF, et al. (1981) Lower gastrointestinal bleeding: diagnostic approach and management conclusions. Am J Surg 141:478–481
16. Welch CE, Athanasoulis CA, Galdabini JJ (1978) Hemorrhage from the large bowel with special reference to angiodysplasia and diverticular disease. World J Surg 2:73–83
17. Britt LG, Warren L, Moore OF (1983) Selective management of lower gastrointestinal bleeding. Am Surg 49:121–125
18. Browder W, Cerise EJ, Litwin MS (1986) Impact of emergency angiography in massive lower gastrointestinal bleeding. Ann Surg 204:530–536
19. Athanasoulis CA, Baum S, Rosch J, et al. (1975) Mesenteric arterial infusions of vasopressin for hemorrhage from colonic diverticulosis. Am J Surg 129:212–216
20. Wright HK, Pelliccia O (1980) Controlled, semi-elective, segmental resection for massive colonic hemorrhage. Am J Surg 139:535–538
21. Turnage RH (1996) Acute gastrointestinal hemorrhage. In: Greenfield LJ (ed) Scientific principles and practice, 2nd edn. Lippincott Williams & Wilkins, Baltimore, pp 1158–1172
22. Bender JS, Wieneck RG, and Bouwman DL (1991) Morbidity and mortality following total abdominal colectomy for massive lower gastrointestinal bleeding. Am Surg 57:536–540
23. Setya V, Singer JA, Minken SL (1992) Subtotal colectomy as a last resort for unrelenting, unlocalized, lower gastrointestinal hemorrhage: experience with 12 cases. Am Surg 58:295–298
24. Keighley MRB, Williams NS (eds) (1999) Surgery of the Anus, Rectum and Colon, 2nd edn, WB Saunders, London
25. Chong J, Tangle M, Barkin JS, Reiner DK (1994) Small bowel push-type fiberoptic enteroscopy for patients with occult gastrointestinal bleeding or suspected small bowel pathology. Am J Gastroenterol 89:2143–2146
26. Berner JS, Mauer K, Lewis BS (1994) Push and Sonde enteroscopy for the diagnosis of obscure gastrointestinal bleeding. Am J Gastroenterol 89:2139–2142
27. Drapanas T, Pennington DG, Kappelman M, et al. (1973) Emergency subtotal colectomy: the preferred approach to management of massively bleeding diverticular disease. Ann Surg 177:519–526
28. Boley SJ, Sammartano R, Brandt LJ, Sprayregen S (1979) Vascular ectasias of the colon. Surg Gynecol Obstet 149:353–358
29. Wright HK, Pelicia D, Higgins EF, et al. (1980) Controlled semi-elective segmental resection for massive colonic hemorrhage. Am J Surg 139:535–538
30. Eaton AC (1981) Emergency surgery for acute colonic hemorrhage – a retrospective study. Br J Surg 68:109–111
31. Gianfrancisco JA, Abcarian H (1982) Pitfall in the treatment of massive lower gastrointestinal bleeding with "blind" subtotal colectomy. Dis Colon Rectum 25:441–445
32. Baker R, Senagore A (1994) Abdominal colectomy offers safe management for massive lower GI bleed. Am Surg 60:578–582
33. Schrock TR, Deveney CW, Dunphy JE (1973) Factors contributing to leakage of colonic anastomoses. Ann Surg 177:513–518
34. Golub R, Golub RW, Cantu R JR, Stein HD (1997) A multivariate analysis of factors contributing to leakage of intestinal anastomoses. J Am Coll Surg 184:364–372
35. Irvin TT, Goligher JC (1973) Etiology of disruption of intestinal anastomoses. Br J Surg 60:461–464
36. Sorensen LT, Jorgensen T, Kirkeby LT, et al. (1999) Smoking and alcohol abuse are major risk factors for anastomotic leakage in colorectal surgery. Br J Surg 86:927–931
37. Karanjia ND, Corder AP, Bearn P, Heald RJ (1994) Leakage from stapled low anastomosis after total mesorectal excision for carcinoma of the rectum. Br J Surg 81:1224–1226

38. Rullier E, Lamment C, Ganelon JL, et al. (1998) Risk factors for anastomotic leakage after resection of rectal cancer. Br J Surg 85:355-358
39. Tadros T, Wobbes T, Hendricks T (1992) Blood transfusion impairs the healing of experimental intestinal anastomoses. Ann Surg 215:276-281
40. Tadros T, Wobbes T, Hendriks T (1993) Opposite effects of Interleukin-2 on normal and transfusion suppressed healing of experimental intestinal anastomoses. Ann Surg 218: 800-808
41. Gonzalez RP, Merlotti GJ, Holevar MR (1996) Colostomy in penetrating colon injury: is it necessary? J Trauma 41:271-275
42. Sasaki LS, Allaben RD, Golwala R, Mittal VK (1995) Primary repair of colon injuries: a prospective randomized study. J Trauma 39:811-812
43. Corwell EE, Velnahos GC, Berne TV, Murray JA, Chahwan S, Asensio J, Denetriades D (1998) The fate of colonic suture lines in high-risk trauma patients: a prospective analysis. J Am Coll Surg 187:58-63
44. Fasth S, Halten L, Palselius I (1980) Loop ileostomy: an attractive alternative to a temporary transverse colostomy. Acta Chir Scand 146:203-207
45. Williams NS, Masmyth DG, Jones D, Smith AH (1986) Defunctioning stomas: a prospective controlled trial comparing ileostomy with loop transverse colostomy. Br J Surg 73:566-570

Invited Comment

HUNTER H. MCGUIRE, JR.

Introduction

The authors of this chapter have correctly identified five controversial questions that must be answered to safely manage acute lower GI bleeding. The following opinions are derived from experiences with diverticular bleeding that we described in 1972 [1], subsequently refined by colonoscopy, scintography, and angiography, and described with revised conclusions in 1994 [2]. As diverticular hemorrhage is often diagnosed by excluding other causes, these remarks will pertain to them as well.

Admit to ICU or Ward?

When the source of acute bleeding is determined to be distal to the ligament of Treitz, the first controversial question is whether to admit to an intensive care unit or to a hospital ward. Most of these patients should be admitted to wards because bleeding from all sources other than diverticula and 75% of diverticula bleeds will be slow, will have stopped, or will stop spontaneously. They can be identified by their hemodynamic stability and their need for less than three units transfusion. Intensive care is needed for the one-quarter of diverticular bleeds that require emergency surgery to prevent fatal exsanguination. These are distinguished from slow bleeders by persistent instability, profuse hematochezia, rapid hemoglobin fall in a short interval, and by their need for over four units transfusion after initial stabilization. Because surgeons are experienced and secure in dealing with these phenomena, it is our rule to admit all patients with acute lower GI bleeds to the surgical services. A surgeon then decides and redecides for each case whether the patient is safe on a ward or needs intensive care. Decisions must be tailored to the resources of the hospital as well as to the stability of the patient.

Which Test?

The second controversial question is which test should be performed? All patients need immediate anoscopy to rule out bleeding hemorrhoids and rectal ulcers. All need their prothrombin times measured. Correction of a prolonged prothrombin time almost always stops bleeding and allows preparation for elective colonoscopy. Colonoscopy is the best test for patients whose bleeding is slow, intermittent or has stopped.

For the 25% of bleeds that might exsanguinate, colonoscopy is of no value. They need their bleeding sites or segments defined by scintigraphy or by angiography in order to guarantee an effective operation. Our policy is to defer these tests until it is clear that an operation will be needed, and then to begin with scintigraphy. We request it when an unstable patient is beginning his or her third transfusion. If scintigraphy shows an immediate extravasation in the right abdomen that moves across the upper abdomen and down the left side to the pelvis, angiography is unnecessary. The patient needs an emergency right colectomy. If extravasation begins elsewhere or fails to move prograde in the colon to the rectum, immediate angiography is needed to locate the site of bleeding. Surgeons who believe scintigraphy can never be trusted have too often ordered it prematurely in patients who have stopped bleeding or have not witnessed its clearly diagnostic results in many right colon bleeds.

Angiographic Therapy?

The third controversial question is whether radiologists should try embolization or vasopressin infusion. Publications supporting these measures do not describe the rates of bleeding before treatment, so we suspect most good results may have been in patients whose bleeding would have stopped spontaneously. We believe the known risks of embolization and of vasopressin exceed their unproved benefits.

"Blind" Subtotal Colectomy?

The fourth controversial question is whether a "blind" subtotal colectomy is safe and effective when a precise bleeding point or bleeding segment has not been identified. In our experience, blind colectomy has been unsafe [3]. Several patients have rebled, presumably from their small bowel, and the challenge of rebleeding superimposed on surgery has been fatal. A cardinal rule of safe surgery is that operations for hemorrhage must succeed. We therefore reserve blind subtotal colectomy for the extremely rare patient who is clearly exsanguinating from a source not defined by scintigraphy and in whom angiography is prevented by allergy to contrast agents, by renal failure, or by arterial occlusion. In this very unusual circumstance, a quick subtotal colectomy is probably safer than an attempt at intraoperative localization of a bleeding point or a bleeding segment.

Primary Anastomosis

The fifth controversial question is whether, after an emergency colectomy for bleeding, a primary anastomosis can be safely performed. The argument in favor of primary anastomosis is that blood is an excellent cathartic for cleansing the colon of feces. The argument against primary anastomosis is more compelling. It is that in an elderly ASA Class 5E patient whose comorbidities may not be discovered until after operation, an unnecessary bowel anastomosis is foolhardy. In our experience, after an emergency right colectomy, anastomoses of ileum to transverse colon have been safe. After emergency left or subtotal colectomies, anastomoses to the proximal rectum have twice leaked and the patients have died. They should have had their rectums closed and colostomies or ileostomies performed.

Careful application of the foregoing rules will prevent fatality due to lower GI bleeding. What it will not prevent is the frustration of dealing with persistent or recurrent slow bleeding from sources not detectable by colonoscopy, bleeding that may require occasional transfusion but will not be fatal. Faced with this dilemma, a surgeon must refrain from a blind resection, knowing that a misdirected operation is more dangerous than slow bleeding.

References

1. McGuire HH Jr, Haynes BW Jr (1972) Massive hemorrhage from diverticulosis of the colon: guidelines for therapy based on bleeding patterns observed in fifty cases. Ann Surg 175:847–855
2. McGuire HH Jr (1994) Bleeding colonic diverticula: a reappraisal of natural history and management. Ann Surg 220:653–656
3. McGuire HH Jr (1998) Preoperative angiography for GI bleeding. Arch Surg 133:781

Editorial Comment

That controversies are unlikely to be definitely settled by extensive reviews of observational, retrospective studies is also evident in this chapter. Thus, for example, Drs. Efron and Wexner in their thorough review suggest that "total abdominal colectomy may be performed with low mortality and morbidity, and without significant postoperative sequelae," while Dr. McGuire, based on his impressive published, personal experience contends that "in our experience 'blind' colectomy has been unsafe."

One of us, working on four continents over 20 years, never had to operate on a colonic bleed which originated from an arteriovenous malformation (angioectasia). He was therefore intrigued with American textbook dogma, claiming that angioectasia is a leading cause for massive rectal bleeding. He is now comforted by the data presented above by Drs. Efron and Wexner, which list arteriovenous malformations as a rare source of bleeding.

The currently prevailing opinion, expressed above by Drs. Leitman and Burpee, maintains that an emergency colonoscopy in a massively bleeding patient is useless, and that colonoscopic therapy of diverticular hemorrhage is difficult and dangerous. Also Dr. McGuire declares that "for the 25% of bleeds that might exsanguinate, colonoscopy is of no value." A recent study, however, by Jensen et al. [1], offers an exciting and potentially promising perspective. The authors subjected their acute lower GI bleeding patients to an emergency colonoscopy after rapid colonic lavage with Golytely. Patients with definite signs of diverticular hemorrhage (i.e., active bleeding, non-bleeding visible vessel, adherent clot) were managed endoscopically with adrenaline injection (for the active bleeders) or by bipolar coagulation (for the nonactive bleeders). Ten patients with definite diverticular hemorrhage, five of whom were actively bleeding, were successfully treated; none had recurrent bleeding or required surgery. It is possible that in the near future, with increased experience and confidence of the endoscopists, lower GI bleeding will be acutely approached like *upper* GI hemorrhage, with surgery reserved for those rare patients who fail endoscopic therapy. In would be interesting to rewrite this chapter 10 years from now.

Reference

1. Jensen DM, Machicado GA, Jutabha R, Kovacs TO (2000) Urgent colonoscopy for the diagnosis and treatment of severe diverticular hemorrhage. N Engl J Med 342:78–82

CHAPTER 14

Morbid Obesity

Gastric Restrictive Operations

ROBERT E. BROLIN

Historical Background

The concept of gastric restriction as treatment for morbid obesity was introduced by Mason in 1967 [1]. At that time these operations were not widely accepted by the surgical community because they were technically difficult to perform and because of the great popularity of jejunoileal bypass. Moreover, the early gastric restrictive operations were associated with a high incidence of early postoperative complications. Complication rates with gastric bypass decreased substantially after Alden introduced the concept of stapling the stomach in continuity rather than dividing it [2]. Incorporation of the Roux-en-Y technique eliminated problems with bile reflux esophagitis, which were common after loop gastric bypass.

In 1979, Pace and Carey introduced stapled gastroplasty, touting its technical simplicity and low incidence of complications relative to gastric bypass [3]. However, an unacceptably high incidence of early staple-line breakdown soon led to a proliferation of other modifications of gastric stapling. Many of these operations were performed in an uncontrolled manner and resulted in poor outcomes. During the past 15 years, three types of gastric restrictive operations, gastroplasty, gastric banding, and Roux-en-Y gastric bypass, have become popular in the treatment of morbid obesity.

All of the current gastric operations are designed to restrict oral intake. The small capacity upper gastric pouch coupled with a calibrated 12-mm diameter outlet effectively limit the quantity of solid food which can be consumed at one time. Conversely, intake of liquids is not limited by these operations. There is no malabsorption associated with either gastroplasty or gastric banding; weight loss results exclusively from reduced caloric intake. Gastric bypass combines gastric restriction with a small amount of malabsorption. However, malabsorption of macronutrients, protein, carbohydrate, and fat has not been reported after conventional gastric bypass. The anatomic parameters of gastric restriction are similar to those of gastroplasty and gastric banding.

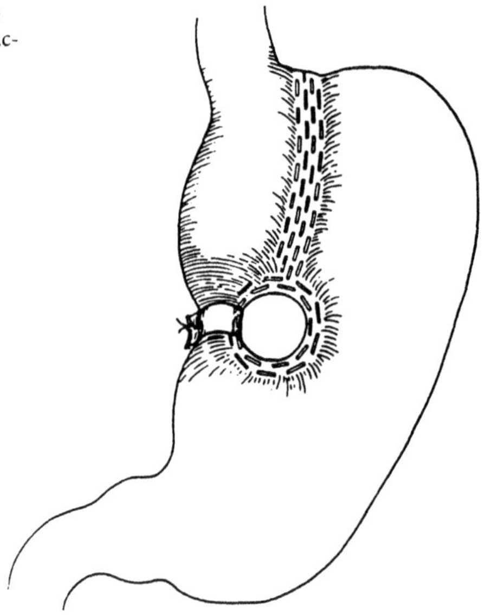

Fig. 1. Vertical banded gastroplasty in which the upper gastric pouch, measured at 15–20 cc capacity, empties into the remainder of the stomach through a calibrated stoma. The stoma is reinforced with a strip of polypropylene (Marlex) mesh measuring 5 cm in circumference. The mesh is placed around the stoma through a "window" created by firing a circular stapling instrument alongside a 32-Fr diameter bougie. The mesh is sutured to itself rather than the stomach. (Courtesy of Churchill Livingstone)

Gastroplasty

In gastroplasty the stomach is partitioned close to the gastroesophageal junction creating a small upper-gastric pouch with a small calibrated outlet leading from the upper pouch to the remainder of the digestive tract. The two most popular techniques of gastroplasty are vertical banded gastroplasty (VBG) and vertical silastic ring gastroplasty (SRG). VBG is shown in Fig. 1. The stoma located at the distal end of the vertically oriented staple-line is reinforced with a prosthetic band to prevent gradual dilatation. Morbidity and mortality rates with both VBG and SRG have been low. Mason and Doherty recently reported an overall morbidity rate of under 10% and a mortality rate of 0.25% in a series of more than 1,200 VGBs [4]. In 1988, Willbanks reported a 3% complication rate with no deaths in a series of 305 SRG patients [5].

Gastric Banding

Gastric banding is a technique that enjoys great popularity in Europe but has received considerably less attention in the United States. The majority of gastric-banding techniques use a premeasured strip of prosthetic material to restrict oral intake (Fig. 2). The circumference of the band is generally in the range of 5 cm, similar to measurements used in VBG. Most gastric-banding techniques lack precision in measuring the volume of stomach above the band. The band is usually sutured to both itself and the stomach to prevent "slipping." Kuzmak introduced the concept of an inflatable Silicone band in which the diameter of the band can be adjusted by infusion of saline through a subcutaneous reservoir [6]. Kuzmak reported that weight loss results and complication rates are better than those observed after the early open banding techniques in which strips of polypropylene or

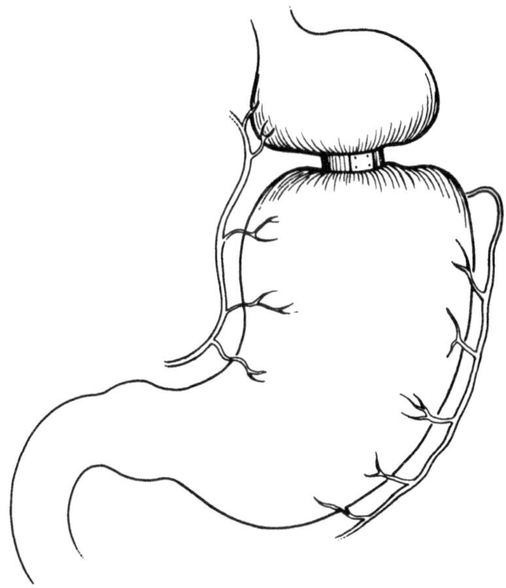

Fig. 2. Gastric banding in which the upper portion of the stomach is encircled by a calibrated prosthetic band. The volume of the stomach above the band is crudely estimated by most surgeons who perform this operation. The band is sutured to the stomach to prevent slipping. (Courtesy of Churchill Livingstone)

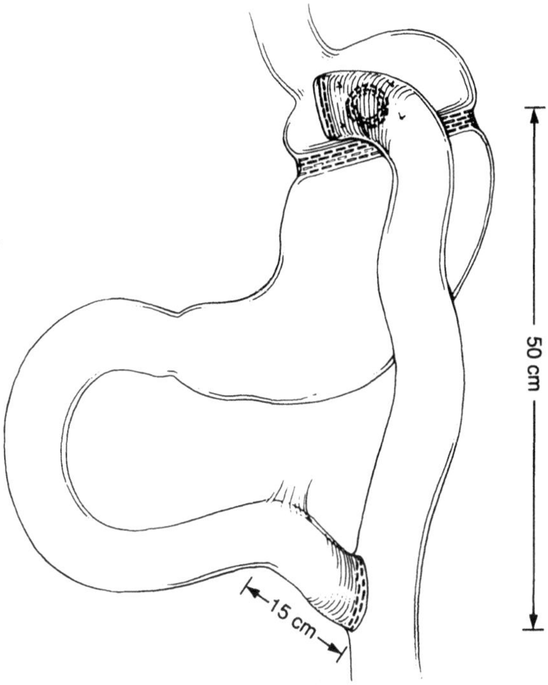

Fig. 3. Roux-en-Y gastric bypass in which the TA 90B stapler (US Surgical Corp., Norwalk, CT) is fired across the cardia of the stomach creating a 20 ± 5 cc upper pouch. The jejunum is divided approximately 15 cm distal to the ligament of Treitz with the distal end anastomosed to the upper stomach using a circular stapler creating an 11×4 cm diameter anastomosis. The proximal end of jejunum is then anastomosed 50 cm below the gastrojejunostomy. (Courtesy of C.V. Mosby Co.)

Teflon are used. Stenosis and/or erosion of the band have been reported in 10–30% of cases [7, 8]. Stenosis and erosion occasionally result in stomal obstruction which frequently requires reoperation. Erosion of the inflatable Silicone bands is quite rare. However, problems with the subcutaneous reservoir are common.

Gastric Bypass

In gastric bypass the upper stomach is closed off, thereby excluding more than 95% of the stomach, all of the duodenum, and 10–15 cm of proximal jejunum from digestive continuity. The Roux-en-Y technique shown in Fig. 3 is currently the preferred method of almost every surgeon who performs gastric bypass. A growing number of surgeons are now transsecting the upper stomach rather than stapling it in continuity. Gastric bypass occasionally produces symptoms of the "dumping syndrome" which include nausea, cramps, bloating, and diarrhea. Dumping is thought to be due to rapid emptying of food from the small gastric pouch directly into the small bowel. Symptoms of "late" dumping including light-headedness, palpitations, and sweating also occur in a smaller percentage of patients. These vasomotor symptoms are the consequence of rebound hypoglycemia and typically occur 1.5–2 h after ingestion of a carbohydrate-laden meal. The incidence and severity of dumping after gastric bypass is variable with some patients reporting no symptoms, others having symptoms associated with eating specific foods such as milk products or sweets. A few patients have troublesome symptoms after almost every meal. Troublesome dumping rarely persists for more than 9–12 months postoperatively.

Controversy 1: The "Procedure of Choice" Among Gastric Restrictive Operations

The early postoperative complication rates with current modifications of the Roux-en-Y gastric bypass (RYGB) are similar to those of gastroplasty and gastric banding. Surgeons who support gastroplasty as the procedure of choice for the treatment of morbid obesity generally cite the lower degree of difficulty in performing the operation and the paucity of long-term metabolic complications relative to gastric bypass. In experienced hands banded gastric restrictive operations can usually be performed in less than 1 h. The duration of ileus is relatively short, so patients usually can be discharged by the third postoperative day. A short length of stay in conjunction with lower operating room cost would seemingly make a strong case in favor of gastroplasty vs. RYGB.

Conversely, surgeons who favor RYGB as the operation of choice cite two issues in support of their position. The primary goal of bariatric operations is to provide sufficient weight loss which would be maintained in the long term. Weight loss and amelioration of medical comorbidities is the primary reason patients seek surgical treatment. Over the years there have been a number of controlled, prospective comparisons of RYGB versus several techniques of gastroplasty. All of these comparative studies have shown significantly greater weight loss after RYGB [9–11]. Although there are conflicting data regarding the correlation between the amount of weight loss and improvement of comorbidities after gastric bariatric operations, the preponderance of these data suggest that medical problems are more likely to improve or resolve with greater weight loss [12, 13].

The second issue favoring RYGB is the rate of surgical revision for either late complications or unsatisfactory weight loss in comparison with stapled gastroplasty or gastric banding. The incidence of unsatisfactory weight loss is at least twice as high after gastroplasty with some series reporting a failure rate greater than 50% [14, 15]. Revisional bariatric operations are associated with perioperative morbidity rates which are five to ten times higher in comparison with primary procedures [16, 17]. Hence, the revision rate may be the most relevant means of assessment of any bariatric operation. Although weight-loss failure following both types of procedure includes cases of late staple line disruption, a substantial number of patients fail after gastroplasty or banding with an anatomically intact operation. Unsatisfactory weight loss is usually the most common reason for revision after banded gastroplasty. The principle complication which leads to surgical revision of banded restrictive procedures is intractable stomal stenosis. Conversely, stomal stenosis after RYGB usually responds to endoscopic balloon dilatation. Marginal ulcer is often cited as the leading indication for revision of RYGB [18, 19]. Most marginal ulcers respond to medical treatment. Disruption of the stapled partition after RYGB is frequently associated with intractable marginal ulcers which require operative treatment.

Controversy 2: Patient Selection Criteria

In 1991, the National Institutes of Health convened a consensus development panel to discuss the current status of gastrointestinal surgery for medically significant severe obesity. This panel recommended guidelines for selection of patients for these procedures which, in large part, have been adopted nationwide by both physicians and third-party payors. These recommendations include minimum weight criteria for uncomplicated obesity [body mass index (BMI) $\geqslant 40\ kg/m^2$] and complicated obesity (BMI $\geqslant 35\ kg/m^2$). The panel also stated that "children and adolescents have not been sufficiently studied to allow a recommendation for surgery..." [20]. The issue of age at both ends of the spectrum remains controversial among bariatric surgeons. Several surgeons have restricted the operation to subjects between ages 18 and 50 [21, 22]. However, there are no convincing data that age restrictions in the field of bariatric surgery are warranted. The limited published experience with bariatric operations in children and adolescents strongly endorse the efficacy of these procedures in this age group [23]. The author affirms these positive results in a personal series of 10 patients age 18 and under. Younger patients generally recover quickly and tend to lose weight faster than older patients. The social benefits of weight loss in this group are profound, characterized by a rapid transition between ridicule and isolation to the mainstream of their peer group.

Although 50 is an old age for morbidly obese patients, the benefits of substantial weight loss are well documented in this group [24]. Successful weight loss frequently results in discarding wheelchairs, walkers, and canes, amelioration of hypertension, cure of type II diabetes, and cancellation of joint replacement operations which were previously contraindicated by the patient's weight. Moreover, bariatric operations are no more physiologically demanding than open-heart procedures which are commonly performed in much older patients. The author suggests that risk/benefit issues in elderly bariatric patients be assessed on a case-by-case basis. Substantial weight loss in patients over 50 years of age usually results in dramatic improvement in qualify of life.

The need for preoperative psychological assessment remains a somewhat controversial issue in large part because several insurance carriers require such evaluation. There is no convincing evidence that routine preoperative psychological evaluation serves any useful purpose in bariatric surgical patients. Although the incidence of depression is somewhat greater in obese patients, there are no hard data supporting the notion that the morbidly obese have significantly more psychological problems than their normal-weight counterparts. Conversely, preoperative psychological evaluation is warranted in patients with a history of suicide attempts or inpatient treatment for mental illness. At the outset of our bariatric surgical program a detailed psychological evaluation was routinely used. We found it to be useless in predicting weight-loss outcome, postoperative complications, or compliance [25].

Ongoing substance abuse in the form of alcohol or drugs is an absolute contraindication for bariatric surgery. However, the issue of past abuse in an allegedly reformed patient has not been addressed in a controlled clinical setting. In the author's limited experience, these "reformed" patients have a high incidence of relapse into their previous problems. Hence, preoperative psychological evaluation is also justified in these patients. However, psychological screening methods may not be sufficiently sensitive to predict relapse in this difficult group.

Controversy 3: Unresolved Technical Considerations

There have been several reports of use of prosthetic bands in RYGB [26, 27]. The rationale for adding a band to the restrictive component of RYGB is to prevent late weight gain which presumably results from dilatation of the gastrojejunostomy. However, there are no well-controlled clinical studies which have addressed this hypothesis. Linner and Drew abandoned the use of silastic reinforcement of the gastrojejunostomy in RYGB, citing a high incidence of late erosion and migration of the ring [27]. Drew currently reinforces the gastrojejunostomy with a strip of fascia from the rectus abdominis and claims a low incidence of anastomotic problems (R.L. Drew, personal communication). The available data suggest that, within a small measurement range, the volume of the upper gastric pouch and the diameter of the gastrojejunostomy do not correlate with weight-loss outcome after RYGB [28].

The need to transsect the stomach after both gastroplasty and RYGB remains a subject of controversy. There has been wide variation in the incidence of late staple-line disruption after both procedures. MacLean et al. have probably performed the most vigilant evaluation of this issue. Their studies concluded that the incidence of breakdown of incontinuity gastric partitions can be virtually eliminated by transsection [19]. Capella has confirmed these results after RYGB [17]. Conversely, Pories et al. abandoned transsection after a controlled study of 100 RYGB patients due to a higher incidence of leaks from the transected stomach [29]. Sugerman et al. use three superimposed firings of the TA90 stapler without transsection and claim a breakdown rate of only 2% [30]. The author has reported a 3% incidence of late staple-line breakdown using one application of the TA 90B [31]. Limitations inherent to the stapling instruments now available for minimally invasive gastrointestinal surgery do not permit stapling of the stomach in continuity during laparoscopic bariatric operations.

During the past several years there have been a number of reports of conventional bariatric operations performed using minimally invasive techniques. Laparoscopic gastric banding using several types of inflatable prostheses has gained great popularity in Europe. In the United States the FDA is overseeing a large multicenter clinical trial using the Lap Band (Bioenterics Corp., Carpinteria, CA) which will be completed by 2000.

Several surgeons have reported large series of patients who have had RYGB via a laparoscopic approach. The weight-loss results of both laparoscopic gastric banding and RYGB are similar to results using open techniques. However, the learning curve is steep. The primary advantages of the laparoscopic approach are a reduction in length of stay of 50% or more and a lower incidence of wound problems. The incidence of leaks is slightly higher after laparoscopic RYGB versus the open approach [32].

Controversy 4: Use of Nutritional Supplements

There is no consensus regarding the use of nutritional supplements after either gastroplasty or RYGB. Because there is no malabsorption after either gastric banding or gastroplasty, many surgeons who perform these procedures do not offer nutritional supplements to their patients. However, there are several studies which show that the RDA of many vitamins and minerals is not reached in the diet of most patients who have gastroplasty or gastric banding [33, 34]. Severe metabolic complications (most notably thiamin deficiency) have been reported after gastroplasty and banding. These deficiencies are extremely rare and are invariably associated with protracted postprandial vomiting [35].

Because nearly all of the stomach and the entire duodenum are excluded from digestive continuity in RYGB, deficiencies in iron, folate, and vitamin B_{12} are quite common. Although prescription of multivitamins is routine for patients who have RYGB, there remains controversy over the need to prescribe other supplements prophylactically. However, there is an emerging consensus regarding the need for folate supplements. Recent reports have shown that folate deficiency is extremely uncommon in RYGB patients who are compliant in taking multivitamin supplements postoperatively [36, 37]. Hence, prescription of multivitamins alone should suffice in the treatment of folate deficiency after RYGB.

Conversely, multivitamin supplements do not consistently provide protection against iron and B_{12} deficiency [37, 38]. Menstruating women are particularly prone to iron deficiency after RYGB. Our group recently showed that prophylactic oral iron supplements consistently protect premenopausal women from developing iron deficiency after RYGB [39]. However, the incidence of postoperative anemia was similar in the iron and placebo groups. Anemia in the absence of measurable micronutrient deficiencies remains a major unsolved problem after RYGB.

The incidence of B_{12} deficiency after RYGB is reported in the range from 30% to 40% [37, 38, 40]. Our group has observed a substantially lower incidence of B_{12} deficiency in patients who regularly take multivitamin supplements. The author has yet to identify a patient with symptoms of B_{12} deficiency in a personal series of nearly 1,000 RYGB procedures. Hence, we do not prescribe prophylactic B_{12} supplements. This practice differs from that of several other experienced bariatric surgeons. Vitamin B_{12} deficiency is easily treated using either oral, aerosol or intramuscular supplements.

Controversy 5: Deep Venous Thrombosis – Prophylaxis

Pulmonary embolism is the leading cause of perioperative death following bariatric operations. Although the need for postoperative deep venous thrombosis (DVT) prophylaxis in bariatric surgical patients is not in dispute, the method(s) of choice is somewhat controversial. Remarkably there are no hard data which show obesity to be an independent risk factor for DVT. However, nearly all surgeons agree that severely obese patients are at greater risk than normal-weight patients for developing pulmonary embolism after major operations. Unfortunately, severely obese patients are resistant to several accepted methods of DVT prophylaxis including compression boots (which frequently do not fit), low dose heparin (absorption inconsistencies), and early ambulation (due to size, physical disabilities). Hence, the controversy is not whether to provide DVT prophylaxis but how. Because there are no data regarding the efficacy of any method of DVT prophylaxis in bariatric surgical patients, there is no established standard of care. Martin et al. have recently shown that recommended doses of Lovinox (low molecular heparin) do not provide adequate levels of anticoagulation in morbidly obese patients [41]. Screening bariatric surgical patients for DVT has been unrewarding both pre- and postoperatively. Improving upon existing methods for DVT prophylaxis is perhaps the most important unresolved problem in bariatric surgery today.

Controversy 6: Assessment of Outcome

There is still no universally accepted methodology for assessment of outcome following bariatric operations. It is almost universally accepted that some measurement of weight loss should be included. However, there is still controversy regarding the preferred method of expressing weight loss outcome. The use of the percentage of excess weight loss is probably the most commonly used method with loss of 50% or more of the excess weight a generally accepted minimum criterion for success. The body mass index (BMI), which is expressed as the ratio of weight in kg over height in square meters, is currently the most acceptable method of expressing weight in humans. The BMI accounts for frame size and has an established range of normalcy for both genders. Use of a mere quantity or percentage of weight loss has fallen into disfavor because of difficulty in correlating these numbers with normal or desirable weight.

Currently there is a growing consensus to include other quality-of-life parameters in outcome assessment. Oria recently introduced a new method which incorporates a combination of outcome criteria entitled Bariatric Analysis and Reporting Outcome System (BAROS) [42]. The BAROS method assigns points to weight loss, medical comorbidity and qualify-of-life categories which are combined to determine an overall outcome score on a scale of 1–9. Although this system includes all of the important categories of outcome assessment for bariatric surgical patients, it has not been subjected to rigorous scrutiny by objective testing methods. The Rand 36 item Health Survey (SF-36) has been used by Choban et al. in a series of bariatric surgical patients [43]. As expected, this study showed that bariatric surgical patients experience remarkable improvement in overall health postoperatively. Both BAROS and the SF-36 are a bit cumbersome for use by practicing surgeons in the office setting. However, it seems likely that some modification of a BAROS-like assessment method will eventually be adopted and utilized by most bariatric surgeons.

References

1. Mason EE, Ito C (1967) Gastric bypass in obesity. Surg Clin North Am 43:1345–1351
2. Alden JF (1977) Gastric and jejunoileal bypass: a comparison in the treatment of morbid obesity. Arch Surg 112:799–804
3. Carey LC, Martin EW Jr, Mojzisik C (1984) The surgical treatment of morbid obesity. Curr Prob Surg 21:10
4. Mason EE, Doherty C, Scott DH, Maher JW, Rodriquez EX (1989) Vertical banded gastroplasty (VBG) for treatment of obesity: an eight year review. Abstract presented at the 75th Clinical Congress of the American College of Surgeons, Atlanta, GA October 17, 1989
5. Willbanks OL (1987) Long-term results of silicone elastomer ring vertical gastroplasty for the treatment of morbid obesity. Surgery, 101:606–610
6. Kuzmak LI (1989) Gastric banding. In: Dietel N (ed) Surgery for the Morbid Obese Patient. Lea & Febiger, Philadelphia, p 225
7. Backman L, Granstrom L (1984) Initial (one-year) weight loss after gastric banding, gastroplasty and gastric bypass. Acta Chir Scand 150:63–67
8. Lorig T, Haffner JFW, Nygaard X, et al. (1987) Gastric banding for morbid obesity: early results. Int J Obes 11:377–384
9. Lechner GW, Callender K (1981) Subtotal gastric exclusion and gastric partitioning: a randomized prospective comparison of one hundred patients. Surgery 90:637–644
10. Naslund I, Wickbom G, Christofferson E, Agren G (1986) A prospective randomized comparison of gastric bypass and gastroplasty: complications and early results. Acta Chir Scand 152: 681–689
11. Sugerman Hi, Starkey JV, Birkenhauer R (1987) A randomized prospective trial of gastric bypass vs. vertical banded gastroplasty for morbid obesity and their effects on sweets vs. non-sweets eaters. Arm Surg 205:613–624
12. Carson JL, Ruddy ME, Duff AE, et al. (1994) The effect of gastric bypass surgery on hypertension in morbidly obese patients. Arch Int Med 154:193–200
13. Brolin RE, Kenler HA, Wilson AC, et al. (1990) Serum lipids after gastric bypass surgery for morbid obesity. Int J Obes 14:939–950
14. Brolin RE, Robertson LB, Kenler HA, Cody RP (1994) Weight loss and dietary intake after vertical banded gastroplasty and Roux-en-Y gastric bypass. Ann Surg 220:782–790
15. MacLean LD, Rhode BM, Forse RA (1990) Late results of vertical banded gastroplasty for morbid and super obesity. Surgery 107:20–27
16. MacArthur RI, Smith DE, Hermreck AS, et al. (1980) Revision of gastric bypass. Am J Surg 140:750–754

17. Capella JF, Capella RF (1995) The weight reduction operation of choice: vertical banded gastroplasty or gastric bypass. Abstract in Obes Surg 5:124
18. Jordan JH, Hocking MF, Rout WR, Woodward ER (1991) Marginal ulcer following gastric bypass for morbid obesity. Am Surg 57:286–288
19. MacLean LD, Rhode BM, Sampalis J, Forse RA (1993) Results of the surgical treatment of obesity. Am J Surg 165:155–162
20. National Institutes of Health Consensus Development Panel (1992) Gastrointestinal surgery for severe obesity. Am J Clin Nutri 55[suppl]: S615–S619
21. Printon KJ, Mason EE (1977) Gastric bypass for morbid obesity in patients more than 50 years of age. Surg Gynecol Obstet 144:192–194
22. Hall JC, Watts JM, O'Brien PE (1990) Gastric surgery for morbid obesity: the Adelaide Study. Ann Surg 211:419–427
23. Rand CSW, MacGregor AMC (1994) Adolescents having obesity surgery: a 6 year follow up. Southern Med J 87:1208–1213
24. MacGregor AMC, Rand CSW (1993) Gastric surgery in morbid obesity: outcome in patients aged 55 years and older. Arch Surg 128:1153–1157
25. Brolin RE, Clemow LPI, Kasnetz KA, et al. (1986) Outcome predictors after gastroplasty for morbid obesity. Nutri Int 2:322–326
26. Fobi MAL, Lee H, Holness R, DeGaulle C (1998) Gastric bypass operation for obesity. World J Surg 22:925–935
27. Drew RL, Linner JH (1992) Revisional surgery for severe obesity with fascia banded stoma Roux-en-Y gastric bypass. Obes Surg 2:349–355
28. Naslund I (1986) The size of the gastric outlet and the outcome of surgery for obesity. Acta Chir Scand 152:205–210
29. Cucchi SG, Pories WJ, MacDonald KG, et al. (1995) Gastrogastric fistulas. A complication of divided gastric bypass surgery. Ann Surg 221:387–391
30. Sugerman HJ, Kellum JM, Engle KM (1992) Gastric bypass for treating severe obesity. Am J Clin Nutr 55(suppl 2):S560–S566
31. Brolin RE (1993) Healing of the stapled stomach in bariatric operations. Surgery 113:484–490
32. Whitgrove AC, Clark GW, Schubert KR (1996) Laparoscopic gastric bypass: technique and results in 75 patients with 3–30-month follow up. Obes Surg 6:500–504
33. MacLean LD, Rhode BM, Schizgal HM (1983) Nutrition following gastric operations for morbid obesity. Ann Surg 198:347–355
34. Andersen T, Laroson U (1989) Dietary outcome in patients treated with a gastroplasty program. Am J Clin Nutri 50:1328–1340
35. Haid RW, Gutman L, Crosby TW (1982) Wernicke-Korsakoff encephalopathy after gastric plication. JAMA 247:2566–2567
36. Mallory GN, MacGregor AMA (1991) Folate status following gastric bypass surgery (The Great Folate Mystery). Obes Surg 1:69–72
37. Brolin RE, Gorman RC, Milgrim LM, Kenler HA (1991) Multivitamin prophylaxis in prevention of post-gastric bypass vitamin and mineral deficiencies. Int J Obes 15:661–668
38. Brolin RE, Gorman JH, Goan RC et al. (1998) Are vitamin B-12 and folate deficiency clinically important after Roux-en-Y gastric bypass? J Gastrointest Surg 2:436–442
39. Brolin RE, Gorman JH Gorman RC, et al. (1998) Prophylactic iron supplementation after Roux-en-Y gastric bypass: a prospective, double-blind, randomized study. Arch Surg 133:740–744
40. Halverson JD, Zuckerman GR, Koehler RE, et al. (1981) Gastric bypass for morbid obesity: a medical-surgical assessment. Ann Surg 194:152–160
41. Martin LF, Finigan KM (1999) Heparin factor XA levels in morbidly obese patients receiving Lovinox R prophylaxis (abstract). Obes Surg 9:128
42. Oria HE, Moorehead MK (1998) Bariatric analysis and reporting outcome system (BAROS). Obes Surg 8:487–499
43. Choban PS, Onyejekwe J, Burge JC, Flancbaum L (1999) A health status assessment of the impact of weight loss following Roux-en-Y gastric bypass for clinically severe obesity. J Am Coll Surg 188:491–497

Malabsorptive Procedures

NICOLA SCOPINARO · FRANCESCO PAPADIA

Since the beginning of the 1980s, biliopancreatic diversion (BPD) [1–3] has become an acceptable malabsorptive approach for the surgical therapy of obesity. BPD represents the only malabsorptive procedure with widespread diffusion. Therefore, controversies in malabsorptive surgery for obesity today are only a question of analysis of the superiority of BPD over the old jejunoileal bypass (JIB), and comparisons of BPD itself and the most used among its many proposed modifications.

Biliopancreatic Diversion

BPD consists of a distal gastrectomy with a long Roux-en-Y reconstruction where the enteroenterostomy is placed at a distal ileal level. A maldigestion is then obtained which results in a selective malabsorption for fat and starch, while the intestinal absorption of the other nutrients is essentially preserved. In the current model of the operation (Fig. 4), called "ad hoc stomach, ad hoc alimentary limb (AHS AHAL)" BPD, the gastric volume and the alimentary limb (AL) length, varying from 200 to 500 ml and from 200 to 300 cm, respectively, are adapted to the

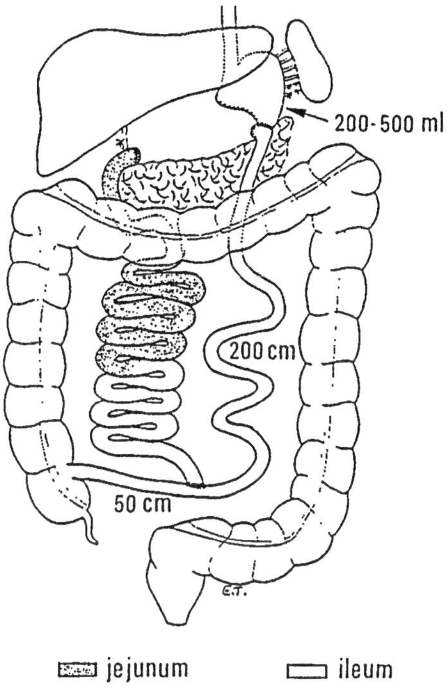

Fig. 4. Ad hoc stomach, ad hoc alimentary limb biliopancreatic diversion. Alimentary limb (*AL*), from the gastroenterostomy to the enteroenterostomy (*EEA*); biliopancreatic limb (*BPL*), from the duodenum to the EEA; common limb (*CL*), from the EEA to the ileocecal valve

patient's individual characteristics in order to obtain maximum of weight loss with minimum complications.

The main feature of BPD is the existence of a threshold intestinal energy transport, which allows a maximum mean daily absorption (in the case of 200 cm AL) of about 40 g of fat and 220 g of starch, for a total of about 1,240 Cal/day. Protein absorption, which, on the contrary, is reduced by about 30% in a sample of our population, accounts for an average of 360 Cal/day. The patient's body weight must then decrease until the body's energy expenditure corresponds to about 1,600 Cal/day and remain constant thereafter, independent of energy intake. The absorption of mono- and disaccharides, short-chain triglycerides, and alcohol (i.e., the energy content of sugar, fruit, sweets, soft drinks, milk, and alcoholic beverages) is undisturbed after BPD, so the intake of these aliments may be varied to counterbalance the interindividual differences in energy absorption capacity and in body composition (which, body weights being equal, determines total energy expenditure). The energy absorption threshold increases with the increase in length of the AL, where starch and protein are absorbed.

The initial weight loss after BPD is caused by temporary food intake limitation due to the decrease of appetite and occurrence of postcibal syndrome consequent to the ileal stimulation by food: this effect being the more intense and long-lasting the smaller the gastric remnant, and thus the quicker its emptying. A small stomach also permanently influences intestinal absorption by reducing intestinal transit time.

Results and Complications

Apart from slightly more than 3% incidence of stomal ulcer and the need for oral calcium and parenteral iron and vitamin D and A supplementation, the only possible major late specific complication of BPD is protein malnutrition, mainly due to the presence of an increased loss of endogenous nitrogen. The incidence of protein malnutrition is greatly influenced by the AL length and the stomach volume. Adapting the latter two to the patient's individual characteristics resulted, in our experience, in a 2.7% incidence of this complication, with a 1% rate of recurrence (the only indication for surgical revision of BPD).

BPD is superior to JIB (Fig. 5) as far as both complications and results are concerned. Generally, all complications of JIB can be attributed to two main defects of the operation, i.e., indiscriminate malabsorption and the presence of a long blind loop, both of which are avoided in BPD. In particular, the absence in BPD of the major complications of JIB is easily explained by the pathogenesis of those complications. Diarrhea and consequent electrolyte imbalance, reported in up to 100% of cases after JIB [5], are due to the irritation of colonic mucosa by bile acids and fatty acids [1]. In BPD, the interruption of the enterohepatic bile salt circulation was calibrated to about 750 mg/day by choosing the appropriate length for the common limb (CL) [4]; moreover, due to the lack of fat digestion, steatorrhea is essentially neutral, the fecal pH being around 7. In fact, studies on intestinal transit time after BPD showed that, in comparison with preoperative transit time, transport speed was unchanged in the large bowel, and even decreased by 50% in

Fig. 5. Jejunoileal bypass. The bypass total length is 45–50 cm in most series, with the ileal length varying between 5 and 20 cm

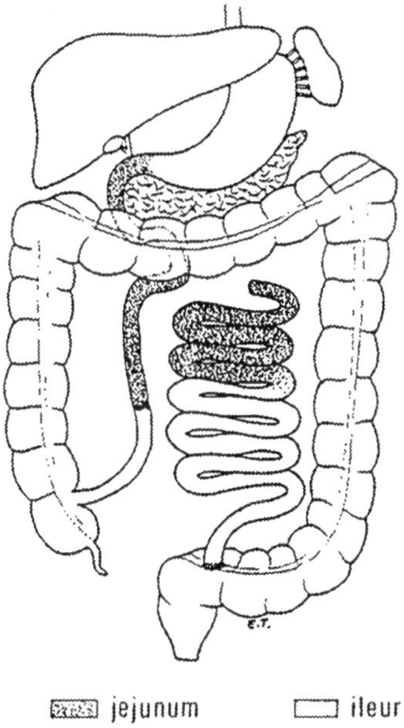

the small bowel [4]. Vitamin deficiencies, reported in up to 88% of cases after JIB [6], are due to the indiscriminate malabsorption. In BPD, hydrosoluble vitamins are normally absorbed in the AL, and the synthesis of vitamin K by the colonic bacterial flora is sufficient to meet the requirement. The pathogenesis of kidney stones, whose incidence may be as high as 50% after JIB [7], is multifactorial. Although the main cause is dehydration secondary to diarrhea [8], other factors related to the indiscriminate malabsorption are also involved, such as hypocitraturia [9] and reduced concentration of other inhibitors of stone formation [10]; hyperoxaluria is obviously a prerequisite factor. Increased urinary oxalate concentration after JIB was attributed to excessive glycoxalate production from unabsorbed glycoconjugated bile salts in the colon [11], to reduced precipitation of oxalate as calcium salt due to sequestration of calcium as soap with unabsorbed fatty acids [12], and to the increased permeability to oxalate of the colonic mucosa due to the presence of excessive bile acids [13]. Since none of these conditions is present in BPD, no hyperoxaluria was found in BPD subjects [13], nor was any difference found between the incidence of kidney stones in AHS BPD subjects (5/1,281, or 0.4%) and in the general population [3].

Some major complications of JIB are to be attributed to the presence of a long, excluded intestinal loop. The so-called bypass enteropathy, besides local manifestations, such as dramatic gas-bloating, voluminous flatulence, and eruptive diarrhea, with possible perforation in the blind loop, may also cause systemic complications [14]. Toxins from the excluded loop [15] and/or protein malnutrition [16] have been advocated as causes for liver damage after JIB, both early [17] and late [6], in up to 29% of cases, with progression towards cirrhosis in up to 7%. There is no blind loop in BPD, and the fact that this operation does not cause any liver damage [18] (only one well-documented case of liver failure reported so far [19] despite more than 10,000 published BPD operations) demonstrates that protein malnutrition is not a sufficient cause for liver injury. In jejuno-ileal bypass, autoantibodies from the excluded loop and immunocomplex deposition are responsible for polyarthritis (up to 20% of cases) [20], and chronic nephritis, with evolution towards renal failure (2% of cases) [21].

In addition to its complications, the main problem with JIB is its narrow "therapeutic interval". In fact, the total length of the small bowel left in continuity is restrained within the range of 40–60 cm, a shorter or longer bypass resulting in life-threatening malabsorption or no weight reduction, respectively. On the other hand, the massive intestinal adaptation phenomena cause an increased absorptive surface leading out of the upper limits of the above range, with ensuing substantial recovery of energy absorption capacity [22]. In fact, both in the past [23, 24] and recently [25] it was demonstrated that the maintenance of a body weight lower than the preoperative one in JIB subjects is at least partly accounted for by a reduction of energy intake postoperatively in comparison with preoperatively. This, in addition to the frequent need of restoration for major complications, ends in a high rate of failure with weight regain [26, 27]. On the contrary, BPD has a wide therapeutic interval, because, by varying the length of the intestinal limbs, any degree of fat, starch, and protein malabsorption can be created, thereby adapting the procedure to the population's or patient's characteristics to obtain the best possible weight-loss results with minimum complications [3]. This extreme flexibility also neutralizes the consequences of intestinal adaptation phenomena.

Modifications of BPD

Among the many proposed modifications of the original BPD, the most commonly used is the so-called "long-Roux-Y gastric bypass" or "distal gastric bypass". Besides the total semantic inadequacy of the naming, these operations essentially consist of a BPD with bypass instead of resection of the distal stomach (Fig. 6), and they meet the necessity of disguising a BPD as a gastric bypass for different opportunistic reasons. If the intestinal lengths and the gastric volumes are correctly used, the results and complications of these operations are exactly the same as in proper BPD, with the exception of a greater incidence of stomal ulcer [28] and the concern for the fate of the bypassed stomach [29]. Actually, many surgeons used this type of operation as conversional surgery after failed gastric restrictive procedures, and kept the original gastric pouch excluding the rest of the stomach. As a gastric volume smaller than 200 ml strongly influences the incidence of early and recurrent protein malnutrition, this policy resulted in a dramatic frequency of this complication in many series [30, 31]. Those surgeons who want to convert a gastric restrictive operation to a BPD should keep in mind how the BPD functions and its rules. For this type of conversion, it is mandatory to restore gastric anatomy first, as far as possible, and then to create a suitable gastric remnant, independently of the volume of the previous gastric pouch.

Certain authors have suggested combining different types of gastric restrictive procedures with a BPD. Reflection on the main mechanism of BPD shows that this

Fig. 6. Biliopancreatic diversion with bypass of the distal stomach

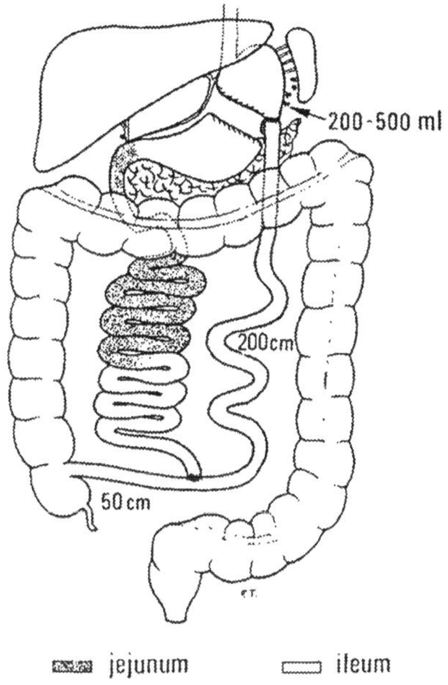

suggestion is unsubstantiated. In fact, should the restrictive component of this combined operation cause the patient to eat less than what he/she can absorb, BPD would be totally useless. The opposite would be true should, on the contrary, the restrictive operation fail. In summary, in the long run only one of the two operations would work and produce results, and the patient would have the risks, complications, and side-effects of both.

The only modification of BPD that deserves to be dealt with is the so-called "biliopancreatic diversion with parietal gastrectomy (or "vertical" or "sleeve gastrectomy") and duodenal switch" (Fig. 7). This operation, introduced by Hess [32] and pioneered by Hess himself [33] and Marceau et al. [34, 35], entails a longitudinal gastrectomy with removal of most of the fundus, and thus the parietal cell mass, and preservation of gastric vagal innervation and of the pylorus with the first portion of the duodenum. Its rationale, apart from prevention of stomal ulcers (whose incidence is null in the series of Hess) is not well understood. The theoretical advantages of saving the pylorus and the first few centimeters of duodenum are an increased iron and calcium absorption, which seems to happen in both series. For the rest, one can imagine that the operation should result in a slower gastric emptying when compared with the distal gastrectomy, and consequently, the gastric volume and the intestinal lengths being equal, an increased intestinal absorption and thus a reduction of all the consequences of malabsorption, e.g., stool frequency, gas problems, and incidence of protein malnutrition, obviously at the expense of weight loss. Since exactly the same can be obtained in the original BPD by simply modifying gastric volume and intestinal lengths, we wonder if the expected benefits are worth the greater technical complexity of the operation. Surprisingly, Marceau [35] compared the results of BPD with distal gas-

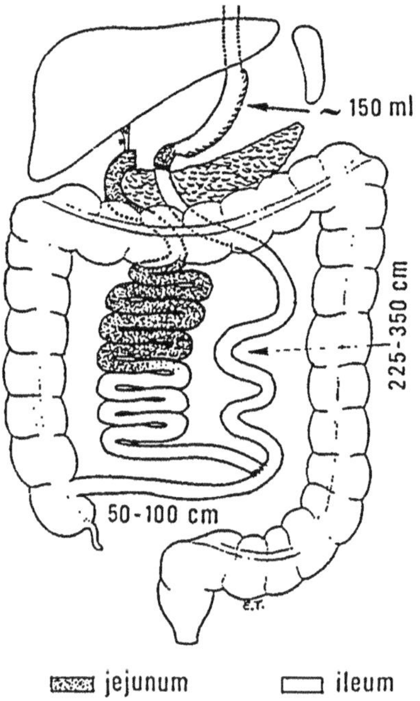

Fig. 7. Biliopancreatic diversion with parietal gastrectomy and duodenal switch according to Hess. The lengths of the AL and the CL approximate 40% and 10%, respectively, of the small bowel total length

trectomy and BPD with sleeve gastrectomy and duodenal switch, and, besides all the above-mentioned beneficial effects, found a weight loss significantly greater following the second procedure. Since he estimates the gastric volume to be equal in the two procedures, and the CL length is double (100 cm) in the second one, it is hard to explain this finding. The only reasonable hypothesis seems to be the greater experience accumulated over the years, which has clear beneficial effects on all results.

Conclusions

In summary, BPD, yielding better results than JIB without its complications, is today the only extensively used malabsorptive procedure for surgical treatment of obesity. Its flexibility allows the surgeon to adapt the operation to the characteristics of the patients in his population for the best possible results with the minimum of complications. The same flexibility is the Achilles' heel of the procedure, as it tempts many surgeons to try their own modifications with no scientific rationale, very often with disastrous consequences. BPD is a very complex procedure, and its many different mechanisms are not easy to understand. Thorough knowledge of these mechanisms and experience in the procedure are the necessary prerequisites to planning a serious rationale for any BPD modification.

References

1. Scopinaro N, Gianetta E, Civalleri D, Bonalumi U, Bach, V (1979) Bilio-pancreatic by-pass for obesity. I. An experimental study in dogs. Br J Surg 66:613–617
2. Scopinaro N, Gianetta E, Civalleri D, Bonalumi U, Bachi, V (1979) Bilio-pancreatic by-pass for obesity. II. Initial experience in man. Br J Surg 66:618–620
3. Scopinaro N, Adami GF, Marinari GM, Gianetta E, Traverso E, Friedman D, Camerini G, Baschieri G, Simonelli A (1998) Biliopancreatic Diversion. World J Surg 22:936–946
4. Scopinaro N, Gianetta E, Civalleri D, Bonalumi U, Friedman D, Traverso E, Adami GF, Bachi V (1987) Biliopancreatic diversion. In: Griffen WO, Printen KJ (eds) Surgical Management of Morbid Obesity. Marcel Dekker, New York, pp 93–162
5. Starkloff GB, Donovan JF, Ramach KR, Wolfe BM (1975) Metabolic intestinal surgery: its complications and management. Arch Surg 110:652–657
6. Hocking MP, Duerson MC, O'Leary JP, Woodward ER (1983) Jejunoileal bypass for morbid obesity. N Eng J Med 308:995–999
7. O'Leary JP, Thomas WC Jr, Woodward ER (1974) Urinary tract stone after small bowel bypass for morbid obesity. Am J Surg 127:53–58
8. Smith LH, Hofmann AF, McCall JT, Thomas PJ (1970) Secondary hyperoxaluria in patients with ileal resection and oxalate nephrolithiasis. Clin Res 18:541
9. Rudman D, Dedonis JL, Fountain MT, Chandler JB, Gerron GG, Fleming GA, Kutner MH (1980) Hypocitraturia in patients with gastrointestinal malabsorption. N Eng J Med 303:657–661
10. Fleisch H (1978) Inhibitors and promoters of stone formation. Kidney Int 13:361–371
11. Wise L, Stein T (1975) Biliary and urinary calculi: pathogenesis following small bowel bypass for obesity. Arch Surg 110:1043–1047
12. Poley JR, Hofmann AF (1972) Role of fat maldigestion in pathogenesis of steatorrhea in ileal resection. Fat digestion after two sequential test meals with and without cholestyramine. Gastroenterology 71:2028–2032
13. Hofmann AF, Schmuck G, Scopinaro N, Laker MF, Sherr HP, Lorenzo D, Meeuse BJD (1981) Hyperoxaluria associated with intestinal bypass surgery for morbid obesity: occurrence, pathogenesis and approaches to treatment. Int J Ob 5:513–518
14. Drenick EJ, Ament ME, Finegold SF, Corrodi P, Passaro E (1976) Bypass enteropathy: intestinal and systemic manifestations following small-bowel bypass. JAMA 236:269–272
15. O'Leary JP, Maher JW, Hollenbeck JI, Woodward ER (1974) Pathogenesis of hepatic failure after obesity bypass. Surg For 25:356–359
16. Moxley RT, Pozefski T, Lockwood DH (1974) Protein malnutrition and liver disease after jejunoileal bypass for morbid obesity. N Eng J Med 290:921–926
17. Brown RG, O'Leary JP, Woodward ER (1974) Hepatic effects of jejunoileal bypass for morbid obesity. Am J Surg 127:53–58
18. Gianetta E, Vitali A, Civalleri D, Friedman D, Adami GF, Traverso E, Scopinaro N (1986) Liver morphology and function after biliopancreatic bypass. Clin Nutr 5 (suppl.):207–214
19. Grimm IS, Schindler W, Haluszka O (1992) Steatohepatitis and fatal hepatic failure after biliopancreatic diversion. Am J Gastroenterol 87:775–779
20. Zapanta M, Aldo-Benson M, Biegel A, Madura J (1979) Arthritis associated with jejunoileal bypass: clinical and immunologic evaluation. Arthritis Rheum 22:711–717
21. Drenick EJ, Stanley TM, Border WA, Zawada ET, Dornfeld LP, Upham T, Llach F (1978) Renal damage with intestinal bypass. Ann Intern Med 89:594–599
22. Scopinaro N (1974) Intervento in Tavola rotonda su trattamento medico-chirurgico della obesità grave. Accad Med 88–89:215–234
23. Pilkington TR, Gazet JC, Ang L, Kalucy RS, Crisp AH, Day S (1976) Explanations for weight loss after jejunoileal bypass in gross obesity. Br Med J 1:1504–1505
24. Condon SC, Janes NJ, Wise L, Alpers DH (1978) Role of caloric intake in the weight loss after jejunoileal bypass. Gastroenterology 74:34–37
25. Su W, Cleator IGM, Phang PT, Birmingham CL (1996) Determinants of weight loss following ileo-gastrostomy. Int J Ob 20:481–487
26. Halverson JD, Scheff RJ, Gentry K, Alpers DH (1980) Jejunoileal bypass: late metabolic sequelae and weight gain. Am J Surg 140:347–350
27. MacLean LD, Rhode BM (1987) Surgical treatment of obesity: metabolic implications. In: Griffen WO, Printen KJ (eds) Surgical Management of Morbid Obesity. Marcel Dekker, New York, pp 205–233

28. Gianetta E, Friedman D, Adami GF, Traverso E, Vitale B, Semino G, Castagnola M, Summa M, Scopinaro N (1987) Present status of biliopancreatic diversion. In: Proceedings of the Third International Symposium on Obesity Surgery, Genoa, Italy, pp 11-13
29. Flickinger EG, Sinar DR, Pories WJ, Sloss RR, Park HK, Gibson JH (1985) The bypassed stomach. Am J Surg 149:151-156
30. Sugerman HL, Kellum JM, DeMaria EJ (1997) Conversion of proximal to distal gastric bypass for failed gastric bypass for superobesity. J Gastroint Surg 1:517-525
31. Fox SR (1991) The use of the biliopancreatic diversion as a treatment for failed gastric partitioning in the morbidly obese. Obes Surg 1:89-93
32. Hess DS (1994) Bilio-pancreatic diversion with a duodenal switch procedure (abstract). Obes Surg 4:106
33. Hess DS, Hess DW (1998) Biliopancreatic diversion with a duodenal switch. Obes Surg 8:267-282
34. Marceau P, Biron S, Bourque RA, Potvin M, Hould FS, Simard S (1993) Biliopancreatic diversion with a new type of gastrectomy. Obes Surg 3:29-35
35. Marceau P, Hould FS, Simard S, Lebel S, Bourque RA, Potvin M, Biron S (1998) Biliopancreatic diversion with duodenal switch. World J Surg 22:947-954

Invited Comment

Walter J. Pories

The section by Brolin on gastric restrictive operations and the contribution by Scopinaro and Papadia provide excellent summaries of bariatric surgery at the start of this new millennium. One can only wonder what our forebears in 1000 a.d., when hunger was widespread and when bread consumed 25% of personal income, would think about operations designed to lose weight. They would certainly be astonished to learn that obesity developed into an epidemic with 15-16% of the English population and 17-19% of the German people exceeding BMI levels of 30.

In the United States, the statistics are grim. From 1960 to 1962, 24.4% of the population was overweight; from 1988 to 1994, in less than one generation, that figure rose to 34.8%, over one-third of the population. Sales of oversized coffins at the nation's largest casket company are up 20% in the last 5 years with the biggest jump over the last year.

The reasons for the explosion in obesity are not clear, although the increased intake of sugar (9% of the calories consumed by teenagers are derived from soft drinks), lack of exercise, increased number of meals consumed away from home, larger portions, and even viral infections are all cited as possible explanations.

What is clear, however, is that the medical therapies for the control of obesity are failing in spite of our expenditures of $68.2 billion each year on diets, drugs, exercise programs, acupuncture, hypnotism, and other programs. The need for better therapies is especially acute for the morbidly obese, those patients that exceed a BMI (kg/m^2) of 35. Every pound of added weight increases their chance for the serious comorbidities of obesity, including diabetes, hypertension, cardio-pulmonary failure, sleep apnea, arthritis of weight-bearing joints, pseudotumor cerebri, stroke, myocardial infarction, depression, stress incontinence, and infertility, as well as cancers of the breast, prostate, and stomach. Further, with each added pound, mortality increases at an asymptotic rate.

Fortunately, the situation is not hopeless for the morbidly obese. The surgical approaches described by our authors are remarkably effective in the control of weight, the associated comorbidities, and can be performed with low mortality and morbidity rates.

Both articles are so well argued and supported by extensive references that I will not plow the same ground again. Instead, I have chosen to present our current approach at East Carolina University where we have not only accumulated a large experience in the surgery of the obese, but where we also have a rigorous database about the outcomes of various procedures.

Controversy 1: Procedure of Choice

The arguments for each of the various procedures are thoroughly reviewed by Brolin. In my opinion, the gastric bypass remains the gold standard procedure for the surgical treatment of morbid obesity. With rigorous follow-up, the operation has been shown to provide long-term weight loss of about 100 lb and excellent control of comorbidities. The operation has been shown to return 87% of Type II diabetics to long-term euglycemia, control hypertension in one-third, and reverses cardio-pulmonary failure in all survivors. Arthritis of weight-bearing joints improves markedly in almost all patients. The operation can be performed with a mortality of 1% for all but the sickest patients. Long-term complications are uncommon and generally easy to manage.

The gastric bypass operation has been sharply improved by the application of laparoscopy, producing less trauma and avoidance of incisional hernias without sacrificing the excellent outcomes of the open procedure. That approach will, I believe, soon be the new gold standard.

My strong opinions about the gastric bypass, however, should not be interpreted as a condemnation of the other procedures. I vigorously applaud the trials of the various alternatives, especially Professor Scopinaro's studies. However, at the present time, I do not believe that any of these operations have attained the success of the gastric bypass and, therefore, should be primarily confined to investigational protocols in bariatric centers.

Controversy 2: Patient Selection Criteria

We agree that the general consensus to limit bariatric procedures to individuals between 18 and 65 is a useful guide that must be somewhat flexible. We have had good outcomes in teenagers as young as 16 and in patients as old as 67.

An evaluation of the patient's emotional and intellectual status is essential, but in most cases can be accomplished by an experienced bariatric team with well-designed instruments. Patients who require more formal consultations, about 10% of our patient population, include those with a history of suicide attempts, alcoholism, drug abuse, psychiatric hospitalizations, severe depression, and an apparent lack of adequate intellectual capacity to understand the procedures. We are also unlikely to proceed if there is any sign of indecision, of a lack of family support, or an unwillingness to participate in long-term follow-up. Unless these matters are resolved, it is usually unwise to proceed.

Patients with severe comorbidities including diabetes that is out of control, cardio-pulmonary failure, ulcerated legs, and crippling arthritis should be regarded as surgical emergencies with early admission, rapid and rigorous correction of metabolic anomalies, and rapid progress to surgical intervention.

Until recently, a significant number of patients were unable to undergo bariatric surgery based on the excuse that insurance carriers did not cover therapy for obesity. Although most of the major carriers now approve these procedures when the indications are clear, there are still some third-party payors who deny coverage. We respond to these unfair decisions with immediate challenges to the highest level with the argument that we do not operate to treat obesity; we perform the surgery to treat the comorbidities. We cite the American Disabilities Act, the NIH Consensus Conference, and our own outcomes data. Copies of the challenge are sent to the patient's employer as well as our state's insurance commissioners. It has been an effective approach.

Controversy 3: Unsolved Technical Considerations

Banding procedures have the advantages of offering minimal interventions but all of these will continue to struggle with erosion of plastic through the walls of the stomach or the intestine as well as slippage of the gastric sac with obstruction. For these reasons, I believe that the use of the bands will remain limited, especially as minimally invasive gastric bypasses are more widely adopted.

There is no perfect way to compartmentalize the stomach. Even triple staple lines break down in 3% of patients. Division of the organ can also be followed by the formation of gastro-gastric fistulas. In our series, such fistulas occurred in 6% of our patients. These breakdowns are not always evident; true outcomes can only be assessed if every patient is subjected to an upper gastrointestinal radio-opaque study. Based on our own work, we prefer the triple staple line for open procedures. For the minimally invasive operations, division is the only choice currently available with present techniques.

Controversy 4: Use of Nutritional Supplement

Although Brolin states that "there is no consensus regarding the use of nutritional supplements," let there be no misunderstanding about the fact that gastric bypass can cause significant malnutrition. Although all patients are not equally affected, there are some who will develop severe deficiencies of calcium, iron, folate, riboflavin, thiamine, and vitamin B_{12}. Further, in rare individuals, these deficiencies can have devastating results with full-blown Wernicke-Korsakoff's syndrome.

The gastroplasties are far less likely to develop problems associated with malnutrition. The other restrictive procedures, especially Scopinaro's bilio-pancreatic diversion and the "duodenal switch", however, may be even more prone to produce serious nutritional problems in Americans than the gastric bypass.

Controversy 5: DVT Prophylaxis

I agree with Brolin that pulmonary embolism is the leading cause of perioperative death following bariatric operations. We use compression stockings during surgery as well as heparin but have not been successful in avoiding either DVT or pulmonary emboli. We need better answers for this controversy. Perhaps, an increase in the dose of heparin may make a difference.

Controversy 6: Assessment of Outcomes

The measurements recommended by Brolin are appropriate. National standards should be set and adopted. Even so, the assessments will only be as good as the follow-up. Our national bariatric surgical association should consider the very tough approach that every lost patient must be recorded as a failure. Until we do so, comparison figures between operations, between centers, and between surgeons will not be very helpful.

Editorial Comment

The excellent contributions by Dr. Brolin and by Drs. Scopinaro and Papadia, followed by the illuminating comments by Dr. Pories leave us, the editors, with almost nothing to add.

What we do wish to add is that morbid obesity, with its increased sagittal abdominal diameter is associated with increased intra-abdominal pressure, which in turn contributes to obesity-related comorbidity. Weight loss reduces intra-abdominal hypertension, thus reversing a few of its systemic cardiovascular and respiratory complications [1].

That a few journals are dedicated to the study of morbid obesity, in which surgeons constantly describe a modification upon a modification of a procedure, is a testimony to the simple truth that no surgical bariatric procedure offers a panacea. A systemic neuro-metablic-endocrine disease treated by surgery? How strange and nonphysiologic. Sooner or later a wonder antiobesity pill will be available – it has to be! At this stage, however, we must realize that morbid obesity is associated with an increased risk of many serious medical complications, including hypertension, coronary artery disease, congestive heart failure, venous stasis, deep vein thrombosis, pulmonary embolism, obstructive sleep apnea, osteoarthritis, gallstones, urinary incontinence, diabetes mellitus, just to name a few. In addition, many of the morbidly obese patients become social outcasts, unable to get appropriate jobs. And although modest weight loss can often be achieved by diet, most of the truly morbidly obese patients are unable to achieve significant long-term weight reduction even with the use of pharmacologic agents. Therefore, at present, bariatric surgical procedures are the best that we can offer to selected morbidly obese patients, unresponsive to conservative therapy.

Reference

1. Sugerman H, Windsor A, Bessos M, Kellum J, Reines H, DeMaria E (1998) Effects of surgically induced weight loss on urinary bladder pressure, sagittal abdominal diameter and obesity co-morbidity. Int J Obes Relat Metab Disord 22:230–235

CHAPTER 15

Surgical Malpractice

The Surgeon's Perspective

Eric R. Frykberg

"Physician: one upon whom we set our hopes when ill and our dogs when well."
Ambrose Bierce
Devil's Dictionary, 1911

Introduction

Perhaps the most disconcerting, disappointing and devastating event in a practicing surgeon's career is to be sued by a patient for malpractice. This turns the surgeon's world upside down. An attempt to fulfill a mission of healing and helping others results in a slap in the face. The patient is no longer a close confidante, but becomes an adversary. The surgeon is no longer in charge as the respected leader of a health care team, practicing a unique skill which is the product of years of training and experience, but becomes a mere subject, and even a villain, who is forced to defend his or her actions to people with no training, understanding, or experience in medicine, and to adhere to unfamiliar rules of conduct in a very threatening environment. In fact, most accusations of surgical malpractice involve cases in which the surgeon did nothing wrong [1].

Of course, there is another view to consider. Adverse outcomes of surgical care do occur, and may be due to a mistake on the part of the surgeon. This may also happen despite appropriate care. How can the patient make this distinction? Should these patients be compensated? Should such compensation come from the treating surgeon? Must there always be blame assigned for less than optimal outcomes regardless of fault? Who should make these decisions?

This chapter will examine these issues in the context of the magnitude and current trends of the surgical malpractice problem in the United States, as well as the structure of the legal system in which malpractice is evaluated and judged.

Magnitude and Nature of the Problem

Over the past 20 years, there has been a substantial increase in the number of medical malpractice suits filed against physicians in the United States. There has also been a progressive increase in the size of monetary awards by the courts [1, 2]. The United States Department of Defense reports a rise in the rate of medical malpractice claims against military physicians from 7.5 per 100 physicians in 1990 to 9.8 per 100 in 1996, compared to rates of physicians in the private sector, which rose from 12.4 per 100 in 1990 to 16 per 100 in 1996. Surgeons accounted for 15.5% of these claims, second only to obstetrics-gynecology specialists, at 23.3%, as the most common specialty against whom claims were filed. Although the number of payments to plaintiffs made by the United States Department of Defense remained constant from 1993 to 1998, the total amount paid rose substantially from $67.29 million in 1992 to $104.16 million in 1998 [3].

The American Medical Association [4] has documented a rise in the incidence of medical malpractice claims against surgeons from 11.4 per 100 physicians in 1990 to 14.9 in 1996, peaking at 18.9 in 1993 [5]. Only obstetrics-gynecology specialists had a higher rate, peaking at 22.5 in 1993 [5].

A 1990 study found that the most common cause of medicolegal claims filed against United States physicians involved surgical procedures and complications [6]. Errors in diagnosis, most commonly involving malignancy, were the second most common cause of medicolegal claims, with a delayed diagnosis of cancer accounting for 19% of all claims related to diagnostic error.

Indemnity payments for cancer misdiagnosis are almost $200 million annually, representing 30% of all liability payments made for medical malpractice in the United States, and almost 8% of the total yearly liability payout by insurers of $2.6 billion [6, 7]. Delayed diagnosis of breast cancer is the most common specific allegation leading to a lawsuit among all errors in diagnosis, and accounts for the greatest number of ongoing litigation claims, the largest proportion of paid claims, and the greatest expense of litigation [3, 7–10]. In a review of claims of breast cancer misdiagnosis, general surgeons were involved in 26.7% of cases, but had the highest proportion of liability payments (42%), and the largest amount of money paid out in awards ($6.2 million total) of all other specialties [11].

This litigation problem has consequences for the surgical profession and for society as a whole. Medical insurance is harder to obtain for the average citizen. Defensive medicine is increasingly practiced by surgeons to reduce the likelihood of a suit, leading to increased costs for the patient and estimated annual expenditures of $60 billion [1, 2]. Malpractice insurance rates are progressively rising, driving surgeons' fees to prohibitive levels in some areas. The average annual professional liability insurance premium for United States surgeons in 1996 was $24,700 [5], ranging as high as $86,000 for general surgeons in some areas [2], and as high as $150,000–200,000 for obstetricians and neurosurgeons [1].

Several factors have contributed to the rising severity of this problem [1, 2, 12]. The advances, sophistication, and complexity of modern medicine is a major factor, allowing treatment of severe illnesses previously considered hopeless. In this setting, complications and human error are quite likely, patient understanding of the medical problem and risks tends to be poor, and there may be disagreements even among physician experts as to whether an adverse outcome could have been prevented. Unrealistic expectations on the part of the patient are another factor, and may be due to poor communication between surgeon and patient, as well as to the abundance of inaccurate information in the media. This leads to the misperception that there must always be someone to blame for any outcome that falls short of perfection. The progressive expansion of tort law has also contributed to the problem of malpractice litigation, with staggering monetary awards providing an incentive for plaintiffs to use the courts as a form of social insurance, and for attorneys (who receive a substantial portion of these awards in lieu of the injured patient) to accommodate and encourage such actions. Of course, the rest of society is burdened with greatly increased health care costs as a result.

The following issues and controversies in this area should serve to clarify the problem and focus on potential solutions.

The "Bad Doctor" Myth

The legal profession, the media, and much of the public believe and promote the concept that the professional liability problem is caused solely by "bad doctors" who should be punished for injuries they inflict upon patients. This harkens back to Hammurabi's Code of 1800 b.c., which provided that physicians whose patients had a bad outcome would have their hands cut off. The obvious corollary of this logic is that the rapidly rising incidence of malpractice litigation in the United States must mean that bad doctors are proliferating at an alarming rate! In fact, there has been no credible evidence to support this self-serving and biased conjecture, and much evidence refutes it [1].

Firstly, medical education in the United States is widely recognized to be the most intense in the world, producing the most highly trained specialists who have the most sophisticated resources available to them. It is quite unlikely that a large and growing portion of these physicians are incompetent and solely responsible for the litigation problem. In fact, substantial study and documentation have revealed that it is the most highly trained, experienced, and board-certified specialists, rather than poorly trained physicians, who are more likely to be sued and to have the highest monetary awards brought against them. This is due to their care of the most complex of illnesses and performance of the most complex procedures which have the highest risks of complication and death [13, 14].

Secondly, the bad doctor myth is frequently supported by its advocates with the fact that each year, only a small number of surgeons are responsible for most lawsuits, monetary awards, and litigation expenses. Again, these tend to be surgeons in high-risk specialties. However, this small group phenomenon is typical of most types of insurance. Only a small percentage of any insurance plan is involved in claims, which does not in itself mean that these few individuals are incompetent [15]. Still another relevant fact, which refutes this myth, is that the few specific surgeons involved in litigation in any one year are different from those involved in other years [1].

Thirdly, several reliable studies have shown that incompetent surgeons make up a very small percentage of all surgeons, which is inconsistent with the rising number of annual malpractice claims. Reviews of true negligence and negligence-prone behavior among thousands of physicians enrolled in physician-owned insurance companies show that less than 1% are incompetent and guilty of actual malpractice [1, 16]. Although efforts to identify and sanction this small number of incompetent physicians must continue, this approach by itself cannot have a significant impact on the overall malpractice problem.

One major consequence of the bad doctor myth is that it promotes the general misperception that any adverse outcome in surgical care must mean that a surgeon is to blame, and that a surgeon who is sued must have done something wrong. This fails to consider that medicine is an inexact science, and that adverse outcomes can and do occur despite the best medical care because many factors which affect outcome are outside the surgeon's control. In fact, the courts clearly and consistently recognize this. The problem of congenital birth defects and neurologic birth injuries clearly illustrates these points. Although the Institute of Medicine has shown that only 8% of such birth problems can be related to poor medical care, and the remaining 92% are due to nonphysician factors [1, 17], staggering jury awards against obstetricians for these events continue due to a perception that perfect babies should be a guaranteed expectation. The state of Florida requires that all physicians pay $250, and that obstetricians pay $5000, every 2 years into a fund that covers the expenses of neurologic birth injuries (including of course attorneys' fees for litigation) as a condition of licensure. This reflects the blatant misperception of the state legislature (made up mostly of lawyers) that physicians automatically are to blame for these largely arbitrary occurrences. Fairness dictates that these expenses be borne by all taxpayers, since the evidence shows this to be a societal and not a medical problem [1].

Other consequences of this myth involve the continued rise in costs of medical care, as more lawsuits and larger monetary awards lead to increased liability insurance costs, increased physicians' fees, increased practice of defensive medicine, and reduced access to medical care due to a greater reluctance of surgeons to care for the sickest patients and to many choosing to abandon their practice altogether. Therefore the concentration of government and medical society resources upon this very small part of the malpractice problem has allowed the major part of the problem (i.e., increased litigation, increased medical costs) to become more severe, resulting in an adverse backlash on society.

Truth, Justice, and the American Way

Tort Law

Surgical malpractice actions are evaluated and judged through civil law, with criminal charges only applicable in rare cases involving deliberately reckless disregard for the patient's welfare. The three grounds on which a civil suit may be filed are lack of informed consent, breach of contract, and malpractice, or negligence. The most common basis for claims against surgeons is negligence, which falls under tort law. A tort is a civil wrong for which the guilty party (the tort-feasor) is held financially responsible for an injury. The underlying rationale is that this not only punishes the tort-feasor (i.e., the surgeon), but also deters this party and others from inflicting future harm. In fact, this deterrent effect has never been credibly demonstrated [1, 18].

Negligence involves four elements, all of which a patient (the plaintiff) must prove by a preponderance of evidence in order to recover damages from a surgeon (the defendant): (1) the surgeon had a duty to treat the patient in accordance with established standards on the basis of an established relationship with the patient, (2) the surgeon deviated from the standard of care, (3) this deviation resulted in an injury to the patient, (4) the patient suffered an actual loss or damage from that injury. Standard of care is defined as how a reasonable and well-qualified surgeon would act under the same or similar circumstances. The law does not require that the best care be given, but that reasonable care be given. There may be valid indications at times to deviate from standard care, but the rationale for such action should be documented clearly in the medical record. The courts currently hold surgeons responsible for adherence to national standards of care, rather than local or community standards (the "locality" rule), since current levels of widespread communication and access to technical advances negate the impact of geographic locale [18, 19].

The Expert Witness

Proof of surgical malpractice usually requires the testimony of another physician "expert", as lay jurors are not expected to properly evaluate the standards of surgical care. The qualifications for an expert are determined by the trial judge, and vary greatly across the United States. Misleading and inaccurate statements by designated experts may unfairly skew the perceptions of a jury. Because experts are paid for their testimony, there is a tendency for them to become active partisans for the plaintiff or defendant, rather than objective purveyors of the truth. Also, it is common for experts for the plaintiff and defendant to provide apparently conflicting testimony, leaving the jury to make their decision more on the basis of subjective impressions of credibility rather than the objective evidence.

Trial by Jury: Inviolate or Inappropriate?

These considerations lead to the question of whether trial by jury, tort law, or the courts in general are the proper venue for evaluating and judging surgical malpractice. Juries in this setting are not truly the peers of the surgeon defendant, as common law intends, in that they do not have the requisite knowledge of surgical practice to make an informed decision. The same is true of attorneys and judges. Thus, the legal system does not deal effectively with the current level of complexity and sophistication of science and surgical practice [20]. The ability of juries to extract exorbitant monetary awards from a surgeon, which may far exceed actual damages or fault, is not only unjust, but becomes an economic burden on the entire health care delivery system. These decisions are too easily influenced by emotional appeals rather than the more appropriate facts of the case and established standards [2, 21]. The foundation of tort law is that the surgeon must be at fault, and if no fault is found, then the injured patient is not compensated. This is unfair to both parties.

Solutions

Several reasonable solutions have been proposed for this growing problem. All solutions should include a mechanism for effectively identifying and sanctioning incompetent or negligent surgeons, preferably through a rigid peer review process within the surgical profession [1].

Patient insurance has been proposed as a more cost-effective, equitable, and prompt mechanism than the courts for compensating patients for adverse outcomes of surgical care. This should work in the same way that automobile, fire, flood, health, or life insurance compensates victims for economic losses, without a presumption of fault [1].

Models already exist outside of the legal system, which effectively deal with determination of fault and appropriate compensation for adverse surgical outcomes through mediation or arbitration. Workmen's Compensation and the medical boards of the United States military are examples, involving an objective panel of medical and lay experts who make these decisions after their own careful review of the medical record. These panels may be hospital-based, or may function on a city, county, or state level. Some have suggested that the hospital, rather than insurance, provide compensation if negligence is determined [22].

Improvements are necessary in the current legal system for assuring that expert witnesses are properly qualified and experienced in the specific specialty involved in a litigated case. Many states still only require that an expert be a licensed physician regardless of training and experience [21]. The American College of Surgeons has taken the position that expert witnesses in surgical cases must be properly trained, experienced, and actively practicing in the relevant area of surgery involved in the litigation, and that they must adhere to acceptable standards of conduct and accuracy in their testimony [23]. Great Britain has adopted the approach of having experts secured by the court, rather than by plaintiff or defendant, in order to prevent experts from becoming biased or partisan in their testimony. This should assure greater objectivity in determining the truth than is currently achieved in the adversarial system of the courts [24].

Several areas of tort reform have shown promise in improving the economic burden of malpractice litigation. Limiting the amount a jury can award for noneconomic damages for "pain and suffering" has been shown to reduce surgeons' malpractice premiums, to reduce the number of malpractice suits, to increase the number of companies willing to provide liability insurance, and to reduce physician fees [2]. Monetary awards to the plaintiff should be offset by the amount paid by the patient's medical insurance. Payouts for medical services should be provided as they are incurred, because lump sum advance payments tend to overestimate actual costs. Contingency fees, large portions of which go to the lawyer rather than the injured patient, should be limited. There should also be reasonable limits on joint and several liability and on statutes of limitations for filing suits.

Finally, many suits can be avoided, and losses minimized, by simple adherence to the principles of compassionate, competent, and thorough care of the patient. Surgeons should treat patients as they would want to be treated. Thorough discussion about the rationale and risks of various forms of management, maintaining communication with the patient and family throughout the course of treatment, comprehensive medical record documentation, and acting honestly and prudently, all reflect diligence and concern for the patient's welfare above all other considerations. Guarantees of outcome should never be made, and the patient and family should be included as an integral part of all decision-making. The best defense against malpractice litigation, and the ultimate mission of physicians, remains the practice of good medicine [22, 25, 26].

References

1. Spencer FC, Halley MM (1990) The harmful effects of the "bad doctor" myth. Bull Am Coll Surg 75:6–12
2. Allen BL, Fischer JE (1999) Caps on malpractice awards: update. Bull Am Coll Surg 84:14–19
3. Granville RL, Williamson J, Guay JD (1999) Characteristics of Department of Defense medical malpractice claims: a quality management tool. In: Legal Medicine. Armed Forces Institute of Pathology, Washington, DC, pp 7–14
4. American Medical Association Center for Health Policy Research (1998) Socioeconomic Characteristics of Medical Practice, 1997–1998 edn. American Medical Association, Chicago
5. Schneidman DS (1999) Trends in medical professional liability claims. Bull Am Coll Surg 84: 8–9
6. Physician Insurers Association of American (1991) Data Sharing Reports, Executive Summary, Cycle 13:1/1/85–6/30/91. Physician Insurers Association of America, Washington DC
7. Kern KA (1994) Medicolegal analysis of the delayed diagnosis of cancer in 338 cases in the United States. Arch Surg 129:397–404
8. Physician Insurers Association of America (1990) Breast Cancer Study. Physician Insurers Association of American, Lawrenceville, N.J.
9. Kern KA (1993) Medical liability and breast cancer diagnosis. Breast Surg Index Rev 1:1–19
10. Kern KA (1994) The delayed diagnosis of breast cancer: biologic, technologic, and sociologic factors. Cont Surg 45:286–289
11. Kern KA (1992) Causes of breast cancer malpractice litigation. a 20-year civil court review. Arch Surg 127:542–547
12. McGill WJ (1976) Report of the Special Advisory Panel on Medical Malpractice. Special Panel on Medical Malpractice, New York
13. Jacobson PD (1989) Medical malpractice and the tort system. JAMA 262:3320–3327
14. Sloan FA, Mergenhagen PM, Burfield WB, Bovbjerg RR, Hassan M (1989) Medical malpractice experience of physicians: predictable or haphazard? JAMA 262:3291–3297
15. Dobson DP (1987) How to put a silver lining in the malpractice cloud. Med Econ Sept 7:173–180
16. Schwartz WB, Mendelson DN (1989) The role of physician-owned insurance companies in the detection and deterrence of negligence. JAMA 262:2342–2346
17. Nelson KB (1989) Relationship of intrapartum and delivery room events to long-term neurologic outcome. Clin Perinatol 16:995–1007
18. Halley MM, Fowks RJ, Bigler FC, Ryan DL (eds) (1989) Medical malpractice solutions: systems and proposals for injury compensation. Charles C. Thomas, Springfield, Ill.
19. Nora PF (ed) (1997) Professional Liability Risk Management: A Manual for Surgeons. American College of Surgeons, Chicago, Ill.
20. Glaberson W (1999) The Courts vs. Scientific Certainty. New York Times, June 27, sect 4:65
21. Spencer FC (1988) The expert witness: one surgeon's opinion. Bull Am Coll Surg 73:11–15
22. Ledgerwood AM (1997) With liberty and justice for all. Bull Am Coll Surg 82:16–26
23. American College of Surgeons (1989) Statement on Physician Expert Witness. Bull Am Coll Surg 74:7–8

24. Friston M (1999) New rules for expert witnesses – the last shots of the medicolegal hired gun. Br Med J 318:1365–1366
25. Spencer FC (1990) The vital role in medicine of commitment to the patient. Bull Am Coll Surg 75:6–19
26. Ferguson EF (1993) For legal reasons. J FL Med Assoc 80:61–62

The Lawyer's Perspective

Seymour Boyers · Anthony H. Gair

At one time, the typical plaintiff's lawyer handling a medical malpractice case would face an experienced and able insurance company lawyer who was well up on his medical-legal knowledge. The plaintiff's lawyer, though well trained in black letter, barrister law on liability issues, would be out maneuvered on his medical feet, and with his morale depressed, have the unenviable task of explaining to his client how, with good liability, the case turned to ashes. Today, however, there are more medically trained and experienced lawyers representing both sides in a seriously contested case.

The Law

What are the significant elements of a medical malpractice case? In a typical medical malpractice case in New York, the judge charges the jury as follows:

> Malpractice is professional negligence and medical malpractice is the negligence of the doctor. Negligence is the failure to use reasonable care under the circumstances, doing something that a reasonably prudent doctor would not do under the circumstances, or failing to do something that a reasonably prudent doctor would do under the circumstances. It is a deviation or departure from accepted practice.
>
> A doctor who renders medical service to a patient is obligated to have that reasonable degree of knowledge and ability which is expected of doctors who (perform, provide) that (operation, treatment, medical service) in the medical community in which the doctor practices.
>
> The law recognizes that there are differences in the abilities of doctors, just as there are differences in the abilities of people engaged in other activities. To practice medicine a doctor is not required to have the extraordinary knowledge and ability that belongs to a few doctors of exceptional ability. However, every doctor is required to keep reasonably informed of new developments in (his, her) field and to practice (medicine, surgery) in accordance with approved methods and means of treatment in general use. The standard of knowledge and ability to which the doctor is held is measured by the degree of knowledge and ability of the average doctor in good standing in the medical community in which the doctor practices.
>
> In performing a medical service, the doctor is obligated to use (his, her) best judgment and to use reasonable care. By undertaking to perform a medical service, a

> doctor does not guarantee a good result. The fact that there was a bad result to the patient, by itself, does not make the doctor liable. The doctor is liable only if (he, she) was negligent. Whether the doctor was negligent is to be decided on the basis of the facts and conditions existing at the time of the claimed negligence.
> A doctor is not liable for an error in judgment if (he, she) does what (he, she) decides is best after careful examination; if it is a judgment that a reasonably prudent doctor could have made under the circumstances.
> If the doctor is negligent, that is, lacks the skill or knowledge required of (him, her) in providing a medical service or fails to use reasonable care and judgment in providing the service, and such lack of skill or care or knowledge or the failure to use reasonable care or judgment is a substantial factor in causing harm to the patient, then the doctor is responsible for the injury or harm caused.
> [Where appropriate, add:]
> A doctor's responsibility is the same regardless of whether (he, she) was paid. (*New York Pattern Jury Instructions* [1998] 1A:650) The law in all jurisdictions is similar to the above charge.

The requisite elements of proof in a medical malpractice case are:

1. A deviation or departure from accepted medical or surgical practice, and
2. Evidence that such departure was a proximate cause of injury or damage

Where plaintiff's expert cannot state with a reasonable degree of medical certainty that defendant doctor's departures were the proximate cause of plaintiff's injuries, plaintiff's malpractice claim does not lie (see in New York, *Evans v Holleran* [198 AD2d 472, 604 NYS2d 958] 2nd Dept. 1993). Likewise, where plaintiff presented no evidence that plaintiff's physical condition would have been any different absent the alleged malpractice, plaintiff's malpractice claim does not lie (see New York, *Bossio v Fiorillo* [210 AD2d 836, 620 NYS2d 596]).

Error in Judgment as Defense to Surgical Malpractice

Pro. A surgeon is entitled to assert the error of judgment defense for injury occurring during surgery.

Con. A surgeon is not entitled to assert the error of judgment defense for an injury occurring during the performance of surgery.

It is accepted law that a doctor is not liable for an error in judgment if it is a judgment which a reasonably prudent doctor could have made under the circumstances. Since medicine is not an exact science, if a surgeon selects one of two courses of treatment he will not be liable for a bad result solely because he, in the exercise of his sound judgment, chose course (a) over course (b). Similarly, if a doctor's course of treatment is based on a misdiagnosis of a patient's condition, he may assert a defense that the misdiagnosis, albeit an error, was predicated upon his considered judgment.

Opinion. The error or exercise of judgment defense is not a valid defense to a claim that a surgical procedure was performed improperly.

Case in Point: *Aiello v Muhlenberg Regional Medical Center,* 159 N.J. 618, 133 A: 2d 433 (Sup Ct New Jersey, 1999). The defendant surgeon performed a tubal ligation on the plaintiff. During the procedure a Verres needle inserted by the surgeon perforated her mesocolon and mesenteric arteries and lacerated her left iliac vein.

The plaintiff asserted that the error or exercise of judgment rule was inapplicable and should not be considered by the jury since the alleged departure from proper practice did not concern the defendant's choices during surgery but rather the manner in which the procedure was performed. The defendant asserted the rule applied arguing she chose from several accepted options in the method she employed during surgery.

The Court held that if a physician's professional conduct implicates only the exercise of reasonable care in the performance of a medical procedure and not the exercise of medical judgment in selecting among acceptable and medically reasonable courses of treatment, the exercise of judgment rule is not applicable.

In medical malpractice cases where the alleged departure is that the surgeon improperly performed a surgical procedure resulting in injury to the patient, the error of judgment rule should not apply. This is so even when the surgeon's expert testifies that the surgeon did not depart from proper and accepted practice. The reason is, of course, because the issue is simply whether her surgery was performed properly, that is in accordance with good and accepted surgical practice. The Court in *Aiello v Muhlenberg Regional Medical Center,* supra, explained this reasoning quite clearly in the context of the case before it.

> Even if we accept the defendant's admission that she made her initial incision too deep, it is clear that she did not employ any judgment when she was incising the skin. Regardless of the method in which she performed the incision, either by elevating the skin prior to the initial incision or by simply holding the skin taut, she simply cut too deep. She did not use her judgment to determine the depth... her incision of the peritoneum was a mistake and cannot be considered an exercise of judgment.

Were the error in judgment defense to be considered a valid defense to surgical malpractice, every injury resulting from a mistake during surgery could be met with the surgeon's response that it was simply a mistake in judgment. It is thus submitted that the error in judgment defense should generally only be involved and the jury instructed as to the defense in two instances. One, where the surgeon chooses, on the basis of his considered judgment one type of surgery rather than another or secondly, where the surgeon, also on the basis of his sound judgment, misdiagnoses the patient's condition and performs unnecessary surgery on the basis of such misdiagnosis or performs no surgery at all. In such cases, while the defense does not immunize the defendant from liability, it may be presented to a jury as a defense for his erroneous diagnosis or incorrect choice of treatment.

Examples of Courtroom Controversies

A classic controversy involved surgery based upon symptoms diagnosed as carpal tunnel syndrome. Plaintiff's expert, a board certified orthopedic surgeon, concluded, with a reasonable degree of medical certainty, that the plaintiff was not suffering from carpal tunnel syndrome at the time she was admitted to the hospital for the surgery in question. A jury ultimately had to decide the question whether the defendant was negligent in failing to conduct proper tests, and whether the defendant performed unnecessary surgery.

The plaintiff, prior to surgery, went to another doctor who performed electromyograph tests and cervical spine x-rays which were negative, and that physician diagnosed the plaintiff's condition as thoracic outlet syndrome and recommended that the plaintiff should have the first rib removed. The defendant doctor agreed that carpal tunnel syndrome and thoracic outlet syndrome could produce similar symptoms. In addition, the plaintiff, prior to surgery, went to a third doctor who performed electromyography and electroconduction studies which led that physician to the clinical impression that the etiology of the plaintiff's problem was scalenus syndrome and not carpal tunnel syndrome, the former condition being described as "thought to be a compression of the blood vessels that course underneath the ... scalenus anticus muscle... a neck muscle that attaches to the clavicle."

The defendant doctor at trial explained that scalenus syndrome could produce symptoms similar to those presented by both thoracic outlet and carpal tunnel syndrome. The plaintiff's expert opined, at trial, that the symptoms exhibited postoperatively resulted from the partial or complete division of the median nerve rather than its entrapment by scar tissue. The trial testimony of defendant doctor's expert, a board certified orthopedic surgeon, controverted that of plaintiff's expert both as to the proper preoperative diagnosis and as to the manner in which the operation was executed.

It was the defendant doctor's expert's conclusion that the defendant had in all respects followed good and accepted medical and surgical practice. Moreover, based upon the expert's review of the medical records, defense counsel elicited testimony regarding a fall plaintiff sustained about a year after undergoing the surgery at issue, which incident had resulted in her hospitalization. X-ray films taken at that time demonstrated, inter alia, a fracture of the navicular (or scaphoid) bone in plaintiff's right wrist. It was the expert's opinion that symptoms referable to such an injury are similar to those of carpal tunnel syndrome and that sequelae of the former were sufficient to constitute the competent producing cause of the injuries complained of. Based upon the above testimony, it was the defendant's position at trial that the plaintiff had failed to produce expert medical testimony sufficient to establish a causal nexus between the alleged malpractice and the plaintiff's alleged injuries.

In a separate controversial case, a medical malpractice action was brought to recover damages for wrongful death and conscious pain and suffering of a pregnant woman in prodromal labor who was administered pitocin and thereafter suffered an amniotic fluid embolism. An amniotic fluid embolism occurs without warning, and is in most instances fatal. The defendants' experts argued that the plaintiff failed to establish a causal connection between the defendants' alleged malpractice or negligence, and the decedent's pain, suffering, and death. This contention rested largely upon the undisputed fact that an amniotic fluid embolism can occur in the absence of any negligence.

The plaintiff's medical malpractice expert testified that the use of pitocin was contraindicated under the facts because the fetal head was unengaged and still floating in the mother's uterus when pitocin was begun, and there was, from the record, inadequate monitoring of the pitocin infusion. Under these conditions, the plaintiff's expert testified that there was an increased risk that the patient's uterus would rupture, and by allowing the amniotic fluid to escape, would permit an amniotic fluid embolism to ensue.

The Court held that because causation is always a difficult issue in medicine "it bears emphasizing that to establish a prima facie case a plaintiff need not eliminate entirely all possibility that a defendant's conduct was not a cause. It is enough that he offer sufficient evidence from which reasonable men might conclude that it is more probable than not that the injury was caused by the defendant."

Informed Consent

The amount of information a surgeon must impart to a patient in order that the patient's consent to the operation be an informed consent is a continuing matter of controversy.

In New York the jury is charged as follows:

> Before obtaining a patient's consent to an operation or invasive diagnostic procedure or the use of medication, a doctor has the duty to provide certain information concerning what the doctor proposes to do, the alternatives to that operation, procedure or medication and the reasonably foreseeable risks of such operation, procedure or medication. It is the doctor's duty to explain, in words that are understandable to the patient, all the facts that would be explained by a reasonable medical practitioner so that when the patient does, in fact, consent, that consent is given with an awareness of (1) the patient's existing physical condition; (2) the purposes and advantages of the operation, procedure or medication; (3) the reasonably foreseeable risks to the patient's health or life which the operation, procedure or medication may impose; (4) the risks involved to the patient if there is no operation, procedure or use of medication; and (5) the available alternatives and the risks and advantages of those alternatives. The first question on this issue that you will be called upon to answer is whether the defendant, before obtaining plaintiff's (decedent's) consent, provided appropriate information. (New York Pattern Jury Instructions [1998] 1B:675)

The following questions must be answered by the jury:

1. Did the defendant provide appropriate information before obtaining the plaintiff's consent to the operation?
2. Would a reasonably prudent person in the plaintiff's position at the time consent was given have given such consent if provided with appropriate information?
3. Was the operation a substantial factor (proximate cause) in causing the injury to plaintiff?

The first two questions must be answered in the negative and the third affirmatively for the plaintiff to prevail.

The plaintiff is required to present the testimony of an expert physician as to the inadequacy of the consent. Failure to do so will result in dismissal of the claim. The controversy is what information must be given to the patient so that his consent may be considered an informal one. The law requires that a physician inform a patient of the material risks involved in the surgery. In reality, very few medical malpractice cases are brought which are predicated solely on a lack of informed consent for the simple reason that such cases are not easily won.

Case Examples

A physician following an examination of a female patient diagnosed a polyp in the sigmoid colon which had to be removed and recommended a colonoscopy and polypectomy. Following surgery a perforation at the polypectomy site was diagnosed which caused peritonitis requiring immediate surgery. The patient brought a medical malpractice action alleging malpractice in the performance of the colonoscopy and polypectomy together with a cause of action based on lack of informed consent.

The patient contended that there were no instructions given at the initial office visit as to after-procedure observations or instructions claiming she thus had insufficient information to understand the risks involved. The physician testified that he advised the patient of the potential risks and explained the procedure. The plaintiff contended that the specific risks such as perforation should be related by the physician while the physician asserted only the general risks had to be given. A jury found for the physician and the verdict was upheld on appeal.

In another case involving a perforated colon during the performance of a colonoscopy, the patient's claim predicated upon lack of informed consent was dismissed by the Court for failing to present the testimony of an expert physician as to the information given not being adequate. In this regard, although many physicians speak of giving informed consent, it is, of course, the physician who gives that information sufficient to allow the patient to make an informed decision.

Invited Comment

ROBERT E. CONDON

> "Legal memory lasted about a day after a trial. You had to forget in order to get along. It made men more enduring: it also made them more brutal, or at least more callous."
> Lord Snow [1]

These two essays, one by a surgeon and the other by two lawyers, illustrate the enormous cultural gap that exists between the two professions. Physicians function in a world in which the vagaries of human biology create variability in nearly everything measurable; boundaries are sometimes indistinct and subject to change. Written records usually are a kind of communication shorthand rather than an exact or complete diary of events. Judgments are made on the basis of probability. Usually, in acute situations, needed information is incomplete or erroneous. Inevitable errors of action and judgment are intrinsic to the practice of medicine. The occurrence of error is not evidence of negligence; the important thing, if possible, is to recognize and correct errors.

Lawyers, in contrast, function in a world that is more orderly and predictable. Detailed and accurate records are routine. Boundaries are usually clear and easily defined. Judgments are made on the basis of written rules and precedents. Error is identified through review on appeal. There are no acute situations in the law comparable to those in medicine. A threat to life or limb as a result of legal error is a vanishingly tiny risk.

Because their cultures are so different, lawyers and physicians often do not understand how members of the other profession think, how they evaluate evidence, or how they define reasonable expectations. As a consequence, they often talk past each other in discussing an issue. I think that is what has happened in the essays by Dr. Frykberg and by Judge Boyers and Attorney Gair. The surgeon identifies malpractice as a problem and offers a solution unlikely to be enacted. The lawyers, on the other hand, see no problem and instead discuss the technicalities of defending or proving a claim.

Medical malpractice is an act by a physician that is outside the standard of care and that results in injury to a patient. The "standard of care" encompasses all judgments and actions that might be employed by any reasonable and prudent physician under a given set of circumstances. It is important to remember that the standard of care is a legal concept, not a medical one. The standard is not defined by optimal behavior, is not a care pathway or a practice guideline, has little to do with quality assurance, and encompasses a wide variety of actions. Meeting the standard only requires behavior by a physician that is acceptable to some, but not necessarily to a majority, of his peers.

Adverse events regularly occur as the result of accepted medical treatment in the absence of any lapse on the part of a physician. The occurrence of an adverse event is not evidence of malpractice. Unfortunately, many lawyers, and many laymen as well, think otherwise. Deciding whether or not an adverse outcome is due to negligence requires evaluation by an expert. Fortunately, many lawyers avail themselves of the opinion of unbiased experts to help them decide whether to file a suit. When they receive such an expert opinion, suits arise only from events involving real malpractice and are usually quickly settled; otherwise, no suit is brought.

Unfortunately, equally many plaintiff's lawyers first develop a theory of negligence about the events surrounding an adverse outcome, and then shop for an "expert" who will support their view. The concurrence of an expert is essential to interdict a claim of malice against the plaintiff's lawyer. Experts who will adopt a lawyer's theory are readily available, frequently from the fringes of the academic community.

Malpractice does occur, but not very frequently. A good estimate of the incidence of malpractice comes from the Harvard Medical Practice Study that reviewed case records of patients discharged from hospitals in New York State [2, 3, 4]. Adverse events of all kinds occurred in 3.7% of hospitalized patients; a similar proportion was found in the recently released (and hyped by the media) report of the Institute of Medicine [5]. In the Harvard–New York study, adverse events were thought to involve any degree of negligence in only 1% of patients. Nearly half of all adverse events arose during surgical operations but were much less likely to result from negligence than were adverse events occurring in other hospital settings.

Interestingly, only a minority of patients injured due to medical negligence actually bring a suit against their doctor. Conversely, nearly half of all medical malpractice actions arise from events in which there is no negligence when the record is objectively reviewed. In other words, in half of the malpractice actions filed against physicians there are no objective grounds for bringing a suit. Nonetheless, in these groundless suits, payments are made to the plaintiff in one case in five [6]. A similar conclusion was reached in another analysis of malpractice claims [7]. The recent rash of malpractice suits involving silicone breast implants is another example.

If real negligence is not the usual motivation and actual negligence is absent in a substantial number of suits, why do patients sue doctors? It is my view that suits are brought primarily because of poor communication by the doctor with the patient and family, especially after an adverse event occurs. Perceptions by the patient and the family of desertion, devaluation of their perspective, and failure to understand their concerns were the motivating forces in 71% of cases reviewed by Beckman and colleagues [8]. Almost as potent a factor in 54% of cases was a suggestion by a health professional of the presence of negligence. In my experience, the involved health professional is often a nurse member or friend of the family. The most effective thing physicians can do, in their self-interest as well as in the interest of their patients, is always to take the time to insure open, effective, and honest communication with patients and their families, particularly when things are not going well.

Are malpractice suits, or the absence of them, any measure of professional competence? Hospitals seem to think so since, based on the advice of their lawyers, they ask for such information in an application for clinical privileges. Many lawyers assert that medical malpractice suits, and the consequences flowing from payment of claims to plaintiffs, serve to improve the quality of medical care by identifying marginal practitioners. Malpractice litigation has even been identified as a pillar of quality assurance [9]. The reality is that marginal practitioners rarely get sued. More often, as pointed out by Dr. Frykberg, it is the best surgeons who face malpractice claims because they assume the care of the most acute and complex cases. That the threat of malpractice suits serves to induce ordering of multiple tests, so-called defensive medicine, is well recognized. That medical malpractice suits serve to improve medical care is a conceit of lawyers with little evidence to support it.

Once a suit for medical malpractice has been lodged, what are the potential outcomes? Sometimes, as evidence accumulates during the pretrial process called "discovery," it becomes obvious that the plaintiff has no case. The suit may then be withdrawn, although the defendant physician and the insurer are never compensated for the time and money spent in mounting their defense. Or, if the accumulating evidence identifies negligence, then a settlement between the parties may be reached. Settlements for "nuisance value," small payments to plaintiffs who had no legitimate claim but that were made to end the suit and reduce overall expenses now occur infrequently because of the adverse consequences of having such a settlement entered into the records of the National Practitioner Data Bank. In the absence of a settlement, the case proceeds to trial.

There are two kinds of trials: criminal and civil. There is a passable understanding among most people of the nature of criminal trials. This understanding arises principally from watching television shows that often include aspects of a criminal trial in the drama. In a criminal trial, the prosecution has to prove its case "beyond a reasonable doubt." The lawyers on both sides in a criminal trial are, at least theoretically, engaged in a search for truth so that justice will be done.

Malpractice actions are not criminal trials. They are civil trials, and they follow rules that are different in critical respects. In contrast to a criminal trial, the plaintiff in a civil trial has only to establish a "preponderance of the evidence" to win. Without wanting to be invidious, it is my view that a civil trial has not so much to do with truth and justice as it does with effective advocacy. While it is not permissible for a lawyer to lie on behalf of a client, it is quite permissible, even expected, that they will not tell the whole truth. All sorts of half-truths and distortions can be uttered by the plaintiff's lawyer, and usually will be ruled admissible by the judge, in an effort to establish the preponderance of evidence. The attorney defending the doctor in a civil malpractice trial clearly has a more difficult task than the defense lawyer in a criminal trial.

In a somewhat cynical view, a malpractice trial can be seen as a kind of theater, the play presented is about a contest between lawyers, each supported by their cast of experts, and supervised by a director-judge who often is also a player. The outcome is decided by an audience-jury composed of ordinary citizens who are by no means the peers of the defendant physician, but who must weigh complex issues which they, inevitably, will only partially comprehend. On this stage, it is the lawyer who is the more effective advocate, who convinces the jury that his interpretation of the evidence is more believable, who will secure a verdict favorable to his client.

Therefore, a doctor on trial for malpractice needs the most effective advocate that can be found. The services of that attorney-advocate should be obtained immediately on receiving notice of a suit. If possible, the effectiveness of the chosen advocate should be assessed by observation in court of other cases in which the advocate is acting. The physician should attend all depositions of the plaintiff's experts for the reasons cogently outlined by Reiling and Gibson [10]. The physician-defendant needs to put feelings of affront and similar emotional reactions aside, be actively engaged in organizing the defense, and assist in objectively interpreting, evaluating, and analyzing the evidence as it develops. Such a stance by the physician will reduce, though nothing can eliminate, the risk of justice going awry.

References

1. Snow, Lord Charles P (1960) Strangers and Brothers. Macmillan Publishing Co, New York
2. Brennan TA, Leape LL, Laird NM, Hebert L, Localio AR, Newhouse JP, Weiler PC, Hiatt HH (1991) Incidence of adverse events and negligence in hospitalized patients. Results of the Harvard Medical Practice Study 1. N Engl J Med 324:370–376
3. Leape LL, Brennan TA, Laird N, Lawthers AG, Localio AR, Barnes BA, Hebert L, Newhouse JP, Weiler PC, Hiatt HH (1991) The nature of adverse events in hospitalized patients. Results of the Harvard Medical Practice Study 2. N Engl J Med 324:377–384
4. Localio AR, Lawthers AG, Brennan TA, Laird NM, Hebert LE, Peterson LM, Newhouse JP, Weiler PC, Hiatt HH (1991) Relation between malpractice claims and adverse events due to negligence. Results of the Harvard Medical Practice Study 3. N Engl J Med 325:245–251
5. Committee on Quality of Health Care in America (1999) In: Kohn L, Corrigan J, Donaldson M (eds) To Err Is Human: Building a Safer Health System. Institute of Medicine, Washington DC
6. Brennan TA, Sox CM, Burstin HR (1996) Relation between negligent adverse events and the outcomes of medical-malpractice litigation. N Engl J Med 335:1963–1967
7. Taragin MI, Willett LR, Wilczek AP, Trout R, Carson JL (1992) The influence of standard of care and severity of injury on the resolution of medical malpractice claims. Ann Int Med 117:780–784
8. Beckman HB, Markakis KM, Suchman AL, Frankel RM (1994) The doctor patient relationship and malpractice. Lessons from plaintiff depositions. Arch Int Med 154:1365–1370
9. Brennan TA (1999) Hospital peer review and clinical privileges actions. To report or not report (editorial). JAMA 282:381–382
10. Reiling R, Gibson GC (1999) A case for the physician defendant at plaintiff's expert witness deposition. Bull Am Coll Surg 84:18–22

Editorial Comment

While Dr. Frykberg provides us with the surgeon's perspective on malpractice, Judge Boyer and Attorney Gair focuses on legal controversies. Dr. Condon – a weathered surgeon himself – looks again at the problem from the surgeon's viewpoint. What we lack here is the voice of the patient.

We know that breeches of "the standard of care" are not uncommon. The Institute of Medicine reported a while ago that between 44,000 and 98,000 hospital patients die each year because of medical errors [1]. A prospective Federal investigation documented almost 3,000 medical mistakes and mishaps in less than 2 years at Veterans Hospitals around the United States and more than 700 patients have died in those cases [2]. Dr. Condon states that "the reality is that marginal practitioners rarely get sued," meaning that the majority of those responsible for "malpractice" continue to walk around unharmed and unrestrained. Dr. Frykberg suggests that "although efforts to identify and sanction this small number of incompetent physicians must continue, this approach by itself can not have a significant impact on the overall malpractice problem." So what should be done with that "minority" of "bad doctors" who continue to practice, unhinged, outside the spectrum of standard of care?

A recent editorial in the British Medical Journal asserted: "Even if all surgeons are equally good, about half will have below average results, one will have the worst results, and the worst results will be a long way below average" [3]. Unfortunately, not a few surgical departments have "one" such surgeon who functions way below average: how do we deal with him or her? Local departmental and hospital-based quality assurance mechanisms are obviously prone to manipulations by the known, ever-present local political and financial circumstances. Consequently, only a small number of "habitually" malpracticing practitioners are eventually referred to the State Medical Boards [4]. It is easy to spot and report sexual or drug-related abuse or misconduct but much more difficult to identify and process a "true medical malpractice". Hence it is estimated that the state authorities deal only with the tip of the iceberg [5].

What should we - you or I - do when encountering misconduct or malpractice which has been ignored by the local authorities for whichever reasons? The policy Compendium of the American Medical Association [6] states that when dealing with knowledge of a colleague's misconduct "a physician should expose it without fear or loss of favor." It calls on the profession to abandon the conspiracy of silence. The Book of Code of Medical Ethics published by the American Medical Association states: "Where the inappropriate behavior of the physician continues despite the initial report, the reporting physician should report to a higher or additional authority" [7].

The present system of whistle-blowing is however unsatisfactory in the United States as it is in the United Kingdom, with the "messenger often being shot" [8]. The quality-assurance system cannot expect people to be heroes because most are not [9]. How to reduce malpractice and patient injury is thus a complex issue requiring an overhaul of how we deliver health care, educate and train physicians, and assess and improve quality [10].

Another issue not mentioned by Drs. Frykberg and Condon, Judge Boyer and Attorney Gair is that surgeons are much more exposed to lawsuits than their non-surgical colleagues. Our mistakes and complications are simply more visible: when a patient dies on a medical ward, it is always the disease, be it pneumonia or arrhythmia, which is to blame, but in the case of any adverse postoperative outcome, the surgeon is the one to attract the accusing eyes of involved parties. Dr. Frykberg writes "...it is the most highly trained... physicians who are more likely to be sued." It is our impression that this is true in particular for surgeons: a well trained and dedicated surgeon who promptly reoperates on a patient whose intestinal anastomosis leaked, is more likely to be sued than the one who failed to diagnose the leak, his patient described as dying from "sepsis".

> "Doctors are just the same as lawyers; the only difference is that lawyers merely rob you, whereas doctors rob you and kill you, too."
> Anton Chekhov

References

1. Preventing Fatal Medical Errors. (1999) New York Times. December 1,
2. Report Outlines Medical Errors in VA Hospitals. (1999) New York Times. December 19
3. Poloniecki J (1998) Half of all doctors are below average. BMJ 316:1734–1746
4. Morrison J, Wickersham P (1998) Physicians disciplined by a State Medical Board. JAMA 279:1889–1893
5. Scutchfield FD (1998) The role of the medical profession in physician discipline. JAMA 279:1915–1916
6. American Medical Association (1997) Policy Compendium. American Medical Association, Chicago, IL
7. American Medical Association (1996) Code of Medical ethics. American Medical Association, Chicago, IL, p 140
8. Treasure T (1998) Present system of whistleblowing is unsatisfactory. BMJ 316:1739–1740
9. Berwick DM (1998) You cannot expect people to be heroes. BMJ 316:1738–1739
10. Chassin MR, Galvin RW, The National Roundtable on Health Care Quality (1998) The urgent need to improve health care quality. JAMA 280:1000–1005

Subject Index

F

G

H

I

J

K

L

M

N

O

P

Q

R

GPSR Compliance

The European Union's (EU) General Product Safety Regulation (GPSR) is a set of rules that requires consumer products to be safe and our obligations to ensure this.

If you have any concerns about our products, you can contact us on ProductSafety@springernature.com

In case Publisher is established outside the EU, the EU authorized representative is:

Springer Nature Customer Service Center GmbH
Europaplatz 3
69115 Heidelberg, Germany

Batch number: 10584518

Printed by Printforce, the Netherlands